AF903108

Total Scar Management

Rei Ogawa
Editor

Total Scar Management

From Lasers to Surgery for Scars, Keloids, and Scar Contractures

Springer

Editor
Rei Ogawa
Department of Plastic, Reconstructive and
Aesthetic Surgery
Nippon Medical School
Tokyo
Japan

ISBN 978-981-32-9790-6 ISBN 978-981-32-9791-3 (eBook)
https://doi.org/10.1007/978-981-32-9791-3

© Springer Nature Singapore Pte Ltd. 2020
This work is subject to copyright. All rights are reserved by the Publisher, whether the whole or part of the material is concerned, specifically the rights of translation, reprinting, reuse of illustrations, recitation, broadcasting, reproduction on microfilms or in any other physical way, and transmission or information storage and retrieval, electronic adaptation, computer software, or by similar or dissimilar methodology now known or hereafter developed.
The use of general descriptive names, registered names, trademarks, service marks, etc. in this publication does not imply, even in the absence of a specific statement, that such names are exempt from the relevant protective laws and regulations and therefore free for general use.
The publisher, the authors, and the editors are safe to assume that the advice and information in this book are believed to be true and accurate at the date of publication. Neither the publisher nor the authors or the editors give a warranty, expressed or implied, with respect to the material contained herein or for any errors or omissions that may have been made. The publisher remains neutral with regard to jurisdictional claims in published maps and institutional affiliations.

This Springer imprint is published by the registered company Springer Nature Singapore Pte Ltd.
The registered company address is: 152 Beach Road, #21-01/04 Gateway East, Singapore 189721, Singapore

Contents

Part I

Basic Science of Scars

Wound Healing and Scarring

1

Adriana C. Panayi, Chanan Reitblat, and Dennis P. Orgill

1.1 Introduction

From the dawn of man to the present day, traumatic injuries have persisted as a major cause of morbidity and mortality. Even as recently as the Civil War in the United States, up to 24% of upper extremity amputations and 88% of amputations just below the hip resulted in death [1]. Over the last 150 years, however, there have been tremendous advances in both the understanding and treatment of wounds that have resulted in fewer amputations and dramatically lowered fatality rates [2, 3]. Despite these strides, chronic wounds and scars left in the wake of trauma continue to physically and emotionally devastate millions of people around the world [4, 5]. Increased insight into the cellular and molecular mechanisms underpinning wound healing holds promise for improving the lives of these individuals and driving the development of new therapies. Accordingly, in this chapter we will focus attention on understanding the mammalian response to injury, basic mechanisms of healing, local and systemic factors affecting healing, and recent advances in the management of chronic wounds and scars.

A. C. Panayi
The Wound Care Center, Brigham and Women's Hospital, Boston, MA, USA
e-mail: apanayi@bwh.harvard.edu

C. Reitblat
Harvard Medical School, Harvard Business School, Boston, MA, USA
e-mail: chanan@hms.harvard.edu

D. P. Orgill (✉)
The Wound Care Center, Brigham and Women's Hospital, Boston, MA, USA

Harvard Medical School, Harvard Business School, Boston, MA, USA
e-mail: dorgill@partners.org

1.2 Mammalian Response to Injury

> "Healing is not a science, but the intuitive art of wooing nature"—W.H. Auden [6]

1.2.1 Basic Concepts in Homeostasis, Growth Adaptation, and Injury

The survival of a living organism depends on its ability to maintain a stable internal environment, known as *homeostasis*. When homeostasis is perturbed by environmental changes, also known as "stressors," complex biological systems within the organism work in tandem to reestablish equilibrium via the process of *growth adaptation* [7].

As a homeostatic regulatory response, growth adaptation depends on the type of stressor, its magnitude, and the type of cell, tissue, or organ affected. Take, for example, the response of skeletal muscle to mechanical stress in the form of strength training. As the mechanical stress increases, muscle cells respond in kind by increasing the number of contractile proteins, myofibrils, and energy stores leading to an overall growth in cell size known as *hypertrophy* [8]. The aggregate effect of cellular hypertrophy can be seen on the tissue level as an enlarged muscle belly now better suited to handle heavier mechanical loads. This is in contrast to *hyperplasia*, the process by which the *number* of cells increases via induction of stem cells in response to increased stress. A classic example is that of liver hyperplasia to compensate for cell loss after hepatic necrosis or resection [9]. The response to increased stress need not be binary, however, as seen in the gravid uterus which undergoes both hypertrophy and hyperplasia in response to mechanical and hormonal stimuli in order to better accommodate a growing fetus.

In contrast to the above processes, tissues experiencing a *decrease* in stress diminish in size, or *atrophy*, due to disuse or withdrawal of trophic factors such as oxygen, nutrients, and hormonal stimulation. Mechanisms of atrophy include a

© Springer Nature Singapore Pte Ltd. 2020
R. Ogawa (ed.), *Total Scar Management*, https://doi.org/10.1007/978-981-32-9791-3_1

decrease in cell size or number. The former occurs via *autophagy* (Ancient Greek for "self-eating"), in which cytoplasmic contents are enzymatically degraded and recycled within lysosomes, as well as the *ubiquitin-proteosome pathway* which targets short-lived (and often damaged) proteins for destruction [10]. A decrease in cell number, on the other hand, can be achieved by an organized program of cell death known as *apoptosis* or the chaotic destruction of large groups of cells in response to injury as seen in *necrosis*.

External changes in mechanical stress can lead to changes in cell size or number, while certain environmental exposures can induce *metaplasia*, a reversible transformation of one differentiated cell type into another type better suited to handle this exposure. The most common forms of metaplasia involve changes in surface epithelium. A classic example is the alteration in the lining of the lower esophagus in the setting of persistent reflux esophagitis, known as Barrett's esophagus. The typical lining of the esophagus is squamous epithelium which can slough off without damaging underlying layers and is, therefore, ideal for overcoming the mechanical friction of a food bolus. When there is chronic inflammation due to persistent acid reflux, however, epithelial stem cells are reprogrammed into mucus-secreting columnar cells like those seen in the small intestine which are better able to withstand an acidic environment. Although this may be beneficial in the short term, this process of cellular reprogramming can be maladaptive if the inciting exposure is not resolved. With time, cellular growth and proliferation becomes disordered, known as *dysplasia*, forming premalignant lesions at increased risk of neoplastic transformation. In the case of reflux esophagitis, 0.5–1% of patients with Barrett's esophagus develop esophageal adenocarcinoma, a highly lethal cancer [11].

Taken together, these adaptations represent but a small fraction of the armamentarium that has evolved to combat injury and maintain homeostasis. Yet, despite an organism's impressive resilience, adaptive measures can also be overwhelmed. Cells can be damaged in a number of ways, including hypoxia, inflammation, nutritional imbalances, physical trauma, genetic derangements, and infectious agents, to name a few, all of which can cause irreversible injury and eventual cell death (Fig. 1.1).

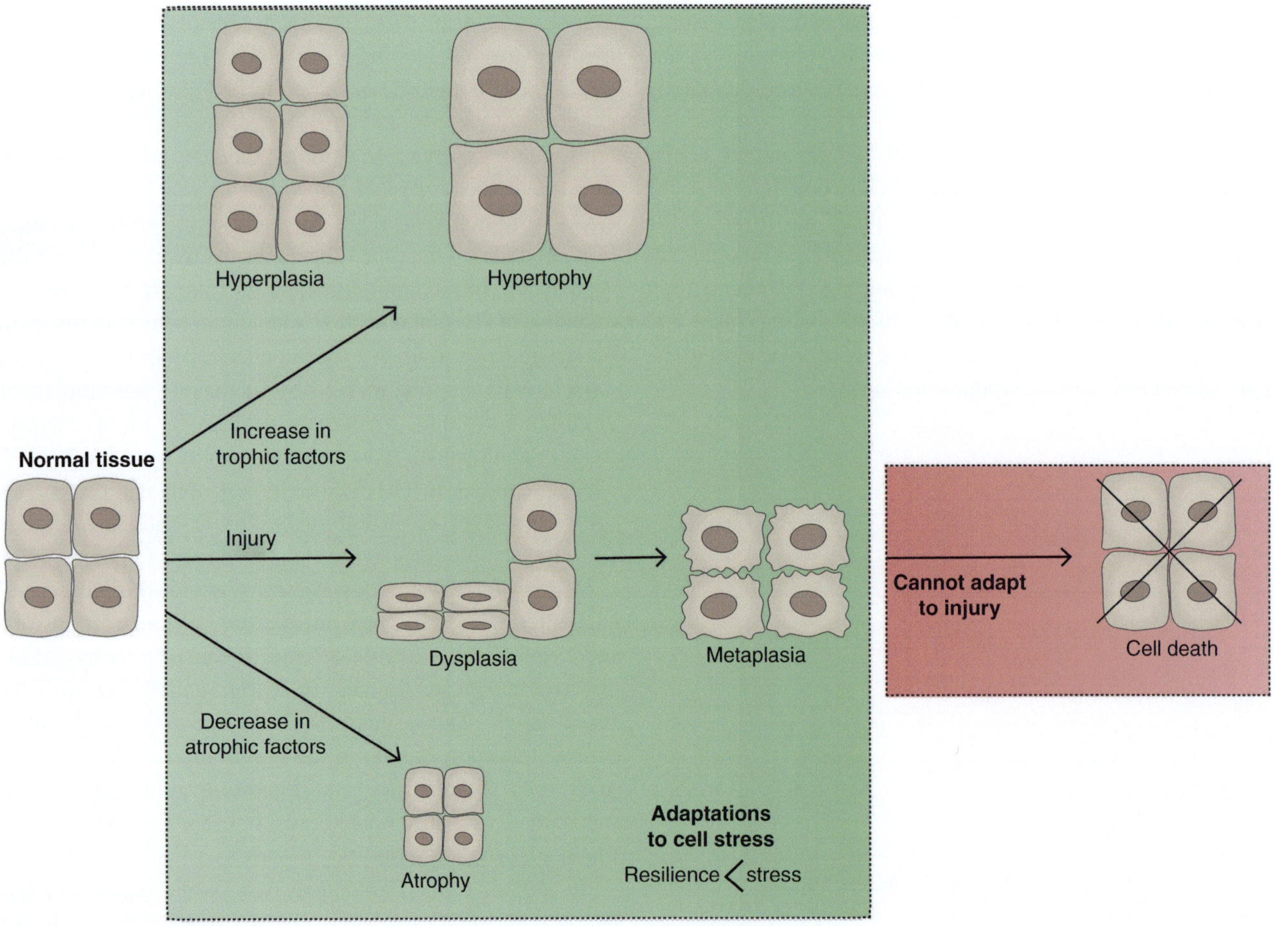

Fig. 1.1 Cells can undergo adaptation when exposed to different factors or injury. When the cells are no longer able to adapt, they undergo cell death via necrosis or apoptosis

1.2.2 Mechanisms of Wound Healing

Wound healing describes the restoration of normal anatomical relationships and physiological integrity of tissues disrupted by injury. This essential response to injury proceeds via a combination of *regeneration* and *repair*, defined as the complete restitution of devitalized tissue or replacement with fibrous scar, respectively. Often occurring simultaneously, the balance between these two processes is dynamic and depends on the proliferative capacity of the tissue involved, as well as the nature and extent of injury.

Tissues can be categorized into three basic groups based on their ability to replace damaged tissue with healthy tissue via the proliferation of stems cells: labile, stable, and permanent. *Labile tissues* such as bone marrow and the epithelial lining of the skin are constantly replicating and produce robust regenerative responses to injury. Less robust are *stable tissues* which comprise stems cells that spend a majority of their life spans in quiescence but can be induced to proliferate. Examples include hepatocytes which regenerate after resection and the epithelium of kidney tubules which divide rapidly following acute kidney injury. *Permanent tissues* such as cardiac myocytes are terminally differentiated and show little to no regenerative capacity. Instead, these tissues heal via repair, explaining why very little cardiac muscle can be regenerated following myocardial infarction.

When repair is the dominant wound healing process, as seen in injury to permanent tissues, but also, injury that results in the loss of stem cells, as in the case of severe burns, the injured tissue is replaced with fibrous scar. Deep within the wound, repair proceeds via the formation of *granulation tissue* which serves to fill the tissue defect, protect the wound bed from further trauma and infection, and lay the groundwork for scar formation. Bright red and granular in appearance, granulation tissue is composed of new blood vessels, fibroblasts, and myofibroblasts that serve to provide nutrients, deposit structural proteins needed for reconstruction, and contract the wound, respectively. On the surface, epithelial cells at the wound margin rapidly proliferate and migrate inwards in order to protect the nascent healing cascade (Fig. 1.2).

1.2.3 Phases of Wound Healing and Beyond

Wound healing is a complex process that begins immediately following tissue injury and proceeds via a well-described sequence of highly regulated and overlapping phases that include hemostasis, inflammation, proliferation, and remodeling (Fig. 1.3).

1.2.3.1 Hemostasis (Immediate)

Immediately following tissue injury and damage to capillary blood vessels, platelets adhere to subendothelial collagen on exposed vessel walls forming a weak *hemostatic plug*. The primary purpose of the plug is to stem blood loss. Circulating coagulation factors subsequently stabilize the plug via an enzymatic cascade that drives platelet aggregation and the formation of a nascent *fibrin scaffold*. In addition to serving as the chief effector cells of hemostasis, activated platelets within the fibrin scaffold secrete growth factors necessary for wound healing. The most well-studied are platelet-derived growth factor (PDGF) and transforming growth factor-β, potent mitogens responsible for the recruitment and proliferation of inflammatory cells that orchestrate subsequent phases of the healing process. Platelets also aid in the revascularization of the wound by releasing vascular endothelial growth factor (VEGF), a proangiogenic factor which facilitates blood flow by restoring the integrity of damaged vessels. Acting in concert, the aforementioned factors lay the necessary groundwork for the initiation of the second phase of wound healing, *inflammation*.

1.2.3.2 Inflammation (Days 0–5)

As hemostasis is achieved, the rudimentary plug is transformed into a complex *extracellular matrix (ECM)* composed of extracellular proteins and carbohydrates that provide physical scaffolding and biochemical support to the healing wound. Among these molecules are chemoattractants derived from platelets, arachidonic acid metabolites, complement system, and bacterial degradation products that attract circulating leukocytes into the wound in a process known as *inflammation*. Neutrophils are first to arrive on scene, phagocytosing invading bacteria as well as necrotic and foreign debris. Neutrophil levels peak within 24 h, at which point macrophages migrate into the ECM and become the dominant mediators of inflammation during days 2–5. While macrophages also fight infection, and remove debris via phagocytosis, their primary function is to recruit the effector cells of repair into the wound bed. This is accomplished by binding to integrin receptors in the ECM such as tumor necrosis factor-α and interleukin-1, enabling the secretion of cytokines which attract fibroblasts, the workhorses of wound healing seen in the proliferative phase.

1.2.3.3 Proliferation (Days 5–10)

With the arrival of fibroblasts by day 5, wound healing transitions into the proliferative phase and typically continues until day 10 post-injury. The hallmark of this phase is the formation of *granulation tissue* comprising

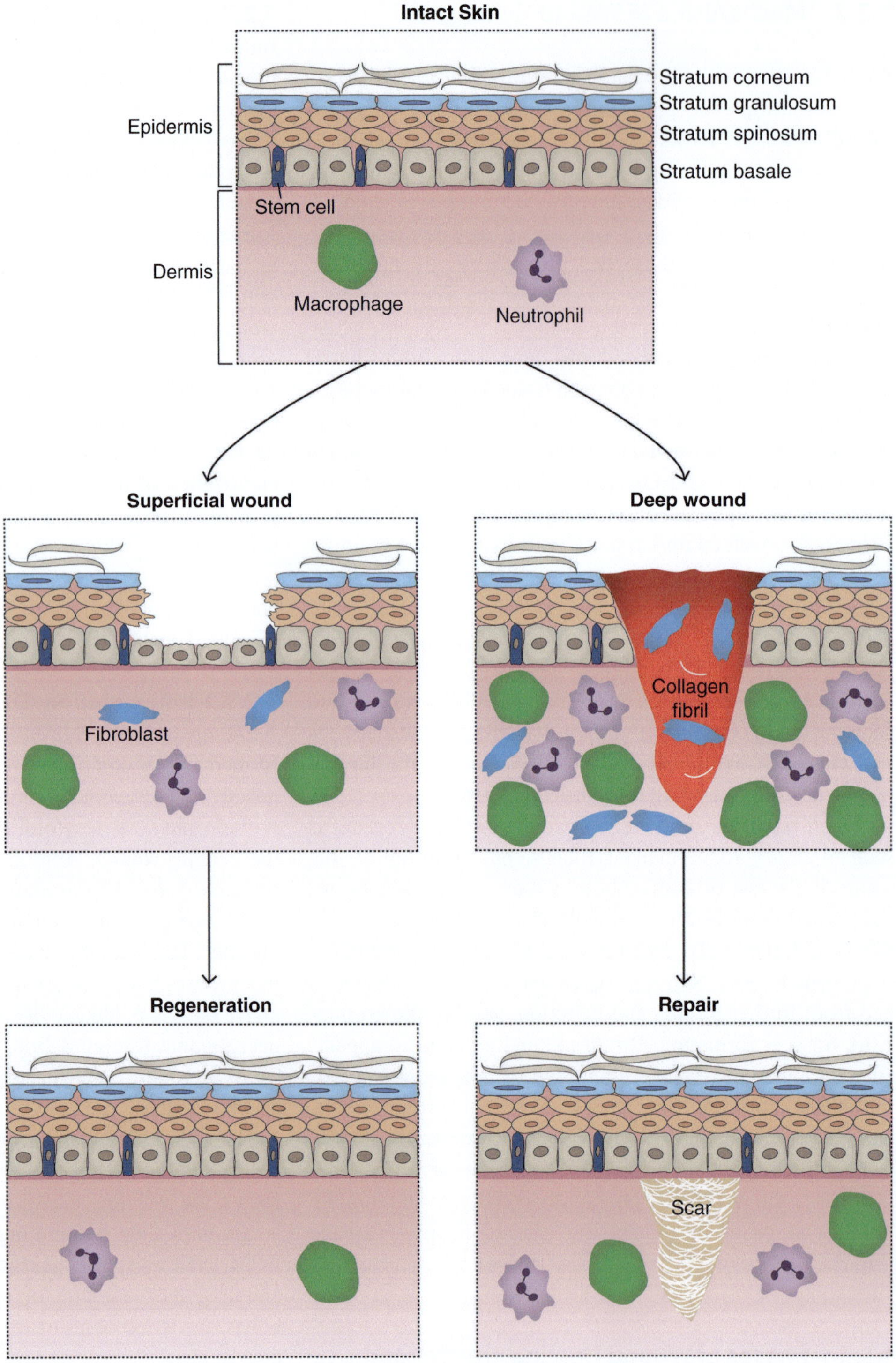

Fig. 1.2 Wound regeneration and repair

capillaries, fibroblasts, myofibroblasts, and loose connective tissue. Early on, the hypoxic wound environment induces the secretion of hypoxia-inducible factor-1 (HIF-1α), a potent stimulator of new blood vessels that deliver nutrients and oxygen to support the metabolically intensive healing process. It is these new blood vessels that are responsible for the erythematous and granular appearance of granulation tissue.

In order to provide structural support for these nascent capillaries and rapidly fill the tissue defect, fibroblasts secrete vast amounts of type III collagen which is weaved into interconnected fibrils. Buried deep within these fibrils are differentiated fibroblasts with muscle-like contractile ability, called myofibroblasts. Actin–myosin complexes within these cells exert a traction force which brings the edges of the wound together in a process known as *wound*

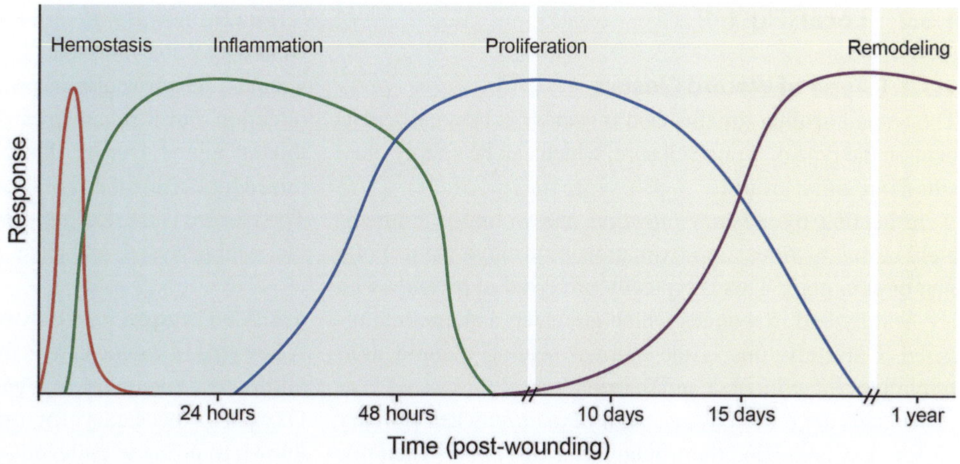

Fig. 1.3 Phases of wound healing

contraction. At the superficial edges of the wound, keratinocytes proliferate and migrate centrally, covering the granulation tissue with a thin layer of protective cells.

The end result of the first three phases of wound healing is an *immature scar*, an evolutionary adaptation critical to the survival of our species after severe injury. As a result, from the moment of trauma we are able to stem blood loss, rapidly restore the structural integrity of gaping wounds, stave off infection, and prevent insensible losses of heat and water. However, immature scars are often unsightly, easily friable, and possess a fraction of the tensile strength of healthy tissue. To overcome these challenges, wounds undergo a long-term *remodeling process* after acute injury, which results in a *mature scar* that more closely resembles the form and function of healthy tissue.

1.2.3.4 Remodeling (Day 10–2 Years)

The final phase of wound healing marks the remodeling of the wound into a mature scar, a process that begins approximately 2 weeks post-injury and can go on for years. Given this prolonged timeline, scar revisions must be delayed until the maturation process is complete.

Within the ECM, remodeling describes the degradation and replacement of weak and disorganized type III collagen with stronger and more organized type I collagen by *matrix metalloproteinases (MMPs)*. This transformation peaks approximately 60 days post-injury at which point the tensile strength of the scar approaches up to 80% of unwounded skin. With time, newly synthesized type I collagen is weaved into stable fibrils, flattening the scar. MMPs also reduce the cellularity and vascularity of wound, giving the scar an appearance that more closely resembles normal tissue.

1.3 Factors Influencing Wound Healing

1.3.1 Introduction

For appropriate wound healing, all four phases—hemostasis, inflammation, proliferation, and remodeling—must be successful, with no sequence or temporal deviations. Factors that can interfere with wound healing kinetics result in inadequate or improper tissue repair. Interfering factors can be classified into non-modifiable and modifiable factors, which can be further subclassified into local and systemic factors.

1.3.1.1 Non-modifiable Factors

Some risk factors for poor wound healing are currently outside the physician's control. These include genetic conditions, such as Down syndrome [12], as well as immune conditions, such as leukocyte adhesion deficiencies [13]. Beyond genetic and immune conditions, the most notable example of a non-modifiable interfering factor is age. Compared to the general population, elderly patients experience slower wound healing and higher rates of chronic non-healing wounds, but the actual quality of the healing is not impaired. The inflammatory phase differs from younger patients, in terms of both the growth factors involved, which decrease with age, and the pro-inflammatory cytokines, such as tumor necrosis factor alpha, which are sustained at a higher level [14]. With increasing age, the expression of angiotensin II in the skin increases, which in turn leads to higher levels of transforming growth factor beta (TGF-β). All these factors in combination are believed to be involved in the inhibition of reepithelialization, ultimately leading to the transformation of acute wounds into chronic wounds [15]. Surgeons should be cognizant of this and work to optimize modifiable factors to ensure proper wound healing in aged patients. When faced with non-modifiable risk factors, the optimization of factors under a surgeon's control gains increased importance [16].

1.3.1.2 Modifiable Factors

Modifiable factors represent preventable parameters that can be altered to facilitate optimal wound healing. These include systemic factors such as nutrition, glucose levels, smoking status, and steroid use. It should be noted that proper management of ischemia and infection is particularly important.

1.3.2 **Local** (Fig. 1.4)

1.3.2.1 Type of Wound Closure

The wound healing timeline and trajectory is heavily dependent on the type of wound closure, which can be simply classified into three groups.

In healing by *primary intention*, the wound is immediately closed by direct approximation, or through the use of a flap or skin graft. This is typically preferred in patients who are healthy and in wounds which are clean and uncontaminated. Currently, this is the optimal healing method as it minimizes infection risk and scarring.

Wounds are closed by *secondary intention* when primary closure has failed and the wound has dehisced, or when primary closure is not possible. In such cases, the wound can be left open to heal by wound contraction and reepithelialization. In order to fill the empty space, the body must produce a granulation tissue matrix that is eventually converted into scar tissue. Epithelialization occurs from the wound edges or from cells around adnexal organs. Contraction results from myofibroblasts exerting a traction force within the wound and laying down an extracellular matrix that contract over time. While *contraction* is a normal part of the secondary intention process, care must be taken to avoid *contracture*. Contracture, which occurs due to excessive contraction, can impair movement around joints resulting in both functional deficits and physical deformity. As wounds treated with secondary intention require more time and energy to heal than in primary intention, they can remain open for extended periods of time rendering them more prone to contamination and subsequent infection.

Finally, *tertiary intention* involves intentionally delaying wound closure. This can be quite useful in contaminated wounds, which if closed primarily will have a high risk of infection, but if dressed, can be safely closed 4–5 days following injury. During this period the wound can be optimized for closure through decontamination and debridement. The closure is carried out once the wound edges appear viable, well perfused, and clean.

1.3.2.2 Oxygen Perfusion

A key goal in wound care is the optimization of blood flow to allow for maximum oxygen delivery to injured tissue. Oxygen is necessary for optimal wound healing as it is known to promote collagen synthesis, fibroblast production, keratinocyte maturation, and epithelial tissue and new vessel formation, but also to inhibit infection [17]. Oxygen is necessary for the proper functioning of a number of enzymes involved in collagen synthesis and cross-linking. For example, the activity of hydroxylase, which hydrolyzes lysine and proline, is directly dependent on the amount of oxygen present in the wound [18, 19]. The strength of a wound is directly proportional to collagen synthesis, and consequently on oxygen [20]. Epithelial tissue formation is optimal in well-perfused, moist wounds with studies having shown that epidermal cells grow best with 10–50% oxygen concentration [21]. The imperative role of adequate oxygen perfusion on the process of angiogenesis can be appreciated by looking at the effect hypoxia has on new vessel formation. When cells become hypoxic, several biochemical pathways trigger the production of various angiogenic transcription factors, such as hypoxia-inducible factor-1 (HIF-1) [22, 23]. It should

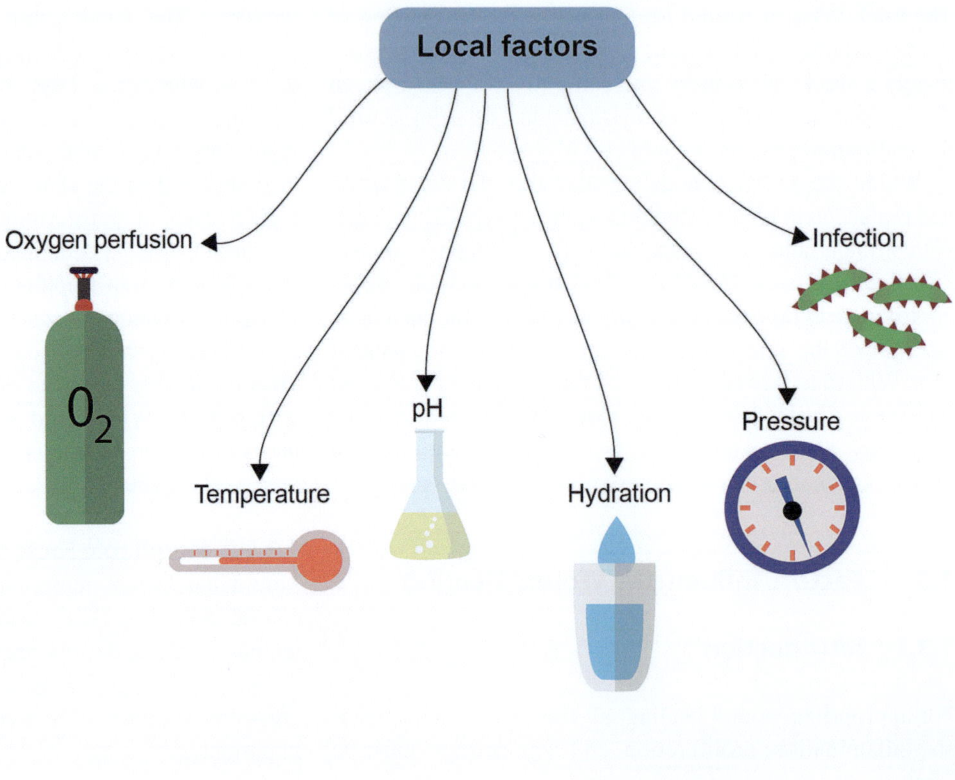

Fig. 1.4 Local factors affecting wound healing include the level of oxygen perfusion and hydration, temperature, pressure, pH, and the presence of infection

be noted that lactate is another factor that appears to collaborate with oxygen in order to induce angiogenesis [17]. Adequate oxygenation and perfusion is critical to fight infection. Cellular antibacterial mechanisms carried out by polymorphonuclear leukocytes directly depend on the availability of free oxygen radicals, such as bactericidal superoxide [17]. Furthermore, inadequate oxygen perfusion has been linked to antibiotic insensitivity, with hypoxic wounds being less sensitive to antibiotics [24]. It should be noted that shortly after injury, hypoxia stimulates wound healing, and it is only after chronic exposure to hypoxia that the wound healing process becomes delayed, with the wound becoming chronic [25]. In other words, hypoxia is necessary for the initiation of wound healing, which should then be sustained with delivery of the required oxygen [26]

1.3.2.3 Hydration

Adequate wound hydration is important for optimal wound healing. Following trauma, the skin barrier is disrupted, resulting in increased loss of fluid from the surface. Desiccation of the wound can result in cell dehydration and death, ultimately leading to scab formation and impairment of wound healing. Ulcers and burns are particularly at risk of desiccation as their rate of fluid loss from the wound surface is tenfold greater than normal skin [27]. Wound hydration allows for faster but also less painful healing [28]. A high moisture environment appears to promote angiogenesis and collagen synthesis [28]. In addition, in comparison to dry wounds, moist wounds have a higher rate of reepithelialization and keratinocyte production [29].

Concurrently, adequate moisture inhibits the degradation of growth factors and proteinases [30] and results in a lower rate of scar formation [31]. Other suggested factors believed to be involved in the improvement of wound healing seen with moist environments is an enhancement of epidermal cell migration [32] and fibroblast production [33]. It should be noted that, contrary to previous beliefs, and in contrast to a dehydrated wound, a moist environment does not increase the risk of infection [34].

1.3.2.4 Temperature

Maintenance of an optimum temperature also influences wound healing. Two factors determine the temperature of the wound, the temperature of the environment and the level of blood supply to the injured area. Blood supply is, in turn, determined by the extent of vasodilation or constriction. In an acute wound environment, an increase in vasoactive mediators results in local vasodilation to enable more efficient oxygen and nutrient delivery. Vasodilation causes an increase in the local temperature [35]. Chronic wounds, such as diabetic foot ulcers, often have poor blood supply networks that results in having a temperature 5 °C lower than the core temperature [36]. Ideally wounds should be maintained at a temperature close to 37 °C to maximize healing. Increased temperature in a wound can be a sign of infection [37].

1.3.2.5 Bioburden/Infection

The presence of excessive bacterial growth in wounds has deleterious effects on the healing process. Bacterial presence can be categorized as contamination, colonization, critical colonization, and invasive infection based on the extent and stage of bacterial growth. Contamination indicates the presence of bacteria without proliferation, whereas colonization indicates that bacteria have begun to multiply but tissue damage has not yet occurred. The critical colonization point is reached when the host immune response becomes overwhelmed by bacterial proliferation. Typically, this coincides with a halt in wound healing. When bacteria continue to proliferate even as the host response occurs, and the bacterial count reaches 10^5 bacteria per gram of tissue, it is considered an infection and subsequent host injury ensues [38]. Bacteria in a wound present a metabolic burden (e.g., bioburden) as they compete with fibroblasts and macrophages for nutrients and interfere with the normal healing process. Consequently, it is imperative to reduce bacterial presence. Contaminated wounds may need simple irrigation and lavage, while infected wounds may require debridement and systemic antibiotics [16]. Systemic antibiotics work best in areas of the wound with adequate perfusion. If, however, decontamination is inadequate, the inflammation phase becomes longer in an effort to clear the microbial burden. If the bacterial level is too high, the wound can become chronic and the healing process may fail. Prolonged inflammation has two sequelae, it promotes the production of MMPs, which as described above are proteases that degrade the ECM, and inhibits the production of naturally occurring protease inhibitors. In combination, these sequelae lead to the degradation of growth factors as the protease function in chronic wounds proceeds unchecked [39].

1.3.2.6 pH

The level of acidity the wound is exposed to can determine the stage of healing, and indeed the pH level varies throughout the healing process [36]. In intact skin, the keratinocytes found in the epidermis secrete acids as a protective function against bacteria and fungi. When this barrier breaks down following injury, the local vasculature can also be injured, resulting in an increase in the pH of the wound surface from a value of approximately 5 to a value of 7.4 [40]. Wounds normally show a pH gradient, with the deepest region of the wound having the highest pH [41]. Studies have shown that acidity promotes wound healing, whereas alkalinity inhibits the wound healing process and promotes chronic wound formation. Acidity aids healing by promoting fibroblast and keratinocyte proliferation and granulation tissue formation

[42]. In addition, acidity inhibits bacterial growth decreasing the risk of infection.

Alkalinity inhibits healing through various mechanisms. First, given that a low pH protects against bacterial growth, bacteria can prevail under alkaline conditions resulting in infection but also biofilm formation [43]. Second, these bacteria can secrete proteases that work optimally under alkaline conditions and can promote proteolysis, resulting in release of toxic products, ultimately inhibiting healing [44].

1.3.2.7 Pressure

Pressure is a fundamental force that is discussed in more detail in Sect. 1.4 later on in this chapter. It is important to maintain the pressure at the site of injury within optimal levels. If pressure is too low, for example, when no external compression therapy is provided, the site of injury and surrounding tissues will experience high levels of edema which can increase the experience of pain [45]. In contrast, excessive pressure or pressure that has been sustained for long periods of time can impede the local vascularity, restricting blood supply to the region, diminishing nutrition and oxygen delivery, and inhibiting the healing process.

1.3.3 Systemic (Fig. 1.5)

The rate and quality of wound healing in patients can be impacted by several systemic factors, including nutrition, alcohol consumption, smoking status, and steroid use.

1.3.3.1 Nutrition

Healing is a metabolically demanding process. Adequate nutrition is required for proper wound healing as macronutrient, micronutrient, and vitamin deficiencies can prolong the healing process. The key role of nutrition in wound healing can be seen in all phases of the wound healing process, with different nutritional deficiencies affecting different processes.

The most important macronutrients required for proper wound healing are proteins and carbohydrates.

Protein is paramount to wound healing, as it is not only required for fibroblast, collagen, and capillary formation, but it is also necessary for proper immune system functioning to prevent infection. Wound healing in patients with protein deficiency has a longer inflammatory phase, caused by decreased production of collagen and other proteins required for healing, and a higher rate of wound dehiscence [46]. The delayed inflammatory phase, in turn, delays the proliferative and remodeling phases. It should be noted that patients with actively healing wounds have a higher daily protein requirement, with one study finding that in order for patients with wounds to maintain adequate nutritional status they require 0.38 g of protein per day higher than patients without wounds [47]. Furthermore, this protein requirement rises even further in multiple, nonhealing wounds with high exudate loss.

Wound healing is a metabolically demanding process which, similar to other processes in the body, utilizes carbohydrates as the primary source of energy. Monosaccharide carbohydrates, such as glucose, are used to produce the

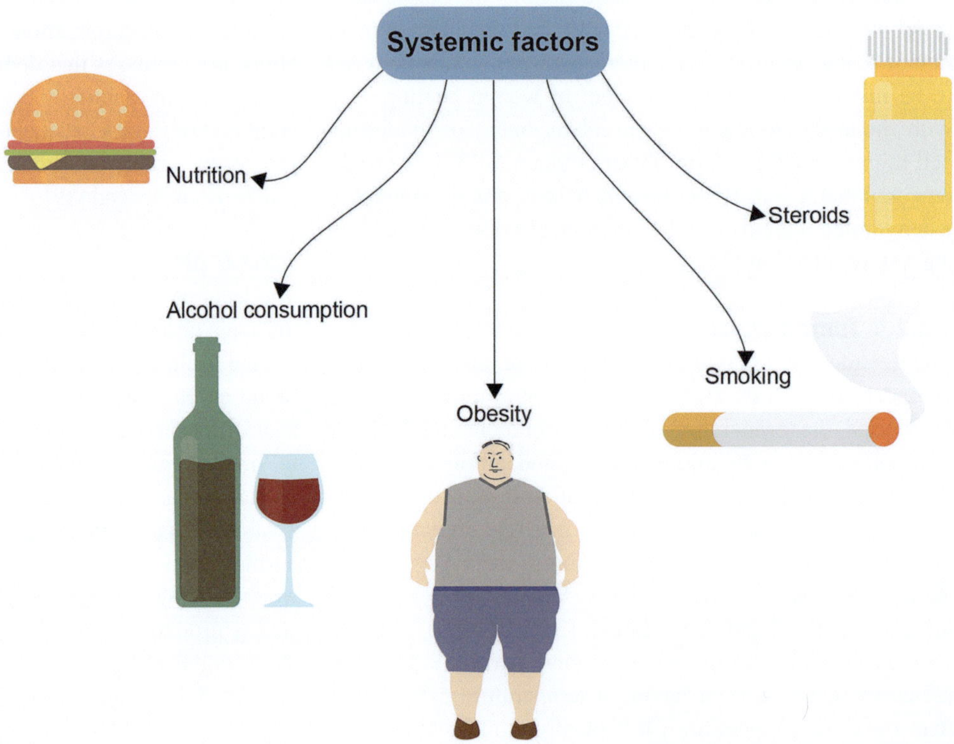

Fig. 1.5 Systemic factors affecting wound healing include alcohol, tobacco, and steroid intake, as well as the state of nutrition and obesity

adenosine triphosphate required to provide energy for processes such as cell proliferation and angiogenesis. In the shortage of glucose, the body is forced to undergo gluconeogenesis, utilizing different sources of energy including amino acids and possibly leading to depletion of the components required for the construction of proteins necessary for efficient wound healing. In contrast, hyperglycemia can also cause major complications in the process of wound healing. Systemic hyperglycemia leads to glycosylation of the microvasculature, which in turn decreases blood flow and reduces the permeability of erythrocytes. This results in hypoxia and nutrient depletion, ultimately impairing wound healing [48].

Certain micronutrients including zinc is strongly correlated to impaired wound healing. This is believed to be due to the fact that zinc is required for the formation of matrix metalloproteinases, which are in turn necessary for adequate wound healing [49]. Iron and magnesium are necessary for collagen formation [50].

Vitamins A, C, and E have the most well-established role in wound healing and deficiencies of either of these vitamins result in impaired wound healing. Specifically, vitamin A and vitamin C deficiencies are associated with decreased angiogenesis, collagen deposition, and fibroblast proliferation. Vitamin A has also been associated with decreased degradation of the ECM while vitamin C has been linked to decreased fragility of capillaries as well as an overall improvement of the immune system, and hence a decreased likelihood of infection. Vitamin E is best known for its role as an antioxidant, and in the process of wound healing it protects the ECM from destruction due to oxidation. Animal research has suggested that vitamin E supplementation is associated with improved wound healing, particularly in terms of decreased scar formation [51].

1.3.3.2 Obesity

Obesity is a significant factor that impairs wound healing, and given the current obesity epidemic, an imperative topic to be discussed in this chapter. The increased risk for various wound complications, including infection, necrosis, dehiscence, seroma occurrence, and ulceration, is well accepted [52]. The proposed mechanism underlying these complications is inadequate perfusion of nutrients and oxygen that occurs in subcutaneous adipose tissue. The theory behind this is that obesity results in hypertrophy and hyperplasia of adipocytes. This leads to metabolic dysfunction and initiation of a low-grade chronic inflammation. Concurrently, M2 macrophages which serve a protective function are replaced with M1 macrophages which are pro-inflammatory. In addition, the rate of adipocyte hypertrophy does not match the rate of angiogenesis, with angiogenesis failing to keep up with the increased need for perfusion. To further add to this unfavorable environment, the adipose tissue in obese individuals releases factors that induce fibrosis and inhibit angiogenesis [53]. Overall, this decreases the perfusion of the area resulting in hypoxia. In terms of infection, hypoperfusion is believed to not only create an environment which is prone to microbial contamination but also the one that hinders antibiotic delivery. Beyond hypoperfusion, wounds in obese individuals are believed to be under higher tension, which not only increases the risk of dehiscence but also adds to the hypoperfusion, via an unfavorable rise in tissue pressure [53]. Obesity also has a general negative impact on the immune system. Adipocytes and macrophages found in adipose tissue release adipokines, which are bioactive molecules which can inhibit the immune system. These molecules which include, but are not limited to, cytokines and hormone-like factors such as leptin and adiponectin are believed to negatively impact wound healing [54].

1.3.3.3 Smoking Status

The negative effects of cigarette smoking on adequate wound healing are well known. In particular, smoking delays wound healing and increases the risk of complications. For example, a study from Wahie and Lawrence found the infection rate following skin biopsies was 64% for smokers compared to 12% for nonsmokers [55]. A different study found that smokers also have a higher risk, three times greater, of necrosis compared to nonsmokers, with this risk further increased for heavier smokers [56]. The exact mechanisms underlying these increased risks are not fully understood, but it is believed that vasoconstriction and tissue ischemia play a role. Following smoke inhalation, peripheral blood flow decreases significantly (30–40%) [57]. In the context of wound healing, this means injured tissue receives less oxygen, impairing its ability to repair. Nicotine, a vasoconstrictor present in tobacco, also has prothrombotic effects. By increasing platelet adhesiveness, nicotine can contribute to tissue ischemia [58]. Tissue ischemia has a deleterious effect on wound healing by inducing tissue hypoxia. Given the negative effects of smoking on wound healing, it is recommended that patients to abstain from smoking for 4–6 weeks prior to surgery.

1.3.3.4 Alcohol Consumption

Wound healing is negatively impacted by both acute and chronic alcohol exposure. This impairment is both due to an increased rate of infection, believed to be owing to the suppression of pro-inflammatory cytokines, neutrophils, and phagocytes, and due to inhibition of the proliferative phase of wound healing [59]. Specifically, acute alcohol exposure has been shown to more than halve the level of angiogenesis, a phenomenon hypothesized to be due to a decline in the expression of the proangiogenic cytokine basic fibroblast growth factor (FGF-2) and vascular endothelial growth factor (VEGF) [60]. Furthermore, animal studies have shown that acute intoxication inhibits the production of collagen, while simultaneously promoting the expression of matrix degrading enzymes and transforming growth factor beta (TGF-β), an immunoinhibitory molecule which impairs monocyte function [61].

1.3.3.5 Steroids

Systemic steroid use is associated with an impaired rate of wound healing through the reduction of angiogenesis, fibroblast proliferation, and collagen deposition. While the mechanisms behind this remain unclear, it has been proposed that systemic steroids lower the levels of TGF-β, insulin-like growth factor-1 (IGF-1), and hypoxia-inducible factor-1 (HIF-1), which in turn causes the aforementioned effects [62, 63]. In addition to the benefits mentioned under Sect. 1.3.3.1, vitamin A may be a useful adjunct for reversing the deleterious effects of systemic steroid usage on wound healing [16]. In addition to their effect on the actual process of wound healing, systemic steroids are also associated with an increased risk of wound infection. It is significant to note that in contrast to systemic steroids, local steroid use has been shown to improve wound healing, particularly through the reduction of hypergranulation tissue formation [64].

1.4 Advanced Wound Healing Strategies

1.4.1 Introduction

Modulating the local and systemic factors described in Sect. 1.2 optimizes wound healing. Through the years a wide armamentarium of wound healing technologies which alter the wound environment have developed. This section will discuss the different options focusing on their advantages and disadvantages.

1.4.2 Debridement

Debridement is the process by which tissue at the wound edge is removed with an ultimate goal to promote wound healing. Debridement can be carried out in order to remove infected tissue and to decrease the biofilm load at the wound edge. Necrotic tissue is also an indication, as nonviable tissue presents a physical barrier to waste removal and oxygen and nutrient delivery, as well as serving as a substrate for bacterial growth. Debridement also assists in removal of extensive hyperkeratosis [65]. In addition, debridement is often carried out in preparation of the wound bed for further treatment, for example, for graft or exogenous factor application.

The remaining tissue, adjacent to the wound edge that has been sharply debrided, is better able to respond to treatment [66]. Studies have shown that the cells at the edge of the wound are less efficient at responding to wound healing stimuli, than the cells from the adjacent, non-ulcerated area. This is believed to be due to a difference in the expression of growth factor receptors in the two areas [67].

Debridement can be performed surgically, mechanically, enzymatically, or through the use of maggots. Surgical debridement, also called sharp debridement, requires a surgeon to selectively remove nonviable tissue using scalpels, scissors, and other instruments. Mechanical debridement uses hydrotherapy, wet-to-dry dressings, and wound irrigation to physically remove nonviable tissue. In contrast, enzymatic debridement and the use of maggots are more biologically driven procedures. Enzymatic debridement entails the application of topical enzymatic agents to the wound. These enzymes break down necrotic tissue. Although not commonly used, maggots have a function similar to enzymatic agents; maggots selectively feed on the necrotic tissue. Regardless of method, debridement must often be performed more than once, as microbial recolonization of the wound is common and often attributed to the formation of biofilms [68].

1.4.3 Dressings

A large number of dressings have been developed to facilitate wound healing. Wound dressings can be subclassified into passive, interactive, and bioactive dressings. Passive dressings, such as gauze, are nonocclusive and act primarily as a cover. Despite its simplicity, plain gauze is still the most widely used dressing. Gauze can itself be impregnated with various substances such as iodine or zinc, offering an inexpensive and easy-to-use option for wound coverage [69]. Passive dressings tend to be favored in clean, dry wounds. Interactive dressings, on the other hand, are either occlusive or semiocclusive and can act as a protective barrier against bacterial contamination. Available options include films, foams, hydrogels, and hydrocolloids. Polyurethane film dressings adhere and conform to the shape of the skin, are transparent, and are semiocclusive allowing gaseous and water vapor transmission. These properties make them best suited for superficial wounds with little exudate. Similarly, foam dressings are semiocclusive. They tend to be made of hydrophobic and hydrophilic foam, which offers the further benefit of being able to absorb wound exudate; consequently, their preferred use is in wounds with high levels of exudate, such as diabetic foot ulcers. Hydrogel dressings are composed of synthetic polymers such as polyvinyl pyrrolidine. They have a high water content being able to create a hydrophilic moist wound environment. They are used commonly in chronic or necrotic wounds which are dry, burn wounds and pressure ulcers. Finally, hydrocolloid dressings offer selective permeability, by allowing some passage of water vapor and gaseous exchange, but preventing the bacterial barrier. Furthermore, they have an inner colloidal layer which allows absorption of exudates [70]. They tend to be used in wounds with moderate amounts of exudate, for example, pressure ulcers and minor burn wounds. Bioactive dressings incorporate biomaterials known to be involved in wound healing, such as collagen, chitosan, and hyaluronic acid, in order to enhance wound healing [71–73]. These can often be combined with growth factors and antimicrobials. Overall, bioactive dressings have been praised to be far superior to other types of dressings particularly because they are biocompatible and biodegradable [70].

1.4.4 Biologics

Cytokines are a group of small secreted proteins involved in the regulation of inflammation and include chemokines, interleukins, and interferons. Growth factors are endogenous proteins that enhance wound healing by promoting cellular proliferation, differentiation, and survival. Many have assumed that topical treatment of wounds with these molecules would revolutionize wound healing. Unfortunately, there is only one growth factor on the market today, PDGF. Becaplermin gel (REGRANEX) was the first recombinant PDGF commercially available in the United States and is approved for the treatment of diabetic foot ulcers [74]. Early mechanistic studies revealed that this topical preparation has the ability to attract neutrophils and macrophages, increase levels of fibroblasts, stimulate production of critical ECM elements, and enhance remodeling, all of which are required for efficient wound healing [75]. In practice, seven clinical trials (total $n = 685$) demonstrated a statistically significant increase in ulcer healing with recombinant PDGF when compared to placebo therapy [76]. Randomized trials of REPIFERMIN, a similar topical treatment containing recombinant isoform of fibroblast growth factor (FGF), have also shown promising results with significant improvement in the healing of chronic venous ulcers. REPIFERMIN is currently in Phase II trials for the treatment of cancer therapy-induced mucositis. Despite the positive results, widespread use of recombinant growth factors has been limited by poor bioavailability and inactivation by wound proteases which render these treatments inefficient [77].

1.4.4.1 Hyperbaric Oxygen

Hyperbaric oxygen therapy (HBOT) has been promoted as an effective treatment for chronic lower limb ulcers. In theory, HBOT reduces local ischemia by promoting oxygen diffusion into the wound bed through an increase in the concentration of dissolved oxygen in the plasma. The evidence on HBOT use is, however, inconclusive. Some research reports that HBOT leads to lower rates of amputation and improved healing at 1 year, albeit the evidence was of poor quality [78]. Another study found that HBOT can have negative results as it increases the risk for both minor and major amputations [79]. Other studies suggest that HBOT neither provides benefits nor induces harm [80]. Overall, the lack of prospective randomized trials of HBOT makes this a controversial area.

1.4.4.2 Skin Substitutes

Skin substitutes can be classified into cellular or acellular products. Cellular products consist of a matrix which contains living tissue, such as fibroblasts or keratinocytes, be it autologous, allogenous, or xenogenous. Acellular products, on the other hand, have a matrix which lacks any cellular tissues. Among the first skin substitutes to become commercially available, Epicel® (Genzyme Biosurgery, Cambridge, MA) is a live epithelial autograft derived from a patient's own keratinocytes that are cultured into large sheet, thereby eliminating donor site morbidity and obviating the need for mesh. Apligraf® (Organogenesis, Canton, MA), an allogenic "skin equivalent" composed of a dermal bovine collagen matrix seeded with neonatal fibroblasts and keratinocytes, has been shown to accelerate healing when applied on chronic wounds [81]. Integra® Dermal Regeneration Template (Integra LifeSciences, Plainsboro, NJ) is a bilayer matrix of epidermal silicone overlying a matrix of dermal bovine collagen and chondroitin-6-sulfate, is commercially available, and has had considerable success in the treatment of life-threatening burns, post-burn contractures, and exposed tendon and joints [82, 83].

1.4.5 Biophysical

1.4.5.1 Negative Pressure Wound Therapy

Negative pressure wound therapy (NPWT), first described 20 years ago, is a broad term used to define any technology designed to form a tight air seal around the wound enabling the application of a vacuum [84]. Negative pressure is a misnomer as all pressure values are positive, and has also been referred to as vacuum assisted closure (VAC), subatmospheric pressure therapy, or microdeformational wound therapy. NPWT has numerous indications, including both acute and chronic wounds, such as burns and diabetic and pressure ulcers [85]. This technology utilizes a porous material, a drainage port, and an adhesive film dressing. The porous material, which can be, but is not limited to, foam or gauze, is used to fill the wound and allows for uniform transmission of pressure. The port is connected to this material and to a vacuum pump which is set to maintain a pressure of −50 to −150 mmHg [86]. The dressing is designed to form an airtight seal around the wound.

NPWT is proposed to work via four main mechanisms. First, the wound edges can be better apposed via macrodeformation, in which the suction applied causes the foam to shrink pulling the wound edges closer together. In addition to this macroscopic change, suction applied to the foam causes microdeformational changes resulting in an undulation of the wound surface. In addition to promoting better apposition of the wound edges, microdeformation stimulates angiogenesis and upregulation of granulation tissue [86, 87]. Third, NPWT can result in fluid removal from the wound, decreasing the compression forces acting at the wound bed and promoting better vascularization and tissue perfusion [84]. Finally, NPWT can cause an overall change in the wound environment. This is not surprising, given that there is fluid removal from the wound and consequently alteration of the local concentration of electrolytes and nutrients. In addition, the packing material and dressing act as insulation, keeping the wound moist and warm [86].

A recent literature review compared the efficacy of NPWT versus standard therapy based on the results of available randomized controlled trials [88]. The overall conclusion was that the technology is both safe and effective in reducing the need for surgical intervention in diabetic patients [89–91], and reducing inflammation and edema when used with split thickness skin grafts, either in preparation for or postoperatively [92–94]. Furthermore, a decreased rate of infection was seen in traumatic wounds [95].

1.4.5.2 Traction-Assisted Dermatogenesis

Traction-assisted dermatogenesis is a noninvasive tissue expansion technique, developed by Daya and Nair a decade ago. In this technique, a series of Micropore (3M, St. Paul, MN) tapes is applied to the skin over a long period of time. Through intermittent tension loading of the skin, the tissue undergoes expansion through the generation of new tissue. Unlike presuturing, tissue expanders, and skin-stretching devices, traction-assisted dermatogenesis is noninvasive and consequently offers the advantages of being easier and cheaper [96].

References

1. Manring MM, Hawk A, Calhoun JH, Andersen RC. Treatment of war wounds: a historical review. Clin Orthop Relat Res. 2009;467(8):2168–91.
2. Feinglass J, Pearce WH, Martin GJ, Gibbs J, Cowper D, Sorensen M, et al. Postoperative and late survival outcomes after major amputation: findings from the Department of Veterans Affairs National Surgical Quality Improvement Program. Surgery. 2001;130(1):21–9.
3. Aulivola B, Hile CN, Hamdan AD, Sheahan MG, Veraldi JR, Skillman JJ, et al. Major lower extremity amputation: outcome of a modern series. Arch Surg. 2004;139(4):395–9. discussion 9.
4. Bayat A, McGrouther DA, Ferguson MW. Skin scarring. BMJ. 2003;326(7380):88–92.
5. Lawrence JW, Mason ST, Schomer K, Klein MB. Epidemiology and impact of scarring after burn injury: a systematic review of the literature. J Burn Care Res. 2012;33(1):136–46.
6. Auden WH, Mendelson E. Collected poems. London: Faber and Faber; 1976. p. 696.
7. Kumar V, Abbas AK, Aster JC. Robbins and Cotran pathologic basis of disease. 9th ed. Philadelphia, PA: Elsevier/Saunders; 2015. xvi, p. 1391.
8. Goldberg AL, Etlinger JD, Goldspink DF, Jablecki C. Mechanism of work-induced hypertrophy of skeletal muscle. Med Sci Sports. 1975;7(3):185–98.
9. Michalopoulos GK. Liver regeneration. J Cell Physiol. 2007;213(2):286–300.
10. Ohsumi Y. Historical landmarks of autophagy research. Cell Res. 2014;24(1):9–23.
11. Wheeler JB, Reed CE. Epidemiology of esophageal cancer. Surg Clin North Am. 2012;92(5):1077–87.
12. Mik G, Gholve PA, Scher DM, Widmann RF, Green DW. Down syndrome: orthopedic issues. Curr Opin Pediatr. 2008;20(1):30–6.
13. Wada T, Tone Y, Shibata F, Toma T, Yachie A. Delayed wound healing in leukocyte adhesion deficiency type 1. J Pediatr. 2011;158(2):342.
14. Gould L, Abadir P, Brem H, Carter M, Conner-Kerr T, Davidson J, et al. Chronic wound repair and healing in older adults: current status and future research. J Am Geriatr Soc. 2015;63(3):427–38.
15. Kurosaka M, Suzuki T, Hosono K, Kamata Y, Fukamizu A, Kitasato H, et al. Reduced angiogenesis and delay in wound healing in angiotensin II type 1a receptor-deficient mice. Biomed Pharmacother. 2009;63(9):627–34.
16. Thorne C, Chung KC, Gosain A, Guntner GC, Mehrara BJ, Rubin JP, Spear SL, editors. Grabb and Smith's plastic surgery. 7th ed. Philadelphia: Wolters Kluwer/Lippincott Williams & Wilkins Health; 2014. xbiii, p. 1030.
17. Gottrup F. Oxygen in wound healing and infection. World J Surg. 2004;28(3):312–5.
18. Prockop DJ, Kivirikko KI, Tuderman L, Guzman NA. The biosynthesis of collagen and its disorders (first of two parts). N Engl J Med. 1979;301(1):13–23.
19. Prockop DJ, Kivirikko KI, Tuderman L, Guzman NA. The biosynthesis of collagen and its disorders (second of two parts). N Engl J Med. 1979;301(2):77–85.
20. Vihersaari T, Kivisaari J, Ninikoski J. Effect of changes in inspired oxygen tension on wound metabolism. Ann Surg. 1974;179(6):889–95.
21. Jonsson K, Hunt TK, Mathes SJ. Oxygen as an isolated variable influences resistance to infection. Ann Surg. 1988;208(6):783–7.
22. Shweiki D, Itin A, Soffer D, Keshet E. Vascular endothelial growth factor induced by hypoxia may mediate hypoxia-initiated angiogenesis. Nature. 1992;359(6398):843–5.
23. Semenza GL. HIF-1 and human disease: one highly involved factor. Genes Dev. 2000;14(16):1983–91.
24. Mader JT, Brown GL, Guckian JC, Wells CH, Reinarz JA. A mechanism for the amelioration by hyperbaric oxygen of experimental staphylococcal osteomyelitis in rabbits. J Infect Dis. 1980;142(6):915–22.
25. Rodriguez PG, Felix FN, Woodley DT, Shim EK. The role of oxygen in wound healing: a review of the literature. Dermatol Surg. 2008;34(9):1159–69.

26. Bishop A. Role of oxygen in wound healing. J Wound Care. 2008;17(9):399–402.
27. Wu P, Nelson EA, Reid WH, Ruckley CV, Gaylor JD. Water vapour transmission rates in burns and chronic leg ulcers: influence of wound dressings and comparison with in vitro evaluation. Biomaterials. 1996;17(14):1373–7.
28. Junker JP, Kamel RA, Caterson EJ, Eriksson E. Clinical impact upon wound healing and inflammation in moist, wet, and dry environments. Adv Wound Care (New Rochelle). 2013;2(7):348–56.
29. Madden MR, Nolan E, Finkelstein JL, Yurt RW, Smeland J, Goodwin CW, et al. Comparison of an occlusive and a semiocclusive dressing and the effect of the wound exudate upon keratinocyte proliferation. J Trauma. 1989;29(7):924–30. discussion 30-1.
30. Svensjo T, Pomahac B, Yao F, Slama J, Eriksson E. Accelerated healing of full-thickness skin wounds in a wet environment. Plast Reconstr Surg. 2000;106(3):602–12. discussion 13-4.
31. Winter GD. Formation of the scab and the rate of epithelization of superficial wounds in the skin of the young domestic pig. Nature. 1962;193:293–4.
32. Eaglstein WH. Moist wound healing with occlusive dressings: a clinical focus. Dermatol Surg. 2001;27(2):175–81.
33. Katz MH, Alvarez AF, Kirsner RS, Eaglstein WH, Falanga V. Human wound fluid from acute wounds stimulates fibroblast and endothelial cell growth. J Am Acad Dermatol. 1991;25(6 Pt 1):1054–8.
34. Field FK, Kerstein MD. Overview of wound healing in a moist environment. Am J Surg. 1994;167(1A):2S–6S.
35. Wilmore DW, Aulick LH, Mason AD, Pruitt BA Jr. Influence of the burn wound on local and systemic responses to injury. Ann Surg. 1977;186(4):444–58.
36. Kruse CR, Nuutila K, Lee CC, Kiwanuka E, Singh M, Caterson EJ, et al. The external microenvironment of healing skin wounds. Wound Repair Regen. 2015;23(4):456–64.
37. Fierheller M, Sibbald RG. A clinical investigation into the relationship between increased periwound skin temperature and local wound infection in patients with chronic leg ulcers. Adv Skin Wound Care. 2010;23(8):369–79. quiz 80-1.
38. Robson MC, Krizek TJ, Heggers JP. Biology of surgical infection. Curr Probl Surg. 1973;10:1–62.
39. Edwards R, Harding KG. Bacteria and wound healing. Curr Opin Infect Dis. 2004;17(2):91–6.
40. Lambers H, Piessens S, Bloem A, Pronk H, Finkel P. Natural skin surface pH is on average below 5, which is beneficial for its resident flora. Int J Cosmet Sci. 2006;28(5):359–70.
41. Schreml S, Szeimies RM, Karrer S, Heinlin J, Landthaler M, Babilas P. The impact of the pH value on skin integrity and cutaneous wound healing. J Eur Acad Dermatol Venereol. 2010;24(4):373–8.
42. Lengheden A, Jansson L. pH effects on experimental wound healing of human fibroblasts in vitro. Eur J Oral Sci. 1995;103(3):148–55.
43. Stewart CM, Cole MB, Legan JD, Slade L, Vandeven MH, Schaffner DW. Staphylococcus aureus growth boundaries: moving towards mechanistic predictive models based on solute-specific effects. Appl Environ Microbiol. 2002;68(4):1864–71.
44. Menke NB, Ward KR, Witten TM, Bonchev DG, Diegelmann RF. Impaired wound healing. Clin Dermatol. 2007;25(1):19–25.
45. Hettrick H. The science of compression therapy for chronic venous insufficiency edema. J Am Col Certif Wound Spec. 2009;1(1):20–4.
46. Pinchcofsky-Devin G. Nutrition and wound healing. J Wound Care. 1994;3(5):231–4.
47. Pompeo M. Misconceptions about protein requirements for wound healing: results of a prospective study. Ostomy Wound Manage. 2007;53(8):30–2. 4, 6–8 passim.
48. Loots MA, Lamme EN, Zeegelaar J, Mekkes JR, Bos JD, Middelkoop E. Differences in cellular infiltrate and extracellular matrix of chronic diabetic and venous ulcers versus acute wounds. J Invest Dermatol. 1998;111(5):850–7.
49. Mirastschijski U, Haaksma CJ, Tomasek JJ, Agren MS. Matrix metalloproteinase inhibitor GM 6001 attenuates keratinocyte migration, contraction and myofibroblast formation in skin wounds. Exp Cell Res. 2004;299(2):465–75.
50. Guo S, Dipietro LA. Factors affecting wound healing. J Dent Res. 2010;89(3):219–29.
51. Burgess C. Topical vitamins. J Drugs Dermatol. 2008;7(7 Suppl):s2–6.
52. Wilson JA, Clark JJ. Obesity: impediment to postsurgical wound healing. Adv Skin Wound Care. 2004;17(8):426–35.
53. Pierpont YN, Dinh TP, Salas RE, Johnson EL, Wright TG, Robson MC, et al. Obesity and surgical wound healing: a current review. ISRN Obes. 2014;2014:638936.
54. Juge-Aubry CE, Henrichot E, Meier CA. Adipose tissue: a regulator of inflammation. Best Pract Res Clin Endocrinol Metab. 2005;19(4):547–66.
55. Wahie S, Lawrence CM. Wound complications following diagnostic skin biopsies in dermatology inpatients. Arch Dermatol. 2007;143(10):1267–71.
56. Goldminz D, Bennett RG. Cigarette smoking and flap and full-thickness graft necrosis. Arch Dermatol. 1991;127(7):1012–5.
57. Jensen JA, Goodson WH, Hopf HW, Hunt TK. Cigarette smoking decreases tissue oxygen. Arch Surg. 1991;126(9):1131–4.
58. Wennmalm A, Alster P. Nicotine inhibits vascular prostacyclin but not platelet thromboxane formation. Gen Pharmacol. 1983;14(1):189–91.
59. Greiffenstein P, Molina PE. Alcohol-induced alterations on host defense after traumatic injury. J Trauma. 2008;64(1):230–40.
60. Radek KA, Matthies AM, Burns AL, Heinrich SA, Kovacs EJ, Dipietro LA. Acute ethanol exposure impairs angiogenesis and the proliferative phase of wound healing. Am J Physiol Heart Circ Physiol. 2005;289(3):H1084–90.
61. Radek KA, Ranzer MJ, DiPietro LA. Brewing complications: the effect of acute ethanol exposure on wound healing. J Leukoc Biol. 2009;86(5):1125–34.
62. Wicke C, Halliday B, Allen D, Roche NS, Scheuenstuhl H, Spencer MM, et al. Effects of steroids and retinoids on wound healing. Arch Surg. 2000;135(11):1265–70.
63. Wagner AE, Huck G, Stiehl DP, Jelkmann W, Hellwig-Burgel T. Dexamethasone impairs hypoxia-inducible factor-1 function. Biochem Biophys Res Commun. 2008;372(2):336–40.
64. McShane DB, Bellet JS. Treatment of hypergranulation tissue with high potency topical corticosteroids in children. Pediatr Dermatol. 2012;29(5):675–8.
65. Steed DL, Donohoe D, Webster MW, Lindsley L. Effect of extensive debridement and treatment on the healing of diabetic foot ulcers. Diabetic Ulcer Study Group. J Am Coll Surg. 1996;183(1):61–4.
66. Schiffman J, Golinko MS, Yan A, Flattau A, Tomic-Canic M, Brem H. Operative debridement of pressure ulcers. World J Surg. 2009;33(7):1396–402.
67. Brem H, Stojadinovic O, Diegelmann RF, Entero H, Lee B, Pastar I, et al. Molecular markers in patients with chronic wounds to guide surgical debridement. Mol Med. 2007;13(1–2):30–9.
68. Baranoski S, Ayello EA. Wound care essentials: practice principles. 4th ed. Philadelphia: Wolters Kluwer; 2016. xiv, p. 593.
69. Murphy PS, Evans GR. Advances in wound healing: a review of current wound healing products. Plast Surg Int. 2012;2012:190436.
70. Dhivya S, Padma VV, Santhini E. Wound dressings: a review. Biomedicine (Taipei). 2015;5(4):22.

71. Ramshaw JA, Werkmeister JA, Glattauer V. Collagen-based biomaterials. Biotechnol Genet Eng Rev. 1996;13:335–82.
72. Ishihara M, Nakanishi K, Ono K, Sato M, Kikuchi M, Saito Y, et al. Photocrosslinkable chitosan as a dressing for wound occlusion and accelerator in healing process. Biomaterials. 2002;23(3):833–40.
73. Doillon CJ, Silver FH. Collagen-based wound dressing: effects of hyaluronic acid and fibronectin on wound healing. Biomaterials. 1986;7(1):3–8.
74. Wieman TJ. Clinical efficacy of becaplermin (rhPDGF-BB) gel. Becaplermin Gel Studies Group. Am J Surg. 1998;176(2A Suppl):74S–9S.
75. Heldin CH, Westermark B. Mechanism of action and in vivo role of platelet-derived growth factor. Physiol Rev. 1999;79(4):1283–316.
76. Greer N, Foman N, Dorrian J, Fitzgerald P, MacDonald R, Rutks I, et al. Advanced wound care therapies for non-healing diabetic, venous, and arterial ulcers: a systematic review. VA evidence-based synthesis program reports. Washington, DC; 2012.
77. Robson MC, Phillips TJ, Falanga V, Odenheimer DJ, Parish LC, Jensen JL, et al. Randomized trial of topically applied repifermin (recombinant human keratinocyte growth factor-2) to accelerate wound healing in venous ulcers. Wound Repair Regen. 2001;9(5):347–52.
78. Duzgun AP, Satir HZ, Ozozan O, Saylam B, Kulah B, Coskun F. Effect of hyperbaric oxygen therapy on healing of diabetic foot ulcers. J Foot Ankle Surg. 2008;47(6):515–9.
79. Londahl M, Katzman P, Nilsson A, Hammarlund C. Hyperbaric oxygen therapy facilitates healing of chronic foot ulcers in patients with diabetes. Diabetes Care. 2010;33(5):998–1003.
80. Kalani M, Jorneskog G, Naderi N, Lind F, Brismar K. Hyperbaric oxygen (HBO) therapy in treatment of diabetic foot ulcers. Long-term follow-up. J Diabetes Complications. 2002;16(2):153–8.
81. Falanga V, Sabolinski M. A bilayered living skin construct (APLIGRAF) accelerates complete closure of hard-to-heal venous ulcers. Wound Repair Regen. 1999;7(4):201–7.
82. Jones I, Currie L, Martin R. A guide to biological skin substitutes. Br J Plast Surg. 2002;55(3):185–93.
83. Fitton AR, Drew P, Dickson WA. The use of a bilaminate artificial skin substitute (Integra) in acute resurfacing of burns: an early experience. Br J Plast Surg. 2001;54(3):208–12.
84. Argenta LC, Morykwas MJ. Vacuum-assisted closure: a new method for wound control and treatment: clinical experience. Ann Plast Surg. 1997;38(6):563–76. discussion 77.
85. Panayi AC, Leavitt T, Orgill DP. Evidence based review of negative pressure wound therapy. World J Dermatol. 2017;6(1):1–16.
86. Huang C, Leavitt T, Bayer LR, Orgill DP. Effect of negative pressure wound therapy on wound healing. Curr Probl Surg. 2014;51(7):301–31.
87. Urschel JD, Scott PG, Williams HT. The effect of mechanical stress on soft and hard tissue repair; a review. Br J Plast Surg. 1988;41(2):182–6.
88. Anghel EL, Kim PJ. Negative-pressure wound therapy: a comprehensive review of the evidence. Plast Reconstr Surg. 2016;138(3 Suppl):129S–37S.
89. Stannard JP, Volgas DA, McGwin G 3rd, Stewart RL, Obremskey W, Moore T, et al. Incisional negative pressure wound therapy after high-risk lower extremity fractures. J Orthop Trauma. 2012;26(1):37–42.
90. Masden D, Goldstein J, Endara M, Xu K, Steinberg J, Attinger C. Negative pressure wound therapy for at-risk surgical closures in patients with multiple comorbidities: a prospective randomized controlled study. Ann Surg. 2012;255(6):1043–7.
91. Gillespie BM, Rickard CM, Thalib L, Kang E, Finigan T, Homer A, et al. Use of negative-pressure wound dressings to prevent surgical site complications after primary hip arthroplasty: a pilot RCT. Surg Innov. 2015;22(5):488–95.
92. Saaiq M, Hameed Ud D, Khan MI, Chaudhery SM. Vacuum-assisted closure therapy as a pretreatment for split thickness skin grafts. J Coll Physicians Surg Pak. 2010;20(10):675–9.
93. Petkar KS, Dhanraj P, Kingsly PM, Sreekar H, Lakshmanarao A, Lamba S, et al. A prospective randomized controlled trial comparing negative pressure dressing and conventional dressing methods on split-thickness skin grafts in burned patients. Burns. 2011;37(6):925–9.
94. Bloemen MC, van der Wal MB, Verhaegen PD, Nieuwenhuis MK, van Baar ME, van Zuijlen PP, et al. Clinical effectiveness of dermal substitution in burns by topical negative pressure: a multicenter randomized controlled trial. Wound Repair Regen. 2012;20(6):797–805.
95. Eisenhardt SU, Schmidt Y, Thiele JR, Iblher N, Penna V, Torio-Padron N, et al. Negative pressure wound therapy reduces the ischaemia/reperfusion-associated inflammatory response in free muscle flaps. J Plast Reconstr Aesthet Surg. 2012;65(5):640–9.
96. Daya M, Nair V. Traction-assisted dermatogenesis by serial intermittent skin tape application. Plast Reconstr Surg. 2008;122(4):1047–54.

Burn Wound Healing and Scarring Pathophysiology

2

Haig A. Yenikomshian and Nicole S. Gibran

2.1 Initial Assessment of Burn Depth

Burn injury results from a variety of insulting factors including thermal and nonthermal mechanisms. Flames, fluids, extreme cold, electricity, and radiation damage affected tissue. Descriptions of burn depth and amount of surface area involved are important for clinicians for resuscitation and nutrition calculations and for operative planning. In 1832, Baron Guillaume Dupuytren described six degrees of burn depth [1]. The first-degree burn involves erythema of the skin without formation of bullae. Second-degree burns involve cutaneous inflammation with loss of the epidermis and the development of vesicles filled with serum. Third-degree burns comprise the entire dermis. Fourth-degree burns involve thermal injury into the subcutaneous tissue. Fifth-degree burns extend into muscle. Finally, sixth-degree burns involve thermal injury down to bone. The International Classification of Disease (ICD) simplifies this into the first-, second-, and third-degree burn system [2]. In this system, a first-degree burn involves the epidermis similar to Dupuytren's stage 1. A second-degree burn is partial thickness through the dermis, which corresponds to stage 2. Finally, a third-degree burn involves thermal destruction of the entire dermis or stages 3–6 in the Dupuytren's original description.

Burns can alternatively be classified by Jackson's three distinct zones of burn injury [3]. The outermost least injured wound is the zone of hyperemia, characterized by vasodilatation, increase blood flow, and inflammation. This zone equates to a first-degree burn and is typically viable and progresses to healing [4]. The middle zone of stasis, also known as the zone of ischemia, has marginal tissue perfusion with potentially salvageable tissue depending on systemic factors such as adequate resuscitation, infection, and comorbidity. This zone initially blanches with pressure, but may appear mottled and red [4]. This zone parallels a second degree of burn injury and may progress to healing or may convert to a full-thickness burn through apoptosis and oxidative stress [5]. The final central zone of coagulation, the area exposed to the most thermal injury, correlate with third- to sixth-degree burn injury. This is the site of protein denaturation and cell breakdown secondary to the initial thermal insult leading to coagulation and tissue necrosis. Generally, this central area will not heal without excision.

2.2 Acute Phases of Wound Healing

Limited research exists on responses to thermal injury compared to other excisional or incisional wounds but the continuum of the phases of healing from coagulation, inflammation angiogenesis, epithelialization, and eventually matrix remodeling are similar [6]. For each phase of healing, cellular migration occurs through a complicated balanced regulation by cytokines growth factors, integrins, and metalloproteases [7]. The initial phase of thermal injury to tissues involves activation of the hemostatic cascade [8]. The coagulation cascade is triggered by tissue factor, which results in the cleavage of fibrinogen to fibrin and the formation of a clot. Concomitantly with initial injury, vasoconstriction of the vessel is mediated by catecholamines to aid in hemostasis and platelet aggregation. Following this, vasodilation of the vessel helps aid in recruitment of inflammatory cells into the wound bed [9]. Migration occurs through a complicated regulation by three main factors: growth factors, integrins, and metalloproteases [10].

Inflammatory cells including neutrophils, macrophages, and fibroblasts migrate to the wound bed and secrete cytokines as part of the second "inflammatory phase" of wound healing, with the further recruitment of inflammatory cells as well as fibroblasts. Neutrophils predominate the early wound bed and

H. A. Yenikomshian (✉)
Division of Plastic Surgery, University of Southern California
Keck School of Medicine, Los Angeles, CA, USA
e-mail: haig.yenikomshian@med.usc.edu

N. S. Gibran
University of Washington Regional Burn Center, Harborview Medical Center, Seattle, WA, USA
e-mail: nicoleg@uw.edu

© Springer Nature Singapore Pte Ltd. 2020
R. Ogawa (ed.), *Total Scar Management*, https://doi.org/10.1007/978-981-32-9791-3_2

macrophages become more dominant by day 3 [11]. Macrophages release a variety of cytokines including platelet-derived growth factor (PDGF), insulin-like growth factor (IGF-1), and transforming growth factor beta (TGF-β) [12]. Macrophages can be subdivided into two types: inhibit-type macrophages (M1) which are involved in primary host defense and heal-type macrophages (M2) which are involved in wound healing [13]. Neutrophils also release cytokines including VEGF to promote angiogenesis in the wound bed [14].

Epidermal regeneration occurs in the proliferative phase of wound healing. Keratinocytes, the main structural and inflammatory cells of the epidermis, derive from the basal layer of the epidermis and epidermal appendages including hair follicles and sweat ducts. Epithelialization involves keratinocyte proliferation and migration from wound edges, hair follicles, sweat glands, and sebaceous glands in partial-thickness wounds; full-thickness wounds depend exclusively on cell migration only from the wound edges [15]. Mechanically, keratinocytes migrate by disassembling of hemidesmosomes and desmosomes and retraction and remodeling of intracellular filaments [16]. Basal keratinocytes then migrate superficially and terminally differentiate into coenocytes losing their nuclei and internal organelles becoming a protective barrier against infection and insensible losses [17]. Throughout the wound healing process, bidirectional keratinocyte and fibroblast regulation modulates wound healing and scar remodeling [18]. Fully epithelized wound beds such as donor sites and healed skin grafts are still prone to blistering because of defective reorganization of the basement membrane zone of the epidermis with defective fibroblast organization [19].

Fibroblasts become the predominant cell in the mesenchymal wound bed in the "proliferative phase." These morphogenetic cells synthesize the collagens and other glycosaminoglycans molecules and coordinate the conversion of an acute wound bed to scar extracellular matrix [20]. The highly vascularized granulation tissue formed during this phase consists of fibroblasts, inflammatory cells, and vascular endothelial cells. Capillaries permeate the granulation tissue into the forming extracellular matrix. Molecules secreted from inflammatory cells including VEGF, TGF-β, and angiopoietin are angiogenic and promote angiogenesis and growth of the vasculature into the wound [21]. Whereas granulation tissue indicates that the wound bed is healthy, the increased inflammatory cell and bacteria populations coupled with a high metalloprotease content require that granulation tissue be excised prior to grafting. Furthermore, this rich metabolic layer probably represents a precursor to fibroproliferative scar formation [22, 23].

The final "remodeling phase" of wound healing where fibroblasts transform the acute wound matrix into a mature scar bed may last for several years depending on the extent of the underlying tissue injury [24]. Fibroblasts acquire a smooth muscle cell-like phenotype, referred to as myofibroblasts [25, 26]. These cells replace Type III collagen with Type I collagen [9]. Through this remodeling, granulation tissue is replaced with scar and the modulation of extracellular matrix results in wound contracture [27]. Despite this repair, tensile strength of the scar will only be approximately 70% strength of the pre-injury state [28].

Our evolving understanding of the role of bone marrow-derived mesenchymal and adipose-derived stem cells in wound healing may change how we consider regenerative healing rather than reparative healing [29]. Bone marrow-derived mesenchymal cells are pluripotent that can convert to different types of tissue including skin, fat, and bone [30]. Injection of bone marrow-derived mesenchymal stem cells in mouse models increases proangiogenic factors [31]. Adipose-derived stem cells have also been shown to activate keratinocytes and dermal fibroblasts [32]. Use of these stem cells for dermal regeneration shows promise but is still unrealized in a practice model.

2.3 Hypertrophic Scarring Pathophysiology

Burn sequelae can be debilitating for individuals living with a burn injury and frustrating for burn team members. One common problem after thermal injuries is the hypertrophic scar: a hard, raised, red, and painful thickened scar. Figure 2.1

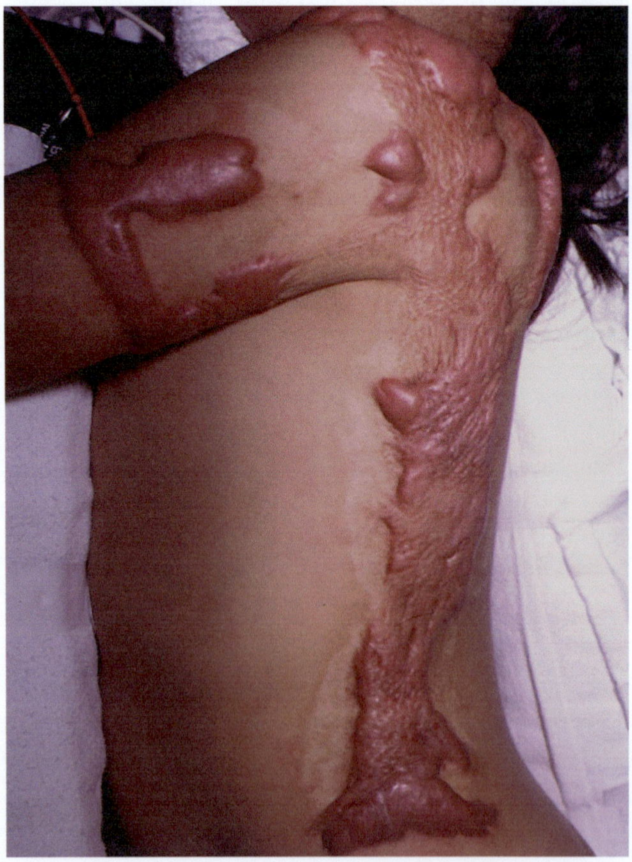

Fig. 2.1 Hypertrophic scar of the left upper extremity and left flank

demonstrates a hypertrophic scar of the left upper extremity and the left flank. The poorly understood pathophysiology of hypertrophic scarring has been an area of intense scrutiny for the past 40 years. The proliferation of fibrous tissue comprises an abnormal response to healing. Both hypertrophic scars and keloids result from this overzealous inflammatory response and may be difficult to differentiate on clinical exam. One main difference is that hypertrophic scars remain within the boundaries of the original wound whereas keloids extend beyond [33]. Histologically, keloids have thick eosinophilic collagen bundles whereas hypertrophic scars do not; however, many scars may present with a mixed picture [34]. Most fibroproliferative scars following a burn injury or donor site constitute hypertrophic scars.

Objective assessment of hypertrophic scar severity challenges clinicians. A reproducible validated measurement tool to determine the degree of scarring would be essential for clinicians and patients to guide treatment and assess therapeutic efficacy over time [35]. Two existing scales include the Vancouver scar scale (VSS) and the patient observer scar assessment scale (POSAS) which combine both objective and subjective measures to rate scars [36]. Whereas these scales are used widely for clinical trials, there is variability in what rating is defined as a hypertrophic scar and the penetrance of the different scales [37, 38].

2.4 Scar Pathophysiology

Fibroblasts, the main cell responsible for the deposition of collagen and remodeling of burn scar over time, vary across individuals as well as by body site and skin depth [39]. Fibroblasts in the deep reticular dermis respond differently to injury than cells in the more superficial papillary dermis, including more systemic release of Il-6 and IFN-gamma [40]. These deep fibroblasts are found early in wound healing in granulation tissue [41]. In normal wound healing, keratinocytes regulate dermal fibroblasts, and with the loss of epithelium this balance is lost with an upregulation of inflammatory cytokines [18]. The more severe the inflammatory response, the more intense the fibroblast response is with a higher risk of hypertrophic scarring [42].

One of the main cytokines involved in hypertrophic scarring is TGF-β, a potent activator of fibroblasts [43]. Hypertrophic scars have increased levels of TGF-β mRNA while fetal wounds which heal without scarring have markedly decreased levels [44]. TGF-β modulates extracellular matrix proteoglycans, and hypertrophic scars have lower levels of decorin but higher levels of versican and biglycan [45]. Production of increased levels of TGF-β may be due to loss of inhibition by other pathways. IFN-α and IFN-γ act to downregulate TGF-β by regulation of mRNA production; aberration in this pathway has also been found to be a cause of hypertrophic scarring [44].

Neural modulation of responses to injury represents an understudied area of research. Neuropeptides regulate several key cellular processes crucial to wound healing, including inflammatory cell migration, angiogenesis, keratinocyte migration, and mast cell degranulation. Substance P, released in acute wounds and inflammation, induces inflammation and mediates angiogenesis [46]. Too little substance P, as found in diabetic wounds, leads to chronic wounds and poor healing, and too much leads to a hyper-inflammatory state and hypertrophic scarring [47]. Aberrant neural modulation of healing processes also manifests as neuropathic pain and itch. Approximately 75% of patients complain of neuropathic-like pain in the months after healed wounds, and patients still complain of pruritus up to 10 years after injury [48, 49]. Related to the neuropathic pain is postburn pruritus, with some studies showing rates of 100% [50]. While the mechanism of action is poorly understood, the mechanism of itch is probably multifactorial. One of the key components is the activation of C fiber transmission of the itch sensation [51]. Tissue injury leads to increase in histamine and xanthine oxidase concentrations and local release of substance P as well as other cytokines [52]. Many of these will bind to C fiber receptors and will upregulate C fiber activation and the sensation of itch. The mechanism behind this is poorly understood and this may last years after initial insult. Treatments like gabapentin have been shown to improve symptoms but a multisite trial is necessary to demonstrate efficacy [53].

Enervated tissue, including diabetic ulcers, has been shown to have less scarring because mechanoreceptors are an integral part of wound healing cascade [54]. Mechanosensitive (MS) ion channels and sensory nerve fibers are stimulated causing activation of afferent sensory neurons and release of neuropeptides, which regulate immune cell function and cytokine production. TGF-β, upregulated by these neuropeptides, causes more hypertrophic scarring [55]. The importance of mechanoreceptors in the formation of hypertrophic scarring and keloid formation explains why certain tension-prone areas of the body are prone to hypertrophic scarring such as the anterior chest and shoulder [56]. Pressure garments are theorized to decrease this mechanical force by applying pressure in the opposite direction to flatten and soften scars [57].

2.5 Animal Models of Hypertrophic Scarring

Animal models have marginally expanded our limited understanding of hypertrophic scarring. The rabbit ear model has been used to measure burn wound healing and hypertrophic scarring showing that deeper burns causes more hypertrophic scarring [58]. Another increasingly recognized animal model has been the female red Duroc pig. Originally described in 1972, this animal has been demonstrated to form thick hypertrophic scars with injury [59, 60]. In comparison to the Yorkshire pig, a same species control that does not form hypertrophic scars, Duroc pigs have fibroblasts with increased collagen contraction and TGF-β1 expression [61]. The model continues to be a useful tool to the understanding of burn wound healing [62, 63].

2.6 Genetic Variability of Hypertrophic Scarring

In the same way that the Duroc and Yorkshire pig heal differently, there is a genetic component of hypertrophic scarring for humans. Children, young adults, and patients with darker skin have a higher prevalence of hypertrophic scarring with little understanding of why [64]. Certain ethnic groups such as Native Americans and Koreans have higher rates of hypertrophic scarring [65]. Variability in expression of immune cells and activity of myofibroblasts effect the formation of hypertrophic scars [66]. In a cohort of patients studied with a genome assay, the CSMD1 gene was found to be protective against hypertrophic scarring [67]. While this gene's function in wound healing is yet to be determined, this may be a promising aspect for prevention of future hypertrophic scarring.

2.7 Contracture Formation

Contractures constitute another complication of burn wound healing. Whereas contraction represents a normal physiologic wound healing process, the pathophysiologic extreme causes tremendous patient disability. Fibrous bands which prevent normal range of motion affect approximately one-third of patients on discharge after a burn injury [68]. Most commonly, contractures involve shoulders/axillae and despite aggressive therapy and skin grafting impaired range of motion persists [68]. Figure 2.2 demonstrates hypertrophic scarring of the neck and shoulders. For pediatric patients, approximately 25% have limited range of motion at discharge, again with the shoulder being the most common contracture [69].

When addressing range of motion in a patient with a major burn injury, heterotopic ossification (HO) represents another debilitating complication from thermal injury. HO is the ectopic formation of lamellar bone after trauma, hip surgery, and spinal cord injury [70]. Around 5% of burn patients develop HO, with the elbow being the most common site [71]. Currently, surgery to remove ectopic bony tissue remains the best option for advanced HO, with other treatment modalities such as radiation and bisphosphonate therapy only serving as adjunct treatments [72]. The pathophysiology of HO remains unclear; possible explanations include altered bone morphogenic protein and insulin-like growth factor-1 signaling pathways [73, 74]. This complication negatively impacts quality of life with higher prevalence in males and younger individuals [73]. Further studies on prevention and treatment are necessary to gain a better understanding of this problem.

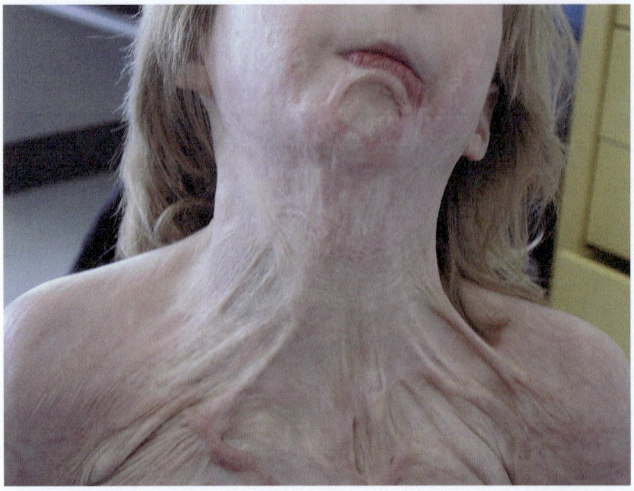

Fig. 2.2 Neck contractures which extend to the lower lip

2.8 Pigmentation

Abnormal pigmentation after burn injury causes significant body image perception problems for patients and providers alike. This complication causes low self-esteem and social isolation, especially in people with color [75]. Both hyper- and hypopigmentation occur in healed burns with unknown mechanism of action. Figure 2.3 demonstrates areas of both hyper- and hypopigmentation on the same patient. After thermal injury, melanocytes proliferate and migrate into the wound from the wound edges and epidermal appendages to produce and transfer melanin to neighboring keratinocytes [76]. A combination of keratinocytic-derived paracrine factors and dermal fibroblasts modulate melanocyte behavior [77]. The fibroblast modulation of melanocytes has been shown to demonstrate significant heterogeneity, which can be a factor for the variable effects of pigmentation [78]. Currently, the options for pigmentary changes are limited [79].

2.9 Marjolin Ulcers

The most notorious complication of burn scar is the Marjolin ulcer. This well-known but rare complication of chronic burn wounds presents as a squamous cell carcinoma in healed burn scar [80]. Patients present with a nonhealing wound in burn scar which arises secondary to chronic inflammation that occurs years after healing [81]. Controversy exists on the proper therapy for this unique, aggressive cutaneous

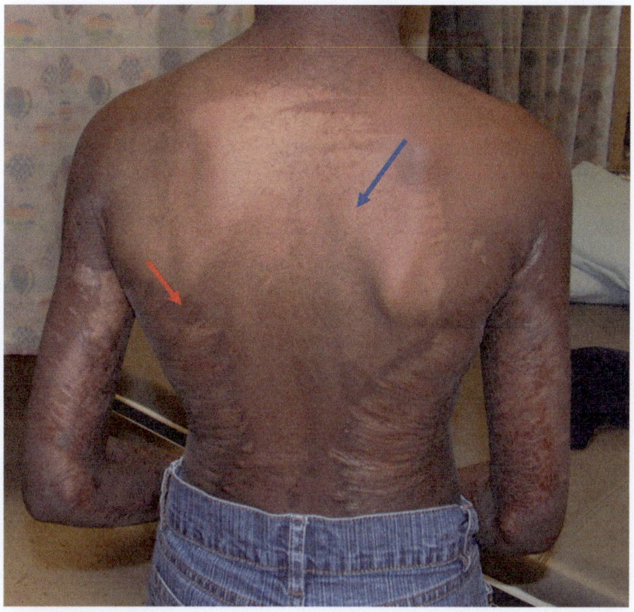

Fig. 2.3 Hyperpigmentation (red arrow) and hypopigmentation (blue arrow)

cancer. Treatment involves wide local excision. Low-grade tumors need lymph node dissection for palpable lymph nodes, but higher grade tumors with more atypia and frequent mitosis require lymph node dissections due to the aggressive nature of the disease [82, 83].

2.10 Psychosocial Recovery

Psychosocial well-being post injury is a growing field of interest for burn care providers. Patients with preexisting psychiatric history have more difficulty in reintegrating into society after discharge. The total body surface of burns may not be directly correlated to poor psychosocial well-being. Two pediatric studies have shown no difference between burn survivors and controls but this is limited to a specific demographic [84, 85]. Despite this data, parents underestimate the amount of stigmatization that children experience [86]. Measuring psychosocial well-being is difficult, a study following women 1 year postburn injury showed that many were hesitant to discuss their feelings and felt conflicted about their recovery [87]. There is little data studying long-term effect of burn scars on psychosocial recovery and requires further research [88].

2.11 Conclusion

With the dramatically reduced mortality after burn injury in the last 50 years, the long-term process of wound healing and associated physical and psychological morbidities embody the next frontier of burn advances in care. Determining when a wound is "healed" no longer equals epithelialization but is now a more difficult task. Functional recovery, body image perception, and neuropathic pain challenge patients for decades. Understanding the continuum of cutaneous responses to injury constitutes the basis for preventing these chronic problems. Thermal injury must be considered a chronic condition rather than a short-term episodic diagnosis. As such, providers must be cognizant of long-term burn complications to identify which patients will benefit from burn specific continuity of care programs.

References

1. Dupuytren G, Doane AS. Clinical lectures on surgery: delivered at Hotel Dieu. Boston: Carter, Hendee; 1832.
2. Center for Disease Control. Release of ICD-10-CM https://www.cdc.gov/nchs/icd/icd10cm.htm#FY%202018%20release%20of%20ICD-10-CM (2018).
3. Jackson D. The diagnosis of depth of burning. J Br Surg. 1953;40:588–96.
4. Jackson D. Second thoughts on the burn wound. J Trauma. 1969;9:839–62.
5. Rowan MP, Cancio LC, Elster EA, et al. Burn wound healing and treatment: review and advancements. Crit Care. 2015;19:243–55.
6. Tiwari VK. Burn wound: how it differs from other wounds? Indian J Plast Surg. 2012;45:364–73.
7. Santoro MM, Gaudino G. Cellular and molecular facets of keratinocyte reepithelization during wound healing. Exp Cell Res. 2005;304:274–86.
8. Zhu Z, Ding J, Shankowsky HA, et al. The molecular mechanism of hypertrophic scar. J Cell Commun Signal. 2013;7:239–52.
9. Gurtner GC, Werner S, Barrandon Y, et al. Wound repair and regeneration. Nature. 2008;453:314–21.
10. Santoro MM, Gaudino G. Cellular and molecular facets of keratinocyte reepithelization during wound healing. Exp Cell Res. 2005;30:274–86.
11. Leibovich SJ, Ross R. The role of the macrophage in wound repair. Am J Pathol. 1975;78:71–95.
12. Ladak A, Tredget EE. Pathophysiology and management of the burn scar. Clin Plast Surg. 2009;36:661–74.
13. Mills CD, Ley K. M1 and M2 macrophages: the chicken and the egg of immunity. J Innate Immun. 2014;6:716–26.
14. Tacchio C, Cassatella MA. Neutrophil-derived cytokines involved in physiological and pathological angiogenesis. Chem Immunol Allergy. 2014;99:123–37.
15. Levy V, Lindon C, Zheng Y, et al. Epidermal stem clels arise from the hair follicle after wounding. FASEB J. 2007;21:1358–66.
16. Martin P. Wound healing: aiming for perfect skin regeneration. Science. 1997;276:75–81.
17. Koster MI. Making an epidermis. Ann N Y Acad Sci. 2009;1170:7–10.
18. Garner WL. Epidermal regulation of dermal fibroblast activity. Plast Reconstr Surg. 1996;102:135–9.
19. Chetty BV, Boissey RE, Warden GD, et al. Basement membrane and fibroblast aberration in blisters at the donor, graft, and spontaneously healed sites in patients with burns. Arch Dermatol. 1992;125:181–6.
20. Sarrazy V, Billet F, Micallef L, et al. Mechanisms of pathological scarring: role of myofibroblasts and current developments. Wound Repair Regen. 2011;19(Suppl):s10–5.
21. Tonnesen MG, Feng X, Clark RA. Angiogenesis in wound healing. J Investig Dermatol Symp Proc. 2000;5:40–6.

22. Hollander DA, Erli HJ, Theisen A, Falk S, Kreck T, Muller S. Standardized qualitative evaluation of scar tissue properties in an animal wound healing model. Wound Repair Regen. 2003;4:150–7.
23. Kischer CW. The microvessels in hypertrophic scars, keloids and related lesions: a review. J Submicrosc Cytol Pathol. 1992;24:281–96.
24. Travis TE, Mino MJ, Moffatt LT, et al. Biphasic presence of fibrocytes in a porcine hypertrophic scar model. J Burn Care Res. 2015;36:e125–35.
25. Ehrlich HP. Wound closure: evidence of cooperation between fibroblasts and collagen matrix. Eye. 1988;2:149–57.
26. Gabbiani G. The myofibroblast in wound healing and fibrocontractive diseases. J Pathol. 2003;200:500–3.
27. Baum J, Duffy HS. Fibroblasts and myofibroblasts: what are we talking about? J Cardiovasc Pharmacol. 2011;57:37–379.
28. Levenson SM, Geever EF, Crowley LV, et al. Healing of rat skin wounds. Ann Surg. 1965;161:293–308.
29. Hocking AM, Gibran NS. Mesenchymal stem cells: paracrine signaling and differentiation during cutaneous wound repair. Exp Cell Res. 2010;316:2213–9.
30. Nambu M, Kishimoto S, Nakamura S, et al. Accelerated wound healing in healing-impaired db/db mice by autologous adipose tissue-derived stromal cells combined with atelocollagen matrix. Ann Plast Surg. 2009;62:317–21.
31. Wu Y, Chen L, Scott PG, et al. Mesenchymal stem cells enhance wound healing through differentiation and angiogenesis. Stem Cells. 2007;25:2648–59.
32. Lee SH, Jin SY, Song JS, et al. Paracrine effects of adipose derived stem cells on keratinocytes and dermal fibroblasts. Ann Dermatol. 2012;24:136–43.
33. Mustoe TA, Cooter RD, Gold MH, et al. International clinical recommendations on scar management. Plast Reconstr Surg. 2002;110:560–71.
34. Ogawa R. The most current algorithms for the treatment and prevention of hyperrophic scars and keloids. Plast Reconstr Surg. 2010;125:557–68.
35. Tyack Z, Simons M, Spinks A, et al. A systematic review of the quality of burn scar rating scales for clinical and research use. Burns. 2012;38:6–18.
36. Tyack Z, Wasiak J, Spinks A, et al. A guide to choosing a burn scar rating scale for clinical or research use. Burns. 2013;39:1341–50.
37. Thompson CM, Sood RF, Honari S, et al. What score on the Vancouver scar scale constitutes a hypertrophic scar? Results from a survey of North American burn care providers. Burns. 2015;41:1442–8.
38. Lumenta DB, Siepmann E, Kamolz LP, et al. Internet-based survey on current practice for evaluation, prevention, and treatment of scars, hypertrophic scars, and keloids. Wound Repair Regen. 2014;22:483–91.
39. Rinkevich R, Walmsley GG, Hu MS, et al. Science. 2015;348:aaa2151.
40. Kwan PO, Tredget EE. Biological principles of scar and contracture. Hand Clin. 2017;33:277–92.
41. Kischer CW, Pindur J, Krasovith P, et al. Characteristics of granulation tissue which promote hypertrophic scarring. Scanning Microsc. 1990;4:877–87.
42. Ogawa R. Keloid and hypertrophic scars are the results of chronic inflammation in the reticular dermis. Int J Mol Sci. 2017;18:606–16.
43. Honardoust D, Varkey M, Marcoux Y, et al. Reduced decorin, fibromodulin, and transforming growth factor: B3 in deep dermis leads to hypertrophic scarring. J Burn Care Res. 2012;33:218–27.
44. Tredget EE, Wang R, Shen Q, et al. Transforming growth factor-beta mRNA and protein in hypertrophic scar tissues and fibroblasts: antagonism by IFN-alpha and IFN-gamma in vitro and in vivo. J Interferon Cytokine Res. 2000;20:143–52.
45. Scott PG, Dodd CM, Tredget EE, et al. Immunohistochemical localization of the proteoglycan decorin, biglycan, and versican and transforming growth factor-beta in human post-burn hypertrophic and mature scars. Histopathology. 1995;26:423–31.
46. Scott JR, Muangman PR, Tamura RN, et al. Substance P levels and neutral endopeptidase activity in acute burn wounds and hypertrophic scar. Plast Reconstr Surg. 2005;115:1095–102.
47. Scott JR, Muangman P, Gibran NS. Making sense of hypertrophic scar: a role for nerves. Wound Repair Regen. 2007;15:S27–31.
48. Malenfont A, Forget R, Papillon J, et al. Prevalence and characteristics of chronic sensory problems in burn patients. Pain. 1996;67:493–500.
49. Carrougher GJ, Martinez EM, McMullen KS, et al. Pruritus in adult burn survivors: postburn prevalence and risk factors associated with increased intensity. J Burn Care Res. 2013;34(1):94–101.
50. Ahuja RB, Gupta R, Gupta G, et al. A comparative analysis of cetirizine, gabapentin and their combination in the relief of post-burn pruritus. Burns. 2011;37:203–7.
51. Brooks JP, Malic CC, Judkins KC. Scratching the surface—managing the itch associated with burns: a review of current knowledge. Burns. 2008;34:751–60.
52. Shimizu S, Tanaka H, Sakaki S, et al. Burn depth affects dermal interstitial fluid pressure, free radical production, and serum histamine levels in rats. J Trauma. 2003;54:683–7.
53. Schneider JC, Harris NL, El Shami A, et al. A descriptive review of neuropathic-like pain after Burn injury. J Burn Care Res. 2006;27:524–8.
54. Yagmur C, Guneren E, Kefeli M, et al. The effect of surgical denervation on prevention of excessive dermal scarring: a study on rabbit ear hypertrophic scar model. J Plast Reconstr Aesthet Surg. 2011;64:1359–65.
55. Ogawa R. Mechanobiology of scarring. Wound Repair Regen. 2011;19(Suppl 1):s2–9.
56. Ogawa R, Okai K, Tokumura F, et al. The relationship between skin stretching/contraction and pathologic scarring: the important role of mechanical forces in keloid generation. Wound Repair Regen. 2012;20:149–57.
57. Kim JY, Willard JJ, Supp DM, et al. Burn scar biomechanics following pressure garment therapy. Plast Reconstr Surg. 2015;136:572–81.
58. Friedrich EE, Niknam-Bienia S, Xie P, et al. Thermal injury model in the rabbit ear with quantifiable burn progression and hypertrophic scar. Wound Repair Regen. 2017;25:327–37.
59. Silverstein, et al. Hypertrophic scarring etiology and control of disabling complications in burned soldiers. Ann Res Progr Rep (US Army Institute of Surgical Research). 1972;37:1–5.
60. Zhu KQ, Carrougher GJ, Gibran NS, et al. Review of the female Duroc/Yorkshire pig model of human fibroproliferative scarring. Wound Repair Regen. 2007;15(Suppl 1):S32–9.
61. Sood RF, Muffley LA, Seaton ME, et al. Dermal fibroblasts from the red Duroc pig have an inherently fibrogenic phenotype: an in vitro model of fibroproliferative scarring. Plast Reconstr Surg. 2015;136:990–1000.
62. Seaton M, Hocking A, Gibran NS. Porcine models of cutaneous wound healing. ILAR J. 2015;56:127–38.
63. Hollander DA, Erli HJ, Theisen A, et al. Standardized qualitative evaluation of scar tissue properties in an animal wound healing model. Wound Repair Regen. 2003;11:150–7.
64. Engrav LE, Garner WL, Tredget EE. Hypertrophic scar, wound contraction, and hyper-hypopigmentaiton. J Burn Care Res. 2007;28:593–7.
65. Thompson CM, Hocking AM, Honari S, et al. Genetic risk factors for hypertrophic scar development. J Burn Care Res. 2013;34:477–82.
66. Santucci M, Borgogni L, Reali UM, et al. Keloids and Hypertrophic scars of caucasians show distinctive morphologic and immunophenotypic profiles. Virchows Arch. 2001;438:457–63.

67. Sood RF, Hocking AM, Muffley LA, et al. Genome-wide association study of postburn scarring indentifies a novel protective variant. Ann Surg. 2015;262:563–39.
68. Goverman J, Mathews K, Goldstein R, et al. Adult contractures in burn injury: a burn model system national database study. J Burn Care Res. 2017;38:e328–36.
69. Goverman J, Mathews K, Goldstein R, et al. Pediatric contractures in burn injury: a burn model system national database study. J Burn Care Res. 2017;38:e192–9.
70. Levi B, Jayakumar P, Giladi A, et al. Risk factors for the development of heterotopic ossification in seriously burned adults: a national institute on disability, independent living and rehabilitation research burn model system database analysis. J Trauma Acute Care Surg. 2015;79:870–6.
71. Orchard GR, Paratz JD, Blot S, et al. Risk factors in hospitalized patients with burn injuries for developing heterotopic ossification—a retrospective analysis. J Burn Care Res. 2015;36:465–70.
72. Schneider JC, Simko LC, Goldstein R, et al. Predicting heterotopic ossficaition early after burn injuries. A risk scoring system. Ann Surg. 2017;266:179–84.
73. Peterson JR, Eboda ON, Brownley RC, et al. Effects of aging on osteogenic response and heterotopic ossification following burn injury in mice. Stem Cells Dev. 2015;24:205–13.
74. Ranganathan K, Peterson J, Agarwal S, et al. Role of gender in burn-induced heterotopic ossification and mesenchymal cell osteogenic differentiation. Plast Reconstr Surg. 2015;135:1631–41.
75. Holavanahali RK, Helm PA, Kowalske KG. Long-term outcomes in patients surviving large burns: the skin. J Burn Care Res. 2010;31:631–9.
76. Chadwick SL, Yip C, Ferguson MW, et al. Repigmentation of cutaneous scars depends on original wound type. J Anat. 2013;223(1):74–82.
77. Park HY, Kosmadaki M, Yaar M, et al. Cellular mechanisms regulating human melanogenesis. Cell Mol Life Sci. 2009;66:1493–506.
78. Sirimahachaiyakul P, Sood RF, Muffley LA, et al. Race does not predict melanocyte heterogenous responses to dermal fibroblast-derived mediators. PLoS One. 2015;10:e0139135.
79. Greenhalgh DG. A primer on pigmentation. J Burn Care Res. 2015;36:247–57.
80. Shen R, Zhang J, Zhang F, et al. Clinical characteristics and therapeutic analysis of 51 patients with Marjolin's ulcers. Exp Ther Med. 2015;10:1364–74.
81. Bozkurt M, Kapi E, Kuvat SV, et al. Current concepts in the management of Marjolin's ulcers: outcomes from a standardized treatment protocol in 16 cases. J Burn Care Res. 2010;31:776–80.
82. Fleming MD, Hunt JL, Purdue GF, et al. Marjolin's ulcer: a review and reevaluation of a difficult problem. J Burn Care Rehabil. 1990;11:460–9.
83. Yanofsky VR, Mercer SE, Phelps RG. Histopathological variants of cutaneous squamous cell carcinoma: a review. J Skin Cancer. 2011;2011:210813.
84. Lawrence JW, Rosenberg LE, Fauerbach JA. Comparing the body esteem of pediatric survivors of burn injury with the body esteem of an age-matched comparison group without burns. Rehabil Psychol. 2007;52:370–9.
85. Pope SJ, Solomons WR, Done DJ, et al. Body image, mood and quality of life in young burn survivors. Burns. 2007;33:747–55.
86. Lawrence JW, Rosenberg L, Mason S, et al. Comparing parent and child perceptions of stigmatizing behavior experience by children with burn scars. Body Image. 2011;8:70–3.
87. Hunter TA, Medved MI, Hiebert-Murphy D, et al. Put on your face to face the world: women's narratives of burn injury. Burns. 2013;39:1588–98.
88. Lawrence JW, Mason ST, Schomer K, et al. Epidemiology and impact of scarring after burn injury: a systematic review of the literature. J Burn Care Res. 2012;33:136–46.

Cellular and Molecular Mechanisms of Hypertrophic Scarring

3

Antoinette T. Nguyen, Jie Ding, and Edward E. Tredget

3.1 Introduction

The skin is the largest organ in the human body. It protects our internal organs from the external environment; therefore it must have an efficient and effective means to heal after sustaining injury. Wound healing and scar formation are a dynamic process that is spatially and temporally regulated. Prenatal and postnatal oral mucosa wounds heal without scarring, whereas postnatal deep dermal injury but not superficial or epidermal injury results in scar formation [1, 2]. Thus, the restorative capabilities of the skin are under intensive research to reveal the cellular and molecular mechanism of wound healing and scar formation. Wound healing occurs in four phases and involves the interaction of several components including the extracellular matrix (ECM) (e.g., collagen, elastin, and proteoglycans), blood-borne cells (e.g., monocytes, T lymphocytes, and fibrocytes), dermal cells (e.g., keratinocytes, endothelial cells, and fibroblast), and signaling molecules (cytokines, chemokines, growth factors, and microRNAs (miRs)) found within the local environmental milieu. Aberrant wound healing can lead to pathological scars such as hypertrophic scars (HTS) and keloids (Fig. 3.1), both of which are considered as dermal fibroproliferative disorders [3].

A. T. Nguyen · J. Ding
Wound Healing Research Group, Department of Surgery, University of Alberta, Edmonton, AB, Canada

E. E. Tredget (✉)
Wound Healing Research Group, Department of Surgery, University of Alberta, Edmonton, AB, Canada

Division of Plastic and Reconstructive Surgery and Critical Care, Department of Surgery, University of Alberta, Edmonton, AB, Canada
e-mail: etredget@ualberta.ca

3.2 Wound Healing and Scar Formation

Wound healing occurs in four phases: hemostasis, inflammation, proliferation, and remodeling. After injury to the epidermis and dermis, platelets and endothelial cells are activated, thereby triggering the clotting cascade to prevent any further loss of blood. During this time, a provisional matrix, the fibrin clot, is formed, and serves as a scaffold for cellular migration. Following vasoconstriction, platelets release a host of factors including cytokines, chemokines, and growth factors that recruit inflammatory mediators such as neutrophils and monocytes to the site of injury. Thus, the initial phase of wound healing is completed within hours from the time of injury [4, 5].

The appearance of polymorphonuclear cells (neutrophils) indicates the transition from hemostasis to the inflammatory phase. These cells can be found between 2 and 5 days after injury [5]. Neutrophils, mast cells, and monocytes release pro-inflammatory mediators to ensure that all foreign products are destroyed and cellular debris is removed. Neutrophils then undergo apoptosis, which are phagocytosed by pro-inflammatory macrophages after differentiation from circulating monocytes chemoattracted to the wound. These pro-inflammatory M1 macrophages are signaled to polarize into anti-inflammatory M2 macrophages, which lead to the transition of inflammation to the proliferation phase [6].

The proliferation phase is characterized by formation of granulation tissue, which subsequently replaces the provisional matrix. Angiogenesis also occurs during this phase of wound healing via activation of several growth factors such as vascular endothelial growth factor (VEGF) [5, 7]. Anti-inflammatory macrophages secrete chemokines, cytokines, and growth factors to stimulate cellular proliferation, migration, adhesion, and differentiation. Surrounding keratinocytes and epithelial stem cells in the adnexal structures of the hair follicles and sebaceous glands and the basal layer of the epidermis carry out re-epithelialization [8]. Granulation tissue formation is the last event in the proliferation phase and consists mostly of fibroblasts among other cell types.

© Springer Nature Singapore Pte Ltd. 2020
R. Ogawa (ed.), *Total Scar Management*, https://doi.org/10.1007/978-981-32-9791-3_3

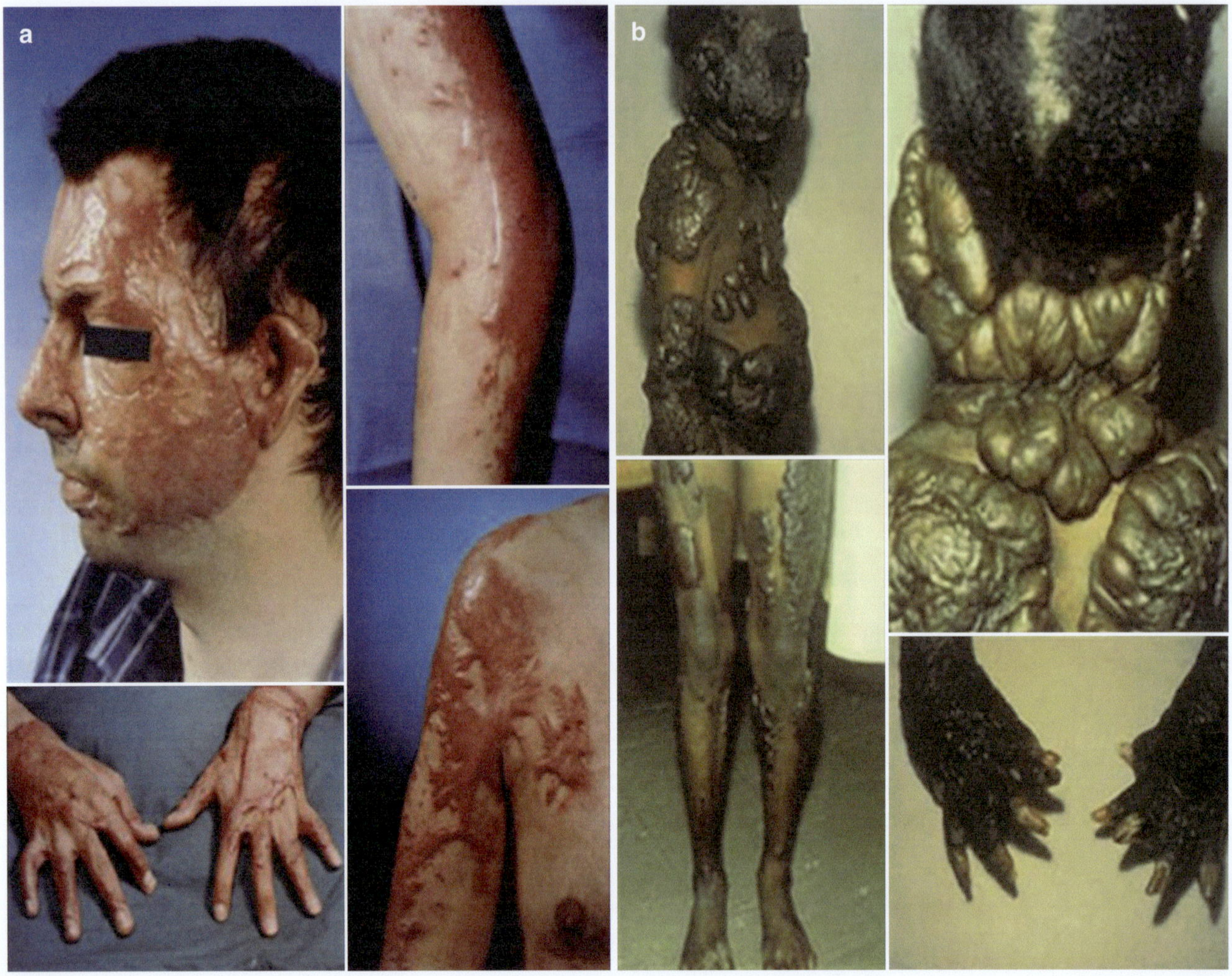

Fig. 3.1 The gross morphology of hypertrophic scars (**a**) and keloids (**b**) [3]. (With permission to reuse, images obtained from Tredget et al. Dec 2014)

Fibroblast cells are responsible for the deposition of collagen and several other ECM components.

The final phase is remodeling, which can extend from months to years. During this phase, modest increase in the ratio of type III to type I collagen is slowly reversed as type I collagen becomes the predominant isoform of mature scars. Wound contraction occurs and is carried out by myofibroblasts. Mature scars appear flat, faded, and are devoid of appendages such as sebaceous glands and hair follicles. As the depth of injury extends deeper into the dermis, scarring ensues, which in the lateral hip this occurs when the laceration is 0.56 ± 0.03 mm deep (Fig. 3.2) [9–11]. This was found using a jig to create a wound of increasing depth, from superficial to deep dermal, on the lateral side of the hip on humans [9]. Moreover, the newly formed scar consists of tissue that is inferior to the original form. For example, the newly formed epidermal layer of the scar cannot protect against ultraviolet radiation as effectively as normal skin and the dermis has reduced tensile strength.

3.3 HTS and Keloids

Fetal and superficial dermal wounds heal without scarring, referring to regeneration, while HTS and keloids represent replacement-based wound healing following deep dermal injuries (Fig. 3.3) [12]. Disruptions in the normal cellular and molecular processes of wound healing can cause an excessive deposition and reduced degradation of ECM components, particularly collagen [12]. Both HTS and keloids are fibrotic disorders, and show features of increased cutaneous thickness, hypercellularity, excessive deposition of disorganized collagen, and increased vascularity. Although both disorders are similar, HTS are erythematous, raised, confined

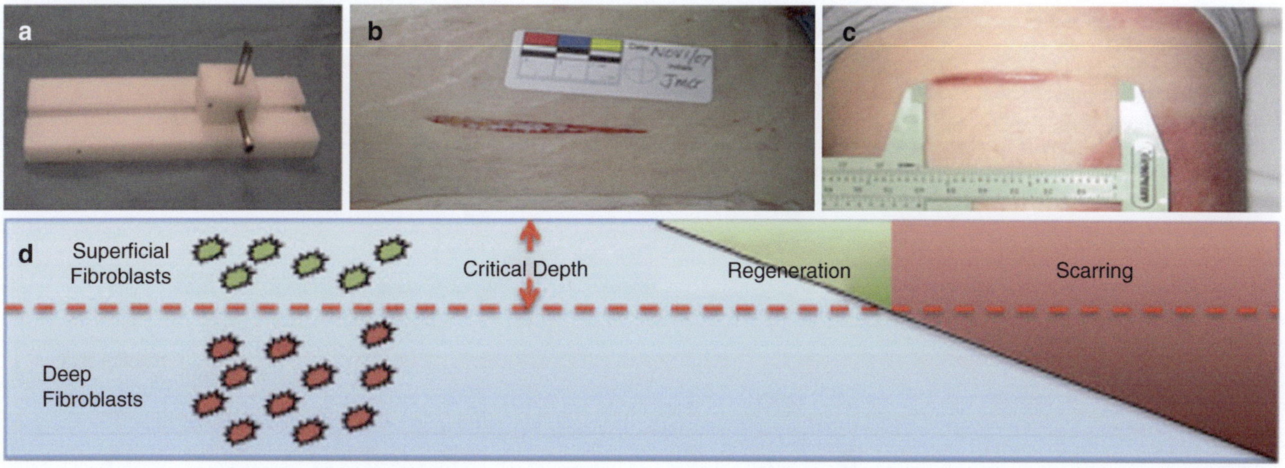

Fig. 3.2 The jig (**a**) is used to make a wound that progressively increases in depth (**b** and **c**) and the wound healed scarless at the superficial end and with a scar at the deeper end [10]. It is suggested that once dermal injury exceeds the critical depth, a hypertrophic scar is formed (**d**) [11]. (With permission to reuse, images obtained from Honardoust et al. 2012 and Kwan et al. 2009)

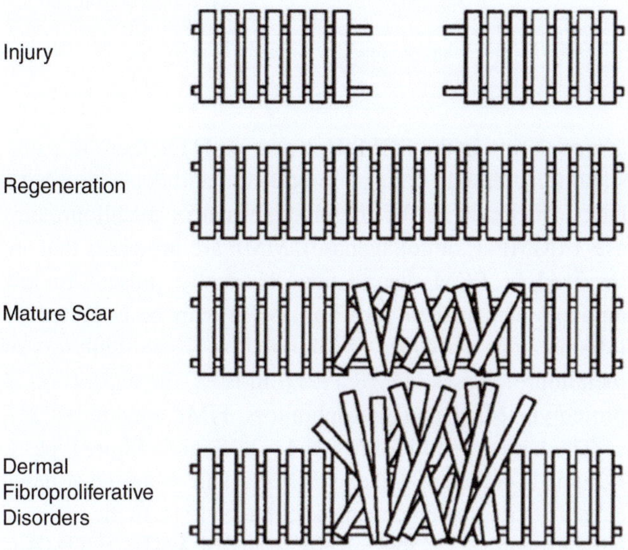

Fig. 3.3 An illustration of wound injury followed by regeneration- and replacement-based wound healing. Regeneration-based wound healing leads to scarless wound healing. Replacement-based wound healing involves replacing lost structures and formation of mature and pathological scars [12]. (With permission to reuse, image obtained from Tredget EE. 1999)

to their boundaries, and can regress overtime. Keloids appear similar, but extend outside of the original wound boundaries, do not regress, and are often more severe. HTS can arise from deep lacerations, surgery, and in individuals suffering from burns. Keloids can arise from major or even minor skin trauma and have a strong as yet unknown genetic predisposition. Development of HTS can lead to contractures due to a high density of myofibroblasts, indicated by positive staining for alpha-smooth muscle actin (α-SMA), a feature not shared by keloids [5]. Pathological scars can arise from prolonged inflammation, delayed wound closure, and infections [13].

3.4 Cellular and Molecular Mechanisms of Pathological Scars

The precise systemic and local cellular and molecular mechanism associated with pathological scar formation is not completely understood (Fig. 3.4) [14]. There are several factors that can influence the outcome of scar formation such as race, genetics, age, medical comorbidities, and depth of injury. Thus, several research investigations are underway to elucidate the cellular and molecular components that are involved with scar formation.

3.4.1 Extracellular Matrix (ECM)

In normal tissue, the ECM is found within the hypocellular dermal layer, providing structural integrity and facilitating cellular signaling. The structural components include collagen, elastic fibers, and glycosaminoglycans. The cellular constituents of the dermis include fibroblasts, myofibroblasts, and endothelial cells. The ECM acts as a reservoir for cytokines, chemokines, and growth factors. The ECM can also function as a scaffold for cellular adhesion and migration, and can stimulate cellular metabolism through signal transduction pathways associated with proliferation, differ-

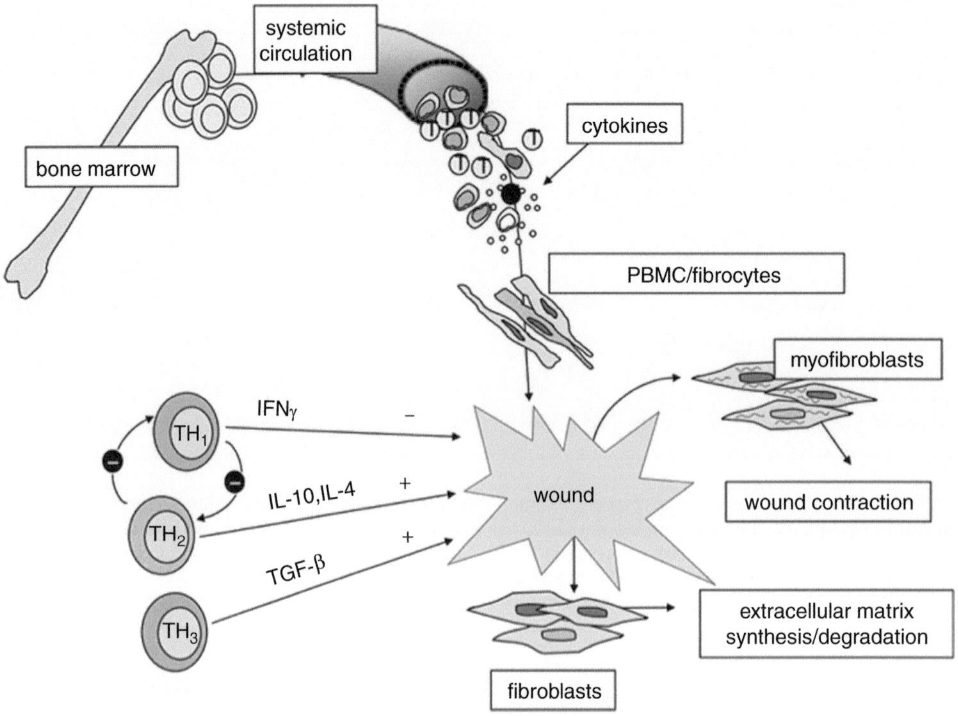

Fig. 3.4 Wound healing and scar formation involve the complex interaction between local and systemic factors [14]. (With permission to reuse, image from Armour et al. 2007)

entiation, and apoptosis. In normal skin and pathological scars, the appearance and composition of the ECM differs. In HTS, the collagen fibers are thin, densely packed, and there is an increased ratio of type III to type I collagen as compared to normal skin [5]. The collagen appears whorl-like and nodular, and is orientated parallel to the surface of the skin in HTS, unlike the typical basket weave-like appearance seen in normal skin architecture [15, 16]. No hair follicles, sebaceous glands, or sweat glands are present in both HTS and keloid scars [15, 16] and the normally undulating rete ridges between the epidermis and dermis is flattened [17]. The hypocellular dermal layer becomes hypercellular due to the increase in proliferation and migration of fibroblasts, myofibroblasts, endothelial cells, and immune cells. The increase in cells also increases deposition of extracellular components, resulting in an unbalanced production of ECM elements.

Collagen, the main component in the ECM, is a triple helical extracellular protein within the dermis. Collagen can be divided into two groups, fibrillary collagen and fibril-associated collagens. Collagen is synthesized by fibroblasts as propeptides and requires enzymatic cleavage. Collagen type I and III, both of which are fibrillary collagen, are commonly found in the dermis. Together, they form a basket weave-like pattern to provide strength and stabilization. The ratio of type I to type III collagen has been shown to be age dependent [18–20]. The type I to type III collagen ratio is higher in normal skin, while in HTS, the ratio of type I to type III collagen is lower [18–20]. In normal skin, the production and degradation of collagen is balanced, avoiding accumulation in the ECM. However, in HTS, there is a substantial increase in collagen production and deposition but a lack of degradation by the enzyme matrix metalloproteinase-1 (MMP-1, or collagenase). MMP are proteases that are involved in ECM degradation. Normally present in low amounts and in their pro-form, MMP can be activated by inflammatory cytokines or inhibited by tissue inhibitors of metalloproteinases (TIMPs) [21]. In HTS, the expression of proteolytic MMP and their inhibitors, TIMP are altered [21].

The target protein for MMP-1, -2, -8, and -13 are types I, II, and III collagen, whereas MMP-2 and -9 are gelatinases capable of degrading denatured collagen [21]. In the tissue of patients with HTS, the mRNA levels of MMP-2, TIMP-1, and TIMP-2 were higher compared to controls; however, no difference was found in MMP-9 expression [21]. Interestingly, in the sera of patients with HTS as a result of burn injury, only TIMP-1 was significantly expressed compared to controls [21]. Thus, improper regulation of the MMP and TIMP ratio may contribute to the excessive collagen deposition found in the ECM [21]. The higher expression of TIMP-1 found in HTS may be contributed by keratinocytes [22]. In a study by Dasu et al., normal and hypertrophic fibroblasts were cultured with IL-6 leading to increases in MMP-1 and MMP-3 mRNA expression and pro-MMP-1 and MMP-3 protein values in normal but not hypertrophic fibroblasts [23]. The lack of changes to MMP expression in HTS fibroblasts may contribute to the excessive collagen deposition observed in the ECM of HTS.

Ghahary et al. examined the expression of collagenase in dermal fibroblasts derived from patients who developed postburn HTS [24]. Punch biopsies of HTS and site-matched normal dermal tissue were taken from the same patients and fibroblast cells were cultured [24]. The authors found a significantly reduced collagenase activity and mRNA expression, with no changes in the enzyme inhibitor TIMP-1 in HTS fibroblasts [24]. These outcomes may, in part, be mediated by increased insulin growth factor-1 (IGF-1) expression found in postburn HTS tissue [24, 25]. The growth factor IGF-1 was also shown to increase both type I and type III procollagen transcripts [25]. Taken together, the data reveals an imbalance between collagen production and degradation observed in patients with HTS. Aside from collagen, another structural protein found in the ECM is elastic fibers, which provides resiliency of the normal skin from contortion. Both elastin and fibrillin-1, elastic fibers, are found to be perturbed in HTS [26]. The volume of both elastin and fibrillin-1 was significantly lower in the dermis of HTS [26, 27]. This aberrant remodeling and reorganization contributes to the loss of tensile strength and increased contraction observed as compared to normal skin [28].

In addition to collagen and elastic fibers, the ECM is also composed of proteoglycans. Proteoglycans are proteins that contain glycosaminoglycan side chains [29]. Small leucine-rich proteoglycans (SLRPs) normally found in the skin include decorin and fibromodulin [30]. Decorin is the predominant form of SLRPs found in the normal skin. The protein core is able to attach to several ECM structures such as collagen, where it can assist in collagen organization and fibrillogenesis. Both mRNA and protein expression of decorin and fibromodulin, negative regulators of transforming growth factor beta 1 (TGF-β1), were significantly reduced in HTS tissue compared to normal [30]. Moreover, Honardoust et al. also found lower expression of these two SLRPs in fibroblast cells from HTS [30]. Scott et al. cultured fibroblast cells from punch biopsies of HTS and normal dermal tissue from the same patient [31]. Decorin mRNA and protein expression from hypertrophic fibroblast cells were significantly less compared to normal fibroblast cells [31]. Treatment of the cells with the growth factor TGF-β1 decreased both protein and mRNA expression of decorin [31]. A time course analyses of decorin expression in postburn patients revealed that decorin levels remained low up to a year, and gradually increased until it reached levels similar to controls by 3 years [32]. In HTS, the reduction in decorin may contribute to the disorganized collagen fibrils and increased TGF-β1 expression observed in patients with HTS.

Fibroblast cells from the deeper layers of the dermis are more similar to fibroblast cells retrieved from HTS tissue [10, 33]. Honardoust et al. evaluated the decorin and fibromodulin in fibroblast cells from the deep dermis using a linear human wound scratch model [10, 33]. Immunofluorescence staining of the SLRPs revealed decorin in the ECM, while fibromodulin co-localized with cells, and both showed less immunoreactivity in the deep wounds compared to the superficial wound [9, 10]. In fibroblast cells, both syntheses of the SLRPs are reduced in deep cells compared to the fibroblast cells extracted from superficial layers [9, 10]. The SLRPs are negative regulators of TGF-β1; thus, TGF-β1 and its receptors were both highly expressed in the deep dermal wounds and in fibroblast cells from the deep dermal layers [9, 10]. In addition to ECM organization and the negative regulatory effect on the pro-fibrotic growth factor TGF-β1, decorin can also stimulate apoptosis in fibroblast cells to prevent hyperproliferation [34]. *In vitro*, deep dermal fibroblasts were shown to have decreased levels of decorin mRNA and protein compared to superficial fibroblasts [34]. Superficial fibroblasts expressing more decorin are associated with apoptotic cell death indicated by increased mRNA expression of histone-1, both caspase-1, and -8, and p53, all of which are proapoptotic molecules [34]. Deep dermal fibroblasts, on the other hand, do not respond to the same extent as superficial fibroblasts, suggesting that the former cells were not as responsive to the apoptotic effects of decorin [34]. A pilot study was next undertaken to assess the systemic levels of decorin in postburn patients [35]. Kwan et al. found that systemic decorin and IL-1β temporally expressed early after burn injury and TGF-β1 in the serum during the later phase was predictive of scar development [35]. Thus, systemic changes in all three markers, decorin, IL-1β, and TGF-β, can potentially be used as markers for later HTS formation [35].

3.4.2 Recruitment of Blood-Borne Cells into Hypertrophic Scars

Blood-borne cells are mobilized and recruited once an injury is detected. The chemokine stromal cell-derived factor 1 (SDF-1), also referred to as CXCL12, and its receptor CXCR4 have been shown to be involved in fibrosis. The levels of both SDF-1 and CXCR4+ positive cells were elevated in the serum and PBMCs, respectively, following burn injury (Fig. 3.5) [36]. *In vitro* analysis of the signaling pathway revealed that deep dermal fibroblasts secreted higher levels of SDF-1, which subsequently increased the motility of CXCR4+ expressing cells [36]. These results suggest that *in vivo*, the expression of SDF-1 recruits CXCR4+ circulating cells that directly (via fibrocytes) or indirectly (via other immune cells such as monocytes and lymphocytes) promote fibrosis [36]. In human burn patients, treatment with interferon α2b reduced SDF-1/CXCR4 expression and subsequent scar formation [36]. The involvement of the SDF-1/CXCR4 signaling axis was further examined by inhibiting CXCR4 in a HTS nude mouse model using a competitive receptor antagonist [37]. Impeding the signaling axis blocked migration of cells to

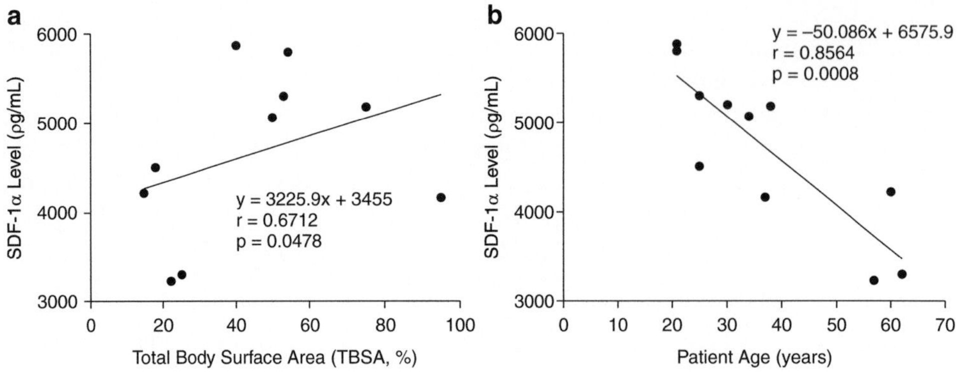

Fig. 3.5 The SDF-1/CXCR4 signaling pathway is involved in hypertrophic scar formation. In burn patients, serum SDF-1 levels were positively correlated with total body surface area (TBSA) (**a**) and negative correlated with patient age (**b**) [36]. (With permission to reuse, images obtained from Ding et al. 2011)

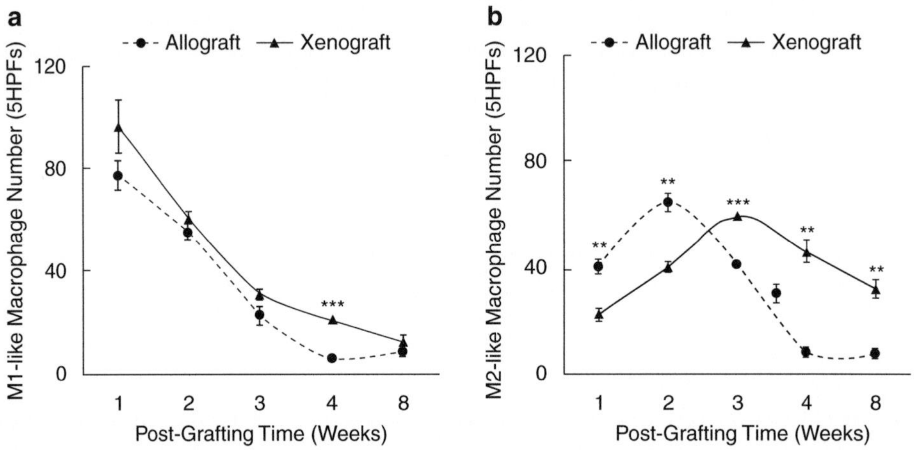

Fig. 3.6 The presence of M1 and M2 macrophages in mice grafted with skin allografts and xenografts. In both models, M1 macrophages showed similar trends, peaking at 1-week post-grafting and decreased gradually (**a**). M2 macrophages peaked in the allograft at 2 weeks post-grafting, however, xenografts models showed a peak at 3 weeks post-grafting (**b**) [46]. (With permission to reuse, images obtained from Zhu et al. 2016)

the wound site, reduced scar formation, and decreased expression of pro-fibrotic mediators [37].

PBMCs are peripheral blood-borne cells arising from the bone marrow that includes monocytes and lymphocytes. Liu et al. collected blood from postburn patients and found a subset of PBMCs that were identified as $CD14^+COL\text{-}1^+$ [38]. To further characterize this subset, the entire $CD14^+COL\text{-}1^+$ population were positive for LSP-1, CD45, while 80% showed CD204, and 70% CXCR4 and TLR-4 [38]. This suggests that the $CD14^+COL\text{-}1^+$ PBMCs population consists of fibrocytes and immature M2 macrophages that are recruited by the SDF-1/CXCR4 chemokine and TLR-4 signaling pathway [38]. Conditioned media from PBMCs induced mRNA and protein expression of the pro-fibrotic factors such as connective tissue growth factor (CTGF) and TGF-β1, and reduced the anti-fibrotic proteoglycan decorin, in dermal fibroblast cells [38]. The conditioned media from PBMCs was also able to increase fibroblast mobility and differentiation into myofibroblasts [38]. Thus, this subset of PBMCs is recruited early during the wound healing process and may mature into fibrotic cells such as fibrocytes or M2 macrophages, contributing to scar formation [38].

Monocytes are recruited to the wound site in part, by monocyte chemoattractant protein-1 (MCP-1), also referred to as the C-C motif chemokine ligand 2 (CCL2), signaling axis [39]. Monocytes are circulating blood-borne cells, which mature into macrophages once they reach their target site in tissues. Macrophages phagocytose debris and foreign materials. Macrophages can also ingest apoptotic neutrophils, which have been suggested to initiate the transition of pro-inflammatory macrophages into the anti-inflammatory phenotype [6, 40, 41]. Once past the inflammatory phase, macrophages secrete anti-inflammatory cytokines, growth factors, and angiogenic factors to provide an environmental milieu that will stimulate proliferation and remodeling. Macrophages are capable of polarizing into different subtypes, M1 and M2. M1 is a pro-inflammatory subtype whereas M2 is referred to as alternatively activated. The expression of either M1 or M2 is complex and the Notch signaling pathway has been implicated in the polarization [42]. M2 macrophages are further subcategorized into M2a, an anti-inflammatory or alternative phenotype, M2b, an immunoregulatory form, M2c, a deactivated type, and M2d, which has an angiogenic role [43, 44]. Because M2 promotes an environment in favor of growth, M2 macrophages have been associated with fibrosis [45].

To evaluate the changes in monocytes and macrophages during scar formation, split-thickness human skin was transplanted onto the dorsum of athymic mice as a model of HTS [46]. Initially, during the first week after grafting, M1 macrophages in the tissue were found in higher quantities, whereas M2 macrophages began to increase in number and peaked 3 weeks post-graft (Fig. 3.6) [46]. Zhu et al. injected the nude mice model of HTS with the macrophage inhibitor clodronate prior to the peak of M2 macrophages [47]. Inhibition of M2 macrophages reduced the thickness of the scar, decreased the number of myofibroblasts, and reduced collagen deposition [47]. In addition, the recruitment of mast cells, which peaked at 4 weeks post-graft, was reduced [47]. *In vitro*, THP-1 cells were differentiated to resting macrophages, M1 and M2 [48]. M2 macrophages that were cocultured with fibroblasts led to an increase in proliferation, collagen synthesis, and myofibroblast differentiation [48]. M2 and fibroblast coculture also reduced the expression of MMP-1 and decorin and increased TGF-β1, COL1A1, and TIMP-1 [48]. These findings support early findings of the critical role of macrophages in wound healing and point to the role of M2 macrophages in HTS.

Two subpopulations of CD4+ T cells recruited to the wound site are T helper cells (Th) 1 and Th2, both of which secrete lymphokines, thereby contributing to the environmental milieu [49]. Th2 lymphocytes secrete interleukin (IL)-4 and IL-13, fibrotic cytokines, which acts on the same receptor and activates the signal transducer and activator of transcription (STAT) 6 pathway [49]. Th1 and Th2 cells have been shown to contribute to wound healing and scar formation. Castagnoli et al. found an increase in CD3+, CD4+, and CD8+ T lymphocytes in the epidermis and the dermal layer of hypertrophic scars [50]. Bernabeia et al. further identified that the T lymphocytes secreted high levels of the pro-inflammatory cytokine interferon (IFN)-γ and low levels of the anti-inflammatory cytokine IL-4 [51]. Wang et al. collected blood from postburn patients and identified a subpopulation of TGF-β1 producing CD4+ T lymphocytes that are elevated 1–2 weeks postburn, peaked at 3–4 weeks, and declined afterwards, albeit remaining higher than controls up to 5 months [52]. These cells were able to infiltrate the skin where it can later mediate its effects [52]. Conditioned medium from TGF-β1 producing CD4+ T lymphocytes promoted fibroblast proliferation, differentiation, and collagen production [52]. Thus, these results suggest that T lymphocytes also contribute to the formation of HTS.

Fibrocytes are derived from the bone marrow and have features similar to fibroblast cells, such as the ability to produce collagen, but to a lesser extent [53]. Yang et al. collected blood from postburn patients where fibrocytes were identified in the PBMC population [54]. Increased serum levels of TGF-β1 were also identified, suggesting that this growth factor may stimulate PBMCs to differentiate into fibrocytes capable of producing type I collagen [54]. Moreover, the authors identified that CD14+ cells were able to differentiate into fibrocytes and this differentiation was inhibited following incubation with the neutralizing anti-TGF-β1 antibody [54]. IL-4 and IL-13 from Th2 lymphocytes are also able to induce the differentiation of CD14+ cells into fibrocytes [49]. An increase in the number of fibrocytes, detected by dual immunostaining with leukocyte-specific protein-1 (LSP-1), a 52 kDa intracellular cytoskeletal protein, and type I collagen was seen in HTS tissue from

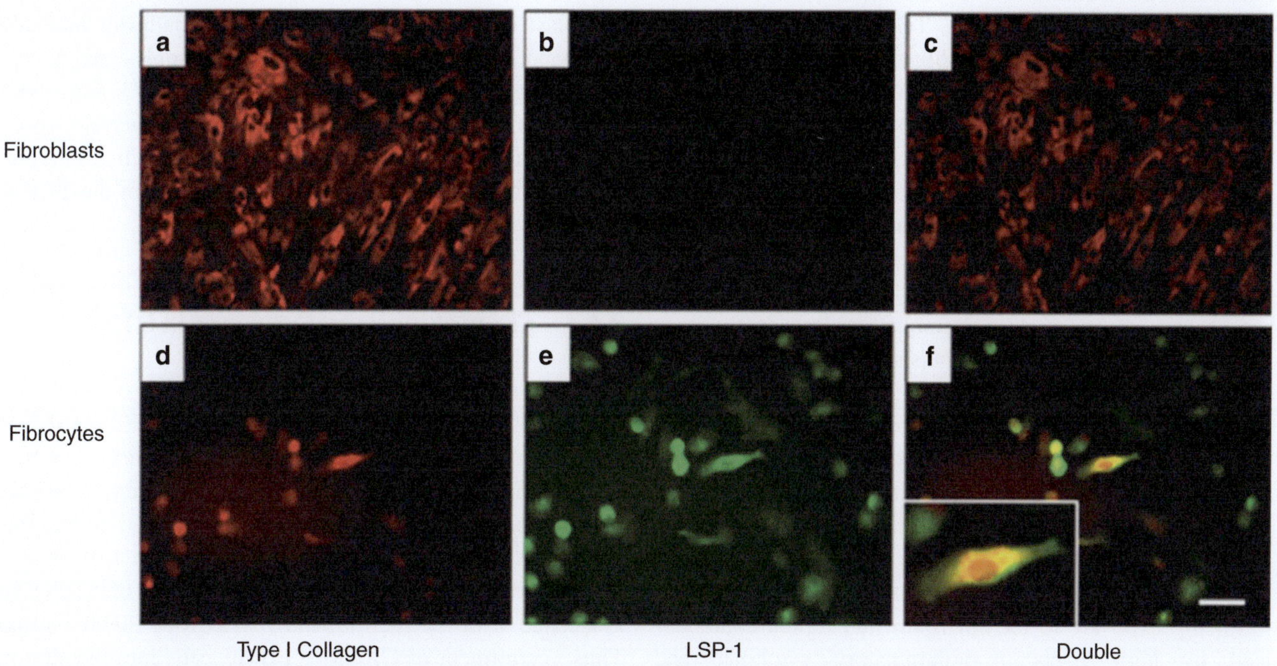

Fig. 3.7 Fibrocyte immunostaining. Fibroblasts expressed type-1 collagen staining (**a**) however, no positive leukocyte-specific protein-1 (LSP-1) staining was detected (**b**). Double immunostaining confirmed that fibroblast only expressed type I collagen (**c**). Fibrocytes on the other hand expressed both type I collagen (**d**), LSP-1 (**e**), and double immunofluorescence confirmed presence of both proteins (**f**) [55]. (With permission to reuse, image obtained from Yang et al. 2005)

burn patients (Fig. 3.7) [55]. Wang et al. collected peripheral blood from postburn patients and normal individuals to isolate fibrocytes and assessed the effects of these cells on modulating the activity of human dermal fibroblast cells [53]. Conditioned media from fibrocytes extracted from postburn patients were able to stimulate fibroblast cells to increase collagen production and proliferative activity, promote migration, stimulate differentiation into myofibroblast cells, and enhance contraction [53]. In addition, increased mRNA expression of both TGF-β1 and CTGF was found in the conditioned media from fibrocytes of postburn patients [53]. The effects of the fibrocyte conditioned media on fibroblast cells were reversed with the addition of TGF-β1 antibody, suggesting an important modulating role of fibrocytes on fibroblast cells [53].

3.4.3 Fibroblasts and Myofibroblasts

Fibroblasts are the primary cells involved in ECM production that is, in part, controlled by TGF-β signaling. In HTS, there is an increase in proliferating and decrease in apoptotic fibroblasts [56]. TGF-β signaling induces fibroblasts cells to produce collagen and differentiate into myofibroblasts. CTGF, a growth factor that is increased downstream of TGF-β signaling, is also suggested to be involved in collagen production through fibroblast signaling. Initially, fibroblasts are recruited into the wound bed by migrating along fibronectin and require the cell surface receptor CD44H [57–59]. Fibroblasts differentiate into myofibroblasts, and this differentiation is activated by PDGF, TGF-β1, and TGF-β2. As mentioned, Wang et al. isolated fibroblasts from normal skin and separated the cells into five layers [33]. The authors found that fibroblasts isolated from the deep dermis were larger, had a slow proliferation rate, and express higher levels of α-SMA, TGF-β1, CTGF, heat shock protein (HSP) 47, collagen, and versican [33]. All of these features are characteristic of HTS fibroblasts. Moreover, bone marrow-derived mesenchymal stem cells were also shown to augment the pro-fibrotic effects of deep dermal fibroblasts [60]. Thus, these results suggest that fibroblasts from the deep dermis contribute to HTS (Table 3.1) [3].

Fibroblasts differentiate into myofibroblasts shortly after tissue granulation formation to facilitate wound closure. Myofibroblasts can also arise from bone marrow-derived sources and mesenchymal stem cells [57]. Myofibroblasts are involved with wound contraction, and remodeling of the ECM [57]. Fibroblasts transition into proto-myofibroblasts following exposure to the environmental milieu characterized by high levels of inflammatory cytokines and chemokines. Proto-myofibroblasts then differentiate into myofibroblasts, which then integrates α-SMA, a marker of myofibroblasts. Under normal conditions, myofibroblasts produce α-SMA and undergo apoptosis once the wound is closed. However, if myofibroblasts persist in the wound bed, contractures can develop. TGF-β1 signaling facilitates myofibroblast differentiation. This signaling pathway includes the ligand TGF-β1, the TGF-β1 receptor complex, and downstream signaling proteins including Smad 2/3 and JNK, referred to as canonical and noncanonical pathways, respectively. In addition, IL-4 and IL-13 can also facilitate myofibroblast differentiation that is independent from the TGF-β pathway.

Table 3.1 Characteristics of human dermal fibroblasts derived from normal skin, hypertrophic scars (HTS), and deep dermis of normal skin [3]. (With permission to reuse, Table 1 obtained from Tredget et al. 2014)

Features of normal, HTS, and deep dermal fibroblasts			
	Normal fibroblasts	HTS fibroblasts	Deep dermal fibroblasts
Cell size	+	+	++
Proliferation rate	++	++	+
Collagen synthesis	+	++	++
Collagenase activity	++++	+	+
α-SMA expression	+	+++	+++
Collagen contraction	+	+++	+++
TGF-β	+	+	+
TGF-β T II receptor	+	+++	+++
CTGF	+	+++	+++
Osteopontin	+	+++	+++
Decorin synthesis	++++	+	+
Fibromodulin	++++	+	+
Biglycan	+	+++	+++
Versican	+	+++	+++
Toll-like receptors	+	+++	?

3.4.4 Chemokines and Cytokines in HTS

Chemokines are chemoattractants, and can be classified as one of four groups: C, CC, CXC, and CX3C [61]. Chemokines are able to recruit inflammatory cells and nearby resident cells by binding to their cognate receptors during wound healing and HTS formation [61]. As mentioned above, the SDF-1/CXCR4+ chemokine pathway plays a role in the development of HTS. Briefly, the expression of SDF-1 is associated with the recruitment of CXCR4+ PBMCs [36]. Thus, recruitment of CXCR4+ PBMC cells into the site of injury can result in differentiation of these cells into fibrocytes, fibroblast, or myofibroblasts, contributing to scar formation [36]. In addition, increased levels of SDF-1α in the serum positively correlated with total body surface area affected by the injury, suggestive of larger burn areas being associated with higher levels of SDF-1α [36]. Moreover, further investigation into this pathway shows that inhibition of this signaling axis improves scar formation [36, 37].

One chemokine pathway of interest is CCL2 (or MCP-1), which binds to CCR2. Murine blood monocytes are subcategorized into one of two groups: C–C chemokine receptor type 2 (CCR2)+/lymphocyte Ag 6C (Ly6C)+ and CCR2−/Ly6C−, reflecting an inflammatory and noninflammatory phenotype, respectively [62, 63]. Using a CCR2-eGFP reporter mouse, wound injury acutely recruited CCR2+/Ly6C+ monocytes to the site of damage [63]. Interestingly, some of these recruited monocytes mature into pro-angiogenic macrophages, thereby contributing to wound healing [63]. In MCP-1 knockout mice, wound re-epithelialization, angiogenesis, and collagen production were all delayed [64]. In a bleomycin model of dermal fibrosis that resembles scleroderma, MCP-1 knockout mice collagen architecture was evaluated following bleomycin injections, and the phenotype resembled wild-type, suggesting a reduced fibrotic response [65]. In another study, CCR2+ human and murine fibrocytes are able to respond to CCL2, leading to an increase in cellular migration and differentiation into myofibroblasts, suggestive of a pro-fibrotic role [66]. These results in regard to wound healing and scar formation suggest that further studies are required to investigate the role of CCL2/CCR2 on HTS formation. Interestingly, this signaling axis may also be involved in keloid formation [67].

The CXC chemokine receptor 3 (CXCR3), a G protein-coupled receptor 9, binds to its respective ligands, including CXCL10 and CXCL11. The chemokine receptor has been shown to be involved with re-epithelialization by promoting keratinocyte and halting fibroblast migration, as well as lessening angiogenesis [68–70]. Yates et al. examined the effects of CXCR3 knockout in mice and found features of scar development characterized as thickened epidermal and dermal layer, increased cellular composition that included fibroblasts, disorganized collagen, higher levels of fibronectin, and a rise in blood vessel formation [69, 71]. Moreover, the presence of inflammatory cells, leukocytes and macrophages, were found in the scar tissue of CXCR3-knockout mice at 6 months after wounding [69, 71]. These features were consistent with HTS, and suggest that, CXCR3 may be a potential therapeutic target to remediate HTS.

The chemokine CX3CL1, or fractalkine, and its receptor CX3CR1, a transmembrane fractalkine receptor or g protein-coupled receptor 13, is involved in wound healing and aberrant signaling and may contribute to HTS formation. CX3CL1 is found in the skin; whereas CX3CR1 is found on inflammatory cells [72]. A transgenic mice line that expressed fluorescently labeled CX3CR1 was used to assess the function of this receptor in wound healing [73]. An increase in CX3CR1+ cells was seen following burn injury, as well as macrophages and endothelial cells [73]. Clover et al. found that CX3CR1 knockout mice resulted in delayed wound healing due to a decreased migration of CX3CR1 positive myeloid cells into the wound bed, as well as reduced angiogenesis [73]. Thus, the results suggest that CX3CR1 signaling contributes to macrophage recruitment and blood vessel formation during wound healing [73]. A full-thickness excisional skin wound was performed on C57BL/6 mice to investigate the role of CX3CL1/CX3CR1 [72]. High gene expression of this signaling axis was identified following injury compared to controls [72]. Moreover, the protein expression of CX3CR1 coincided with macrophages, fibroblasts, and endothelial cells, whereas CX3CL1 was expressed in macrophages and endothelial cells [72]. In CX3CR1 knockout mice, there was a delay in wound closure as well as reduced macrophage infiltration, and decreased mRNA expression of type I collagen [72]. Additionally, absence of CX3CR1 reduced the expression of TGF-β1 and angiogenesis [72]. Thus, these results suggest a role of CX3CL1/CX3CR1 in wound healing.

Cytokines are small signaling molecules, ranging between 4 and 60 kD in size, and influence cell growth, migration, differentiation, proliferation, polarization, and function. In wound healing, both forms of IL-1, IL-1α and IL-1β, appear important. IL-1α has been associated with anti-fibrotic activities while the IL-1β is pro-fibrotic. The expression of IL-1α was found to localized to keratinocytes and dermal neutrophils in a wound healing mice model, suggestive of a role in re-epithelialization and chemotaxis, respectively [74]. Shephard et al. cocultured keratinocytes with fibroblasts, and found an increase in α-SMA, indicative of myofibroblasts observed beginning on day 4 [75]. The transformation from fibroblast to myofibroblast is mediated, in part, by TGF-β, which was expressed within the first two days of culturing, and thus applying the TGF-β neutralizing monoclonal antibody decreased myofibroblast differentiation [75]. The expression of IL-1α in the coculture also reduced the expression of α-SMA, whereas inhibition of this cytokine promoted α-SMA expression, suggestive of a negative regulatory role of IL-1α on TGF-β1 via activation of the transcription factor NF-κB between days 2 and 4 of culturing [75]. However, the TGF-β1 and IL-1 pathway has been shown to share downstream signaling molecules such as interleukin-1 receptor-associated kinase (IRAK) and myeloid differentiation primary response 88 (MyD88), further complicating the signaling mechanism of IL-1 and TGF-β on HTS formation [76]. In HTS, a high level of IL-1β and low IL-1α were detected most notably in the epidermis [77, 78]. HTS fibroblasts stimulated with IL-1β decreased the gene expression of NF-κB, p53, and cyclooxygenase-2 (Cox-2); thus, the reduction in inflammation and apoptosis favors fibroblast proliferation [79]. Interestingly, endothelial cells were also able to differentiate into myofibroblasts following stimulation with IL-1β, identified by an increase in α-SMA and collagen expression [80]. On the contrary, a study by Mia et al. identified IL-1β as anti-fibrotic [81]. IL-1β in combination with TGF-β1 reduced myofibroblast differentiation and collagen production via downregulation of the transcription factor glioma-associated oncogene homolog 1 [81]. Furthermore, fibroblasts stimulated with IL-1β and TGF-β1 promoted expression of MMP, leading to degradation of the ECM [81]. Thus, IL-1β may act as both a pro- and anti-fibrotic factor that may be temporal and spatially dependent.

IL-4 and IL-13, both acting on the same receptor, have been suggested to induce collagen production in human dermal fibroblasts [82]. The cytokines stimulate the extracellular signal-regulated kinase (ERK)1/2 pathway, which then activates the transcription factor ETS domain-containing protein (Elk-1) [82]. The contribution of the signaling pathway to collagen production was confirmed by transfecting fibroblasts cells with dominant negative plasmids of ERK1/2 and Elk-1, which resulted in a decrease in collagen production [82]. Thus, in burn patients, the levels of IL-4 are increased compared to controls, suggesting a role of IL-4 on scar formation via increased collagen production [83, 84].

IL-6 can modulate HTS formation by binding to the IL-6 receptor, followed by associating with the glycoprotein 130 receptor, leading to phosphorylation of the STAT3 transcription factor, which then binds to its cognate DNA sequence encoding the gene suppressor of cytokine signaling 3 (SOCS3) [85]. Thus, an increase in phosphorylated STAT3 as well as an increase in downstream mRNA procollagen and fibronectin was observed in HTS fibroblasts [85]. Gene expression analyses in HTS and normotrophic fibroblasts revealed that MMP-1 and MMP-3 were increased in normotrophic fibroblasts following IL-6 stimulation, and this upregulation was not observed in HTS fibroblasts, suggesting a lack of ECM degradation [23]. HTS fibroblasts were also assessed for changes in gene expression stimulated with and without IL-6 [23]. The highly expressed genes (greater than threefold) included periplakin, tenascin XB, KIAA0306 protein, and latent TGF-β binding protein 1 [23]. On the other hand, greatly reduced genes (greater than threefold) included KIAA077 protein, serum/glucocorticoid regulated kinase, CTGF, pregnancy specific β-1 glycoprotein, and thromospondin-1 gene [23]. Thus, treatment of hypertrophic fibroblasts with IL-6 is able to modify gene expression of components involved in the ECM and epidermal barrier [23].

IL-10 is an anti-inflammatory and anti-fibrotic cytokine. Fetal wounds heal without scarring, and this may be attributed to a lack of an inflammatory response. Thus, IL-10, an anti-inflammatory cytokine, has been shown to be associated with a lack of scarring when overexpressed in an adult mouse model of scars induced by a punch biopsy [86]. In support of this, skin grafts from IL-10 knockout fetal mice developed scars [2]. IL-10 reduced α-SMA and both type I and III collagen via phosphorylation of the transcription factor STAT3 and protein kinase B (AKT) [87]. Inhibition of the signaling pathway and IL-10 receptors reversed the effects of IL-10 confirming the anti-fibrotic outcomes [87]. Interestingly, serum levels of IL-10 were found to increase in burn patients [84] suggesting a role for IL-10 in HTS formation or remodeling.

An increase in tumor necrosis factor (TNF)-α type I receptors is found in HTS [77]. TNF-α was shown to promote the differentiation of endothelial cells to myofibroblasts, and the myofibroblast were confirmed by an increased expression of α-SMA and collagen [80]. TNF-α also has an anti-fibrotic role [88]. Goldberg et al. showed that TNF-α decreased α-SMA expression, and therefore reduced fibroblast to myofibroblast differentiation [89]. Moreover, TNF-α was also able to reduce genes that are normally increased by TGF-β1 such as collagen and fibronectin [89]. The anti-fibrotic effects of TNF-α on α-SMA were mediated by mRNA destabilization, activation of the c-Jun N-terminal kinase (JNK) pathway, and TGF-β1 by preventing phosphorylation of the Smad3 pathway [89]. Thus, TNF-α also influences scar formation.

The effects of IFN-γ, produced from T lymphocytes were assessed in human postburn HTS fibroblast cells [90]. Treatment of normal and HTS fibroblast cells with IFN-γ resulted in a reduction in cell numbers, collagen protein production, and type I and type III procollagen mRNA levels in HTS fibroblast [90]. Another type of IFN, IFN α2b, which is produced by leukocytes, has also been investigated [91]. Tredget et al. also found reductions in collagen protein and type I procollagen mRNA production [91]. Thus, these effects are opposite of what is observed when cells are treated with TGF-β1, which results in hyperproliferation and increased collagen mRNA and protein production. Further investigations into IFN on collagenase and TIMP-1 expression revealed opposing results [92]. Treatment of fibroblast cells with IFN-γ resulted in reduced collagenase and increased TIMP-1 mRNA expression [92]. Treatment with IFN α2b on the other hand increased both collagenase and TIMP-1 mRNA expression levels [92]. Therefore, the use of IFN α2b as a therapeutic intervention was next evaluated [93–95]. Burn patients treated with IFN α2b had a reduced number of fibroblast and myofibroblast cells compared to their baseline [95]. The effects of IFN α2b treatment were also assessed on fibrocytes [93, 94]. Wang et al. found a reduction in fibrocyte number in control and HTS tissue after treatment with IFN α2b *in vivo* [93, 94]. The authors also found a reduction in all of the following parameters: PBMCs differentiation into fibrocytes, α-SMA expressing fibrocytes, and fibrocyte proliferation in culture [93, 94]. Wang et al. also identified reduced VEGF expression, and therefore angiogenesis in HTS tissue following treatment with IFN α2b [94]. Moreover, burn patients

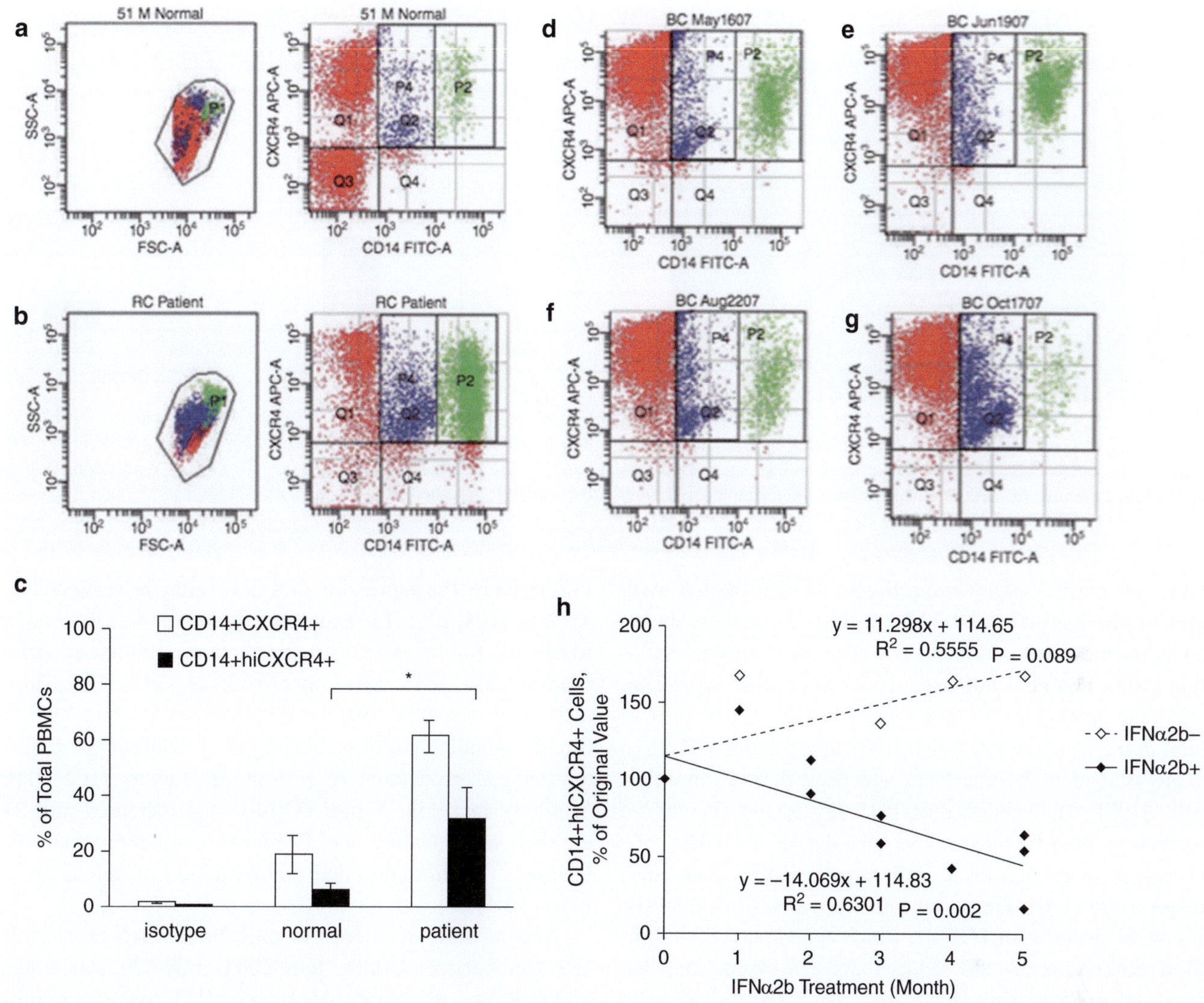

Fig. 3.8 The effects of interferon α2b (IFNα2b) treatment on CD14+hiCXCR4 expressing cells in burn patients. Peripheral blood mononuclear cells (PBMCs) were collected from the blood of normal (**a**) and burn (**b**) patients for detection of CD14+ and CXCR4+ cells by flow cytometry. Total number of CD14+CXCR4+ and CD14+hiCXCR4+ cells was greater in burn patients compared to normal (**c**). Intervention with IFNα2b was then tested and CD14+CXCR4+ cells were investigated before treatment began (**d**), 1 month post-treatment (**e**), 3 months post-treatment (**f**), and 5 months post-treatment (**g**). Patients receiving IFNα2b had a reduction in CD14+hiCXCR4+ cells overtime compared to those that did not (**h**) [36]. (With permission to reuse, image obtained from Ding J et al. 2011)

treated with IFN α2b had reduced SDF-1 expression and CD14+ expressing CXCR4+ cells in the bloodstream (Fig. 3.8) [36]. *In vitro*, conditioned media from dermal fibroblast cells treated with LPS increased PBMCs mobility, and this was reduced when fibroblast cells were treated with IFN α2b [36]. Thus, IFN α2b is an attractive potential therapeutic intervention to treat HTS as it shows reduction in chemotaxis and characteristic features of HTS.

3.4.5 MicroRNAs (miRs) in HTS

MicroRNAs (miRs) are noncoding, endogenous, RNA molecules, capable of regulating post-transcriptional activity of protein expression. miRs are involved with normal physiological wound healing and HTS formation. Several miRs have been implicated in the formation of HTS such as miR-98, miR-29b, miR-185, and miR-145 [96–99]; however, we will only review four miRs and their involvement in HTS formation. miR-181b was identified as a pro-fibrotic factor [100]. The miR-181 family comprises miR-181a, miR-181b, miR-181c, and miR-181d. Kwan et al. investigated potential miRs regulators of decorin expression in both HTS and deep dermal fibroblasts [100]. Tissue from postburn patients and dermal (superficial and deep dermal) fibroblast cells from patients undergoing abdominoplasty were collected [100]. Decorin expression was less in tissue collected from HTS and deep dermis compared to normal and superficial dermal

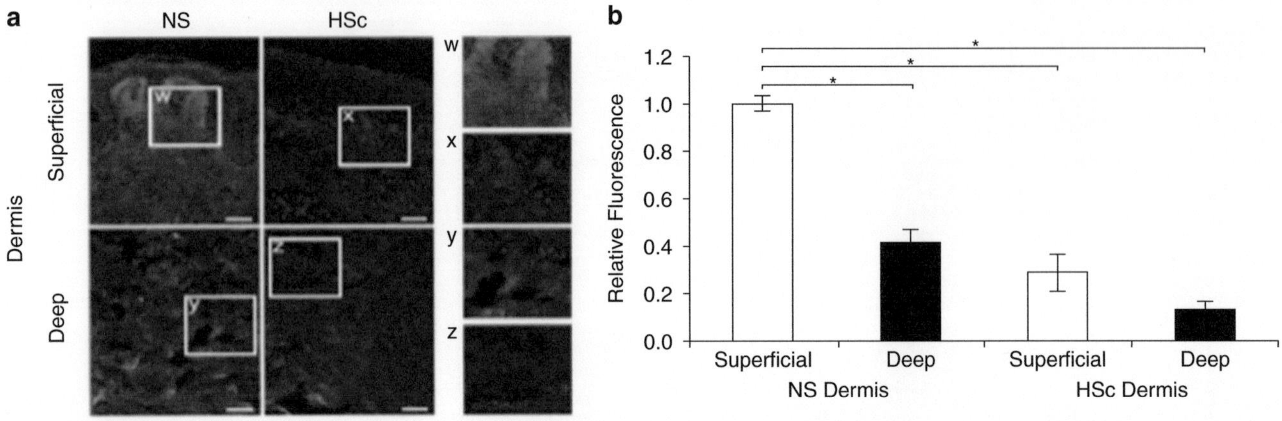

Fig. 3.9 The expression of decorin was evaluated by immunofluorescence in normal skin (NS), hypertrophic scars (HTS), superficial dermis, and deep dermis (**a**). Decorin expression is reduced in deep dermis as compared to the superficial dermis in NS samples and in HTS compared to the normal superficial dermis (**b**) [100]. (With permission to reuse, image obtained from Kwan et al. 2015)

layer of normal skin, respectively, in accordance with previous findings (Fig. 3.9) [31, 33, 100]. The authors speculated that these differences may be attributed to miRs regulation [100]. Potential miRs regulators of decorin expression were narrowed down to miR-181b since its expression was high in the deep dermis and TGF-β1 upregulated miR-181b expression in both superficial and deep dermal fibroblast cells [100]. Analysis of miR-181b expression showed an increase in both HTS tissue and deep dermal fibroblast cells compared to normal tissue and superficial fibroblast cells, respectively [100]. Fibroblast cells harvested from HTS tissue were treated with TGF-β1, which upregulated myofibroblast differentiation and reduced decorin expression, and these effects was reversed when cells were treated with antagomiR-181b, a miR-181b antagonist [100]. These results support the role of miR-181b in decorin regulation and scar formation [100]. Interestingly, increased expression of miR181a has been shown to be associated with keloid formation [101].

Guo et al. performed a microarray analysis and showed 152 miRs abnormally associated with HTS, and found both HTS tissue and fibroblasts to exhibit an increase of miR-21 expression [102, 103]. Inhibition of miR-21 decreased pro-fibrotic factors such as type I collagen gene expression, promoted apoptosis, and decreased both scar area and elevation [102]. Thus, this study revealed that miR-21 is a pro-fibrotic factor and may be an efficacious therapeutic target. MiR-21 targets the phosphatase and tensin homolog deleted on chromosome ten (PTEN) leading to downregulation [102–104]. This led to activation of the phosphoinositide 3-kinase (PI3K)/Akt signaling pathway, and subsequent increased human telomerase reverse transcriptase (hTERT) production in hypertrophic fibroblasts, which may in part explain the mechanism associated with increased proliferation [103]. Furthermore, the expression of miR-21 may be regulated by TGF-β1 [104, 105]. The expression of Smad7 was reduced in fibroblasts following TGF-β1 stimulation, and this coincided with an increased expression of miR-21 [104, 106]. Thus, miR-21 is involved with the PTEN/PI3K/Akt and TGF-β/Smad7 signaling pathway, leading to HTS fibroblast proliferation and production of pro-fibrotic factors [102–104]. Similarly in keloid tissue, TGF-β1 also increases miR-21 expression, activating the PTEN/Akt signaling pathway, leading to proliferation and differentiation of keloid fibroblasts [105].

Another miR of interest is miR-200, which consists of five members: miR-200a, miR-200b, miR-429, miR-200c, and miR-141. Microarray analysis of HTS tissue and fibroblasts also showed a significant downregulation of miR-200b [107]. To confirm that miR-200b plays a role in HTS formation, a transfection study with pre-miR-200b and anti-miR-200b was performed [107]. Transfection with pre-miR200b promoted cellular apoptosis and reduced proliferation by increasing caspase3 and caspase8 while downregulating the expression of proliferating cell nuclear antigen (PCNA) and TGF-β1, respectively [107]. The opposite effects were observed when the hypertrophic fibroblast cells were transfected with anti-miR-200b [107]. Furthermore, the features of HTS, α-SMA, type I collagen, and fibronectin were decreased following pre-miR200b transfection [107]. Expression of TGF-β1 was shown to downregulate miR-200 by regulating expression of the transcription factor zinc finger E-box-binding homeobox1 (zeb1) [104]. Overall, the results suggest that miR-200 is an anti-fibrotic factor.

MiR-29b was identified as a possible player in scar formation. MiR-29b was identified as a candidate through computation analysis, and was shown to regulate the expression of type I collagen [108]. Cheng et al. identified miR-29b to be a negative regulator of collagen such that an increase in miR-29b resulted in a decrease in collagen production and vice versa [108]. MiR-29b may be regulating collagen production in fibroblasts through post-transcriptional modification of the heat shock protein (HSP) 47 [109]. HSP are involved with protein biosynthesis and HSP47 is involved with collagen production [109, 110]. Zhu et al. found that TGF-β1 inhibited miR-29b, which resulted in an increase in HSP47 and, subsequently, collagen [109]. The effect of TGF-β1 on HSP47 is mediated through the Smad signaling pathway [109], and since TGF-β1 is able to reduce the expression of miR-29b, the proinflammatory cytokines IL-1β and TNF-α can increase its expression via NF-κB [109]. In support of miR-29b having an anti-fibrotic role, a scald model in mice injected with miR-29b decreased scar formation and this effect may have been mediated through repression of the TGF-β1 signaling pathway and subsequently CTGF [99].

3.4.6 Growth Factors in HTS

TGF-β is the most studied pro-fibrotic growth factor and is known to play an important role in postnatal HTS formation and scarless wound healing in fetuses. It has three isoforms: TGF-β1, TGF-β2, and TGF-β3 [111]. The TGF-β1 and TGF-β2 are associated with HTS formation; whereas, TGF-β3 is highly expressed in fetuses. TGF-β is first secreted in a precursor form that is inactive [111]. The precursor form is a large complex composed of the latency-associated peptide (LAP) and the latent TGF-β-binding protein (LTBP), together forming the large latent complex (LLC) [111]. MMPs (MMP-2 and MMP-9), among other enzymes, can cleave TGF-β from this complex, freeing it to bind to its receptors [112]. The released TGF-β binds to two receptors, TGFβRI and TGFβRII [111]. Once bound, the phosphorylated receptor induces a signaling cascade. This signaling cascade leads to phosphorylation of the transcription factors Smad 2 and 3 [111]. The Smad 2/3 combines with Smad 4, forming a Smad 2/3/4 complex and initiates transcription of pro-fibrotic genes such as collagen types I and III [111].

TGF-β regulates aspects of wound healing. Thus, perturbations in TGF-β expression or signaling can lead to scarring. Hypertrophic fibroblasts cells produces significantly more TGF-β compared to controls from site-matched normal skin, leading to upregulation of pro-fibrotic factors [113]. Wang et al. assessed the mRNA expression of TGF-β1 and found approximately a fivefold increased expression in HTS compared to normal skin, and that this increase was also observed in fibroblasts cells extracted from HTS compared to normal fibroblasts [113]. Moreover, the receptors TGFβRI and TGFβRII were found in low levels in dermal fibroblasts of normal skin; however, HTS fibroblasts exhibited high levels of TβRI and TβRII [114]. Overall, there is an increase in the mRNA, protein, and receptor expression for TGF-β. TGF-β leads to activation of CTGF via Smad and STAT signaling pathways [115, 116]. CTGF expression is also stimulated by neuregulin-1, and promotes fibroblast proliferation and myofibroblast differentiation through PI3K- or Src-mediated and JAK1 and STAT1 activation [57, 117–120]. Scar tissue exhibits high CTGF expression [119]. Thus, blockade of TGF-β1 production and signaling is an attractive therapeutic target. Inhibition of the TGF-β signaling pathway has been shown to decrease HTS formation [121]. Wang et al. transfected HTS fibroblasts with TGFβRI siRNA [122]. This resulted in a decrease in proliferation of HTS fibroblasts and subsequently a reduction in both collagen and fibronectin production [122]. Thus, HTS formation was reduced following TGFβRI inhibition [122]. Inhibition of CTGF by delivering antisense oligonucleotides in a rabbit model of HTS resulted in a decrease in myofibroblasts, TIMP-1 expression, and both types I and III collagen [123]. Overall, inhibition of the TGF-β pathway can reduce scar development.

VEGF (VEGF-A), a pro-angiogenic growth factor, is implicated in HTS since one of the features of HTS is hypervascularity. VEGF is involved with stimulating angiogenesis, predominantly during the proliferation phase, and is secreted by several different cell types, including fibroblasts, macrophages, and endothelial cells [7]. VEGF also increases blood vessel permeability and recruits inflammatory cells to the site of injury [124, 125]. The increase in blood vessel formation provides oxygen and nutrients to the highly metabolic cells that are undergoing proliferation, migration, and differentiation. During wound healing, a high density of blood vessels is observed during the formation of the granulation tissue that eventually regresses as the wound matures. VEGF binds to the VEGF receptors VEGF-1 and VEGF-2, leading to a cascade of downstream signaling. VEGF can also bind to a soluble receptor, sVEGFR-1, a negative regulator of angiogenesis. Unregulated VEGF expression and signaling can contribute to formation of HTS since VEGF increases angiogenesis, recruits inflammatory cells, and assists in delivering oxygen and nutrients to maintain cellular metabolism. Kwak et al. investigated whether inhibition of VEGF with the monoclonal antibody, bevacizumab, would reduce HTS [126]. Using an ear wound model in New Zealand white rabbits, the authors found less erythema, reduced scar thickness, and less collagen packing [126]. The protein level of VEGF and vessel number was reduced in treatment groups, suggesting that a reduction in VEGF may reduce HTS formation [126]. Furthermore, to confirm the role of VEGF in scar formation, studies of fetal wound healing revealed a low level of VEGF in scarless healing and the addition of VEGF led to scar formation [127].

PDGF is involved with multiple aspects of HTS such as promoting chemotaxis, cellular proliferation, and collagen production. There are five isoforms of PDGF, AA, AB, BB, CC, and DD. PDGF can stimulate cyclooxygenase-2 and PI3K/JNK pathway. PDGF mediates its effects by binding to the tyrosine kinase receptors termed PDGF-αR and -βR. By binding to the receptor, it activates the transcription factor extracellular signal-regulated kinases (ERK). PDGF is also involved with osteopontin production by macrophages, which promotes chemotaxis, collagen attachment, and myofibroblasts differentiation [128]. Thus, PDGF may play a role in HTS since it is released from platelets, and initially acts as a chemoattractant for monocytes and fibroblasts, as well as regulating fibroblast proliferation and subsequent collagen production.

Epidermal growth factor (EGF) binds to the epidermal growth factor receptor (EGFR), leading to phosphorylation of the intracellular component of the receptors by the protein tyrosine kinase. EGF has been shown to be involved in ECM remodeling by regulating MMP-1 expression through ERK, JNK, and p38 [57, 129]. Basic fibroblast growth factor (bFGF) is a member of the FGF family and may be involved with HTS formation [130]. bFGF has been shown to be antifibrotic, since administration of the growth factor reduced scar formation, and decreased expression of the fibrotic factors α-SMA, collagen, fibronectin, and TIMP-1 via the TGF-β1/Smad pathway [131]. FGF has also been shown to increase the expression of the proteolytic enzyme MMP-1 through activation of the ERK and JNK signaling pathway [132]. Overall, FGF may be a potential therapeutic intervention to prevent HTS.

3.5 Human and Animal Models to Study the Mechanism of Scarring

The mechanism of HTS is difficult to study in human patients. Animal models would provide an opportunity to study the temporal and spatial changes of HTS formation [133]. The athymic nude mouse model of HTS was initially established by Yang et al. [134]. Our laboratory had investigated a modified dermal fibrotic nude mouse model that has morphological and cellular changes that are representative of human HTS. Briefly, full-thickness and split-thickness human skin is grafted onto the dorsum of the nude mice (refer to citation for methodology) [135]. The nude mice are athymic, and therefore the lack of T cells prevents rejection of human tissue.

Wang et al. evaluated both full-thickness and split-thickness human skin grafted onto nude mice and the mechanism associated with HTS formation [133]. One month post-grafting, both model grafts harden, the top layer (epidermis and upper layer of the dermis) sloughed off, and the remaining skin graft became swollen, red, and elevated [133]. By 4 months post-graft, the scar was thickened, which then began to slowly regress (Fig. 3.10) [133]. Both full-thickness and split-thickness graft had increased collagen deposition, vascularity, mast cells, fibrocytes, macrophages, and myofibroblasts [133]. The mRNA levels of COL1α1 and HSP 47 were also elevated post-grafting, which both peaked at 2 months post-graft and decreased thereafter [133]. Both mRNA and protein levels of TGF-β1 and CTGF were also increased in both full-thickness and split-thickness skin grafts [133]. In this study, both full-thickness and split-thickness skin grafted onto nude mice induced a HTS very similar to that seen in humans [133]. Further characterization of the split-thickness model also revealed that the HTS formed with an absence of both adnexal structures and hair follicles and a loss of the rete pegs, as well as reduced decorin and higher biglycan production at 30 and 60 days post-graft [136]. Moreover, the changes in proteoglycans were reversed by 180 days post-graft, which suggests remodeling and maturation [136]. Survival of the human cells in the skin graft up to 180 days post-grafting was confirmed with the immunofluorescent stain HLA-ABC [136].

Alrobaiea et al. investigated a deep dermal scratch model of HTS with full-thickness skin grafts transplanted onto nude mice (Fig. 3.11) [137]. Scratches on the full-thickness human skin grafts were made before and after grafting at a depth of >0.6 mm and a control skin graft with no scratch were also evaluated [9, 137]. Both scratch grafts were thickened and peaked at 2 months, which thereafter began to decline [137]. Moreover, there was an increase in thin collagen fibers, myofibroblast cells, and macrophage cells infiltration [137]. Thus, in this deep scratch model, a scratch made before or after the skin is grafted produced similar results and survived for upwards to a year [137]. Human split-thickness skin grafts also developed scars in another three kinds of immunodeficient knockout mice, including recombination activating gene (RAG)-1−/−, RAG-2−/− γc−/−, T-cell receptor (TCR) αβ−/−γβ−/−, which lacks mature B, T, and natural killer cells [138]. This suggests that nonspecific immune cells play critical roles in scarring. There are limitations in the use of animal models. Dermal scars do not develop in animal skin and current HTS research models include rabbit ear and the dorsum of red Duroc pigs [138]. These models are limited because in the rabbit ear model, the ear cartilage also becomes hypertrophied and in the red Duroc pig, the scars become depressed [138].

To overcome these animal model limitations, the dermal human scratch model is another model that can be used to assess the pathophysiology and effects of therapeutic interventions (Fig. 3.12). Linear wounds were made on the hips

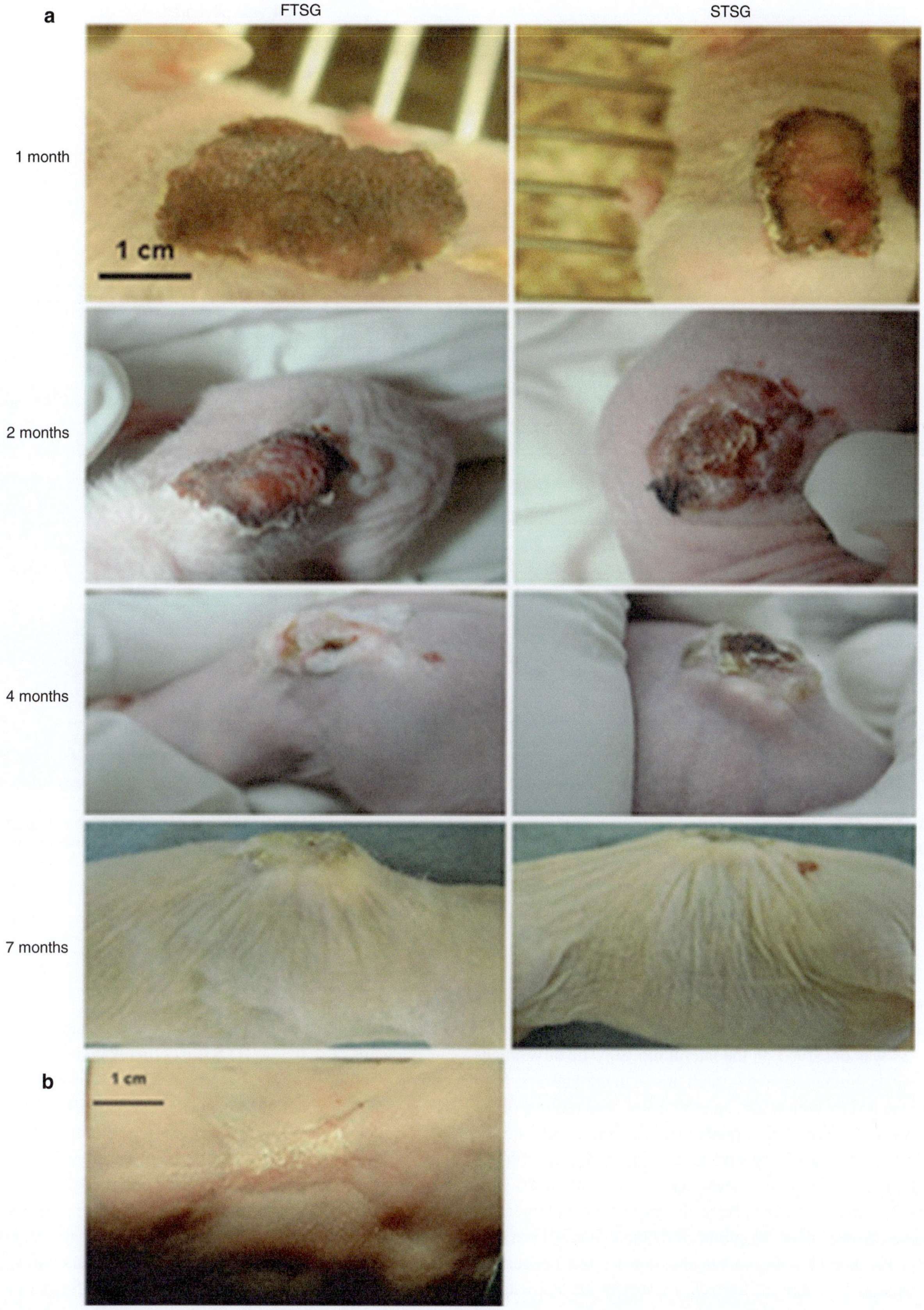

Fig. 3.10 Both human full-thickness (FTSG) and split-thickness skin grafts (STSG) were grafted onto the dorsum of athymic nude mice and the progression of scar formation was imaged at 1 month, 2 months, 4 months, and 7 months post-graft (**a**). Rat skin transplantation was also grafted however, no scar was formed (**b**) [133]. (With permission to reuse, image obtained by Wang J et al. 2011)

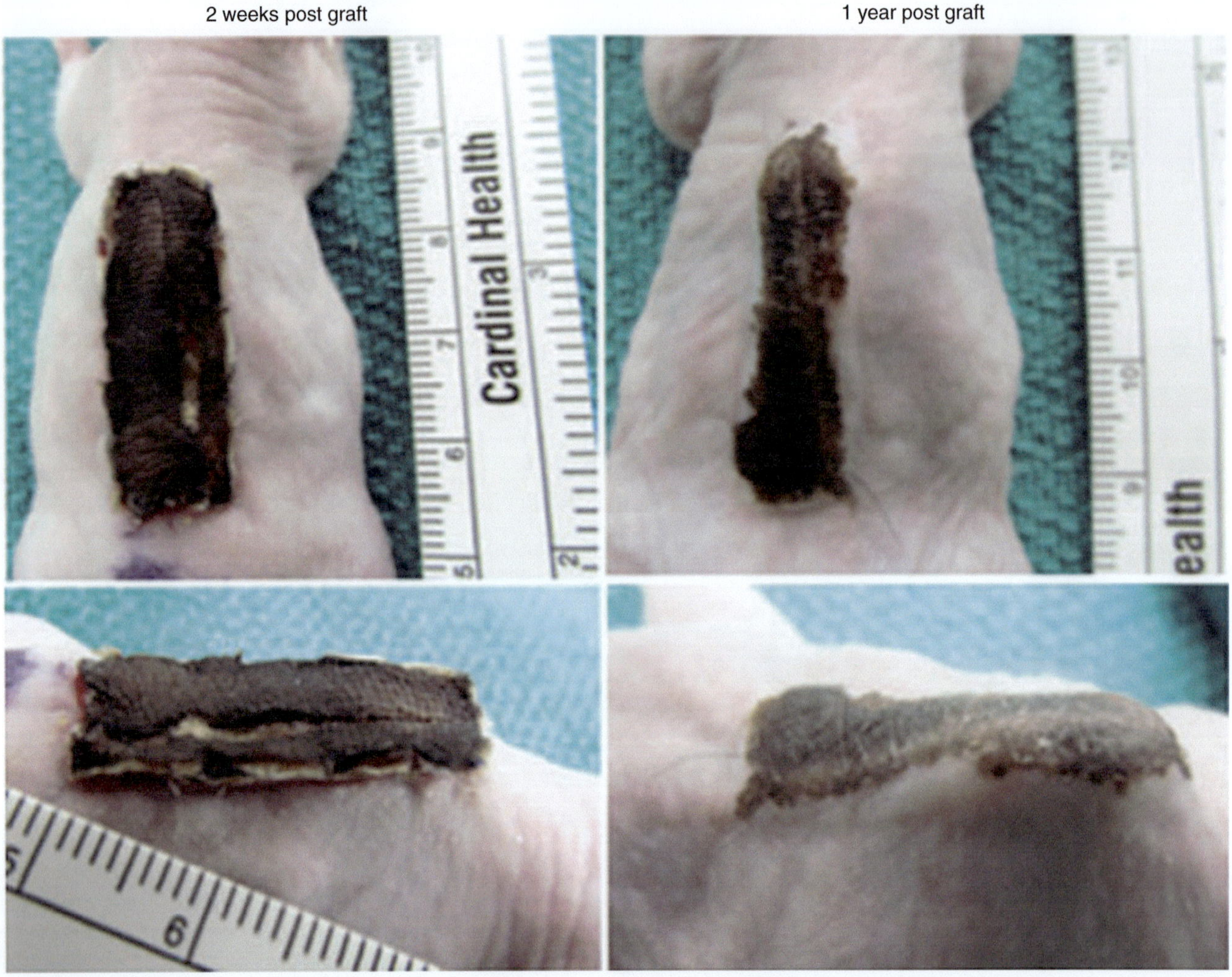

Fig. 3.11 A modified dermal scar mouse model. Full-thickness human skin grafts (FTSG) with a deep wound were transplanted onto nude mice, which were collected from pigmented human skin tissue. The grafted skin survived and developed HTS with morphological and cellular features similar to human HTS at 2 weeks and 1 year post-grafting [137]. This provided the evidence that human skin tissue can survive in the mouse model upwards to one year. (With permission to reuse, image obtained from Alrobaiea et al. 2016)

that were initially superficial and became progressively deeper, resulting in HTS. As mentioned, human wounds exceeding 0.5 mm in depth can result in the formation of a HTS, as was observed on the lateral hip [9]. The advantages of using the human dermal scratch model in humans are: both mature and HTS within the superficial and deep regions of the same wound are created, reproducible and consistent, and the possibility of creating a wound on each hip to test the efficacy of a drug and placebo, thereby reducing inter-individual variability. Overall, in order to fully understand the pathogenesis of human dermal fibrosis, animal and human models are necessary. The use of both models can support and further our understanding of dermal fibrosis. Furthermore, understanding the pathogenesis of HTS will assist in the development of potential therapeutic interventions.

3.6 Conclusion

In this review, we discussed the cellular and molecular mechanisms of scarring. HTS is a complex and dynamic process, involving several different cells and downstream signaling pathways that are temporally and spatially regulated. The mechanisms of scars are further complicated with comorbidities such as diabetes. Furthermore, translation from bench to bedside poses as a challenge because *in vitro* and *in vivo* models of scars and wound healing may not fully resemble the human condition. Thus, further investigations on the cellular and molecular pathways of scars and species differences may provide insights into scar formation and wound healing, thereby enabling the development of effective treatments.

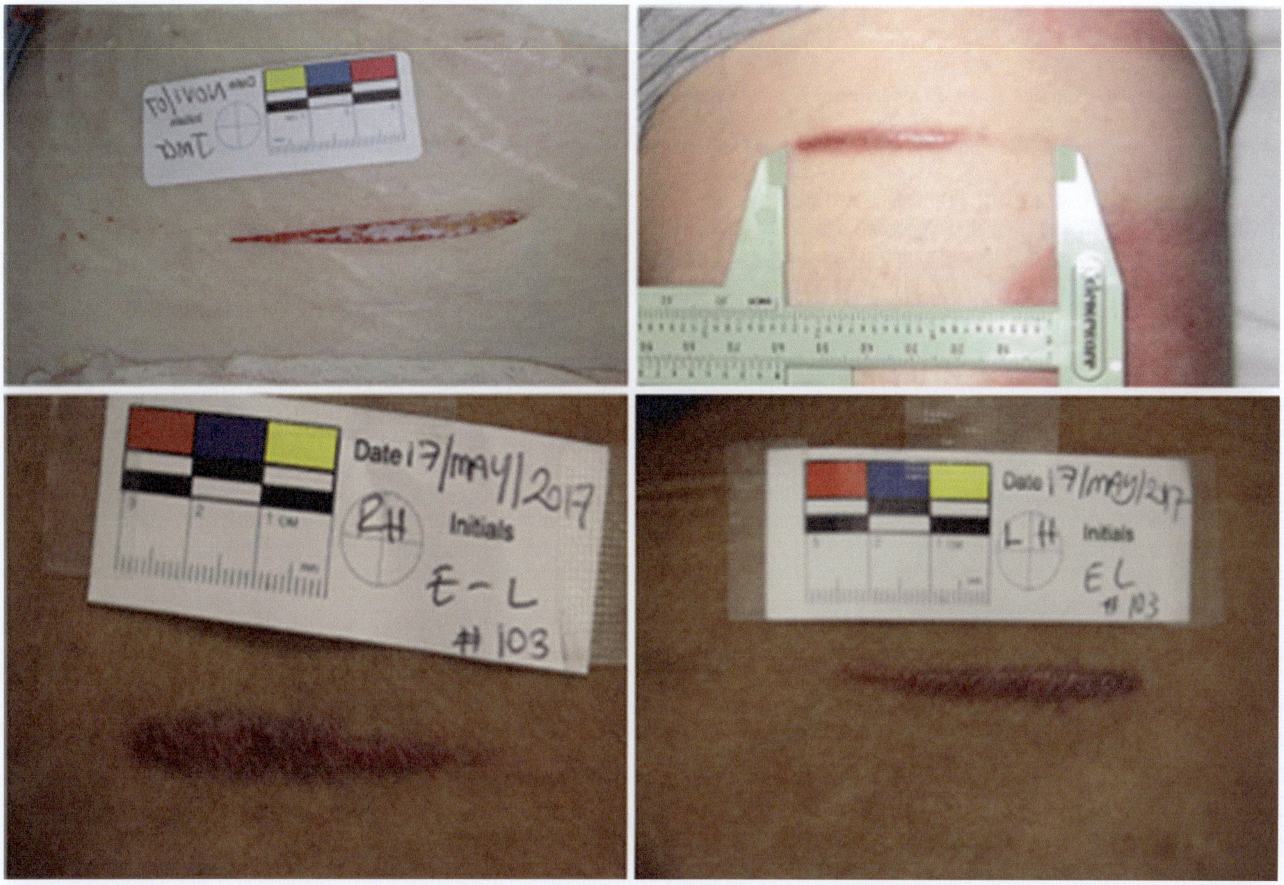

Fig. 3.12 Human dermal scratch wound model. A reproducible and consistent wound of increasing depth can be made using a jig. This model allows assessing superficial to deep wounds, as well as therapeutic interventions

References

1. Soo C, Beanes SR, Hu FY, Zhang X, Dang C, Chang G, et al. Ontogenetic transition in fetal wound transforming growth factor-beta regulation correlates with collagen organization. Am J Pathol. 2003;163(6):2459–76.
2. Liechty KW, Kim HB, Adzick NS, Crombleholme TM. Fetal wound repair results in scar formation in interleukin-10-deficient mice in a syngeneic murine model of scarless fetal wound repair. J Pediatr Surg. 2000;35(6):866–72. discussion 872-3.
3. Tredget EE, Levi B, Donelan MB. Biology and principles of scar management and burn reconstruction. Surg Clin North Am. 2014;94(4):793–815.
4. Robson MC, Steed DL, Franz MG. Wound healing: biologic features and approaches to maximize healing trajectories. Curr Probl Surg. 2001;38(2):A1–140.
5. Zhu Z, Ding J, Tredget EE. The molecular basis of hypertrophic scars. Burns Trauma. 2016;4:2-015-0026-4. eCollection 2016.
6. Fadok VA, Bratton DL, Konowal A, Freed PW, Westcott JY, Henson PM. Macrophages that have ingested apoptotic cells in vitro inhibit proinflammatory cytokine production through autocrine/paracrine mechanisms involving TGF-beta, PGE2, and PAF. J Clin Invest. 1998;101(4):890–8.
7. Bao P, Kodra A, Tomic-Canic M, Golinko MS, Ehrlich HP, Brem H. The role of vascular endothelial growth factor in wound healing. J Surg Res. 2009;153(2):347–58.
8. Santoro MM, Gaudino G. Cellular and molecular facets of keratinocyte reepithelization during wound healing. Exp Cell Res. 2005;304(1):274–86.
9. Dunkin CS, Pleat JM, Gillespie PH, Tyler MP, Roberts AH, McGrouther DA. Scarring occurs at a critical depth of skin injury: precise measurement in a graduated dermal scratch in human volunteers. Plast Reconstr Surg. 2007;119(6):1722–32. discussion 1733-4.
10. Honardoust D, Varkey M, Marcoux Y, Shankowsky HA, Tredget EE. Reduced decorin, fibromodulin, and transforming growth factor-beta3 in deep dermis leads to hypertrophic scarring. J Burn Care Res. 2012;33(2):218–27.
11. Kwan P, Hori K, Ding J, Tredget EE. Scar and contracture: biological principles. Hand Clin. 2009;25(4):511–28.
12. Tredget EE. Pathophysiology and treatment of fibroproliferative disorders following thermal injury. Ann N Y Acad Sci. 1999;888:165–82.
13. Rowan MP, Cancio LC, Elster EA, Burmeister DM, Rose LF, Natesan S, et al. Burn wound healing and treatment: review and advancements. Crit Care. 2015;19:243-015-0961-2.
14. Armour A, Scott PG, Tredget EE. Cellular and molecular pathology of HTS: basis for treatment. Wound Repair Regen. 2007;15(Suppl 1):S6–17.
15. Verhaegen PD, van Zuijlen PP, Pennings NM, van Marle J, Niessen FB, van der Horst CM, et al. Differences in collagen architecture between keloid, hypertrophic scar, normotrophic scar, and normal skin: an objective histopathological analysis. Wound Repair Regen. 2009;17(5):649–56.

16. Linares HA, Kischer CW, Dobrkovsky M, Larson DL. The histiotypic organization of the hypertrophic scar in humans. J Invest Dermatol. 1972;59(4):323–31.
17. Limandjaja GC, van den Broek LJ, Waaijman T, van Veen HA, Everts V, Monstrey S, et al. Increased epidermal thickness and abnormal epidermal differentiation in keloid scars. Br J Dermatol. 2017;176(1):116–26.
18. Oliveira GV, Hawkins HK, Chinkes D, Burke A, Tavares AL, Ramos-e-Silva M, et al. Hypertrophic versus non hypertrophic scars compared by immunohistochemistry and laser confocal microscopy: type I and III collagens. Int Wound J. 2009;6(6):445–52.
19. Bailey AJ, Bazin S, Sims TJ, Le Lous M, Nicoletis C, Delaunay A. Characterization of the collagen of human hypertrophic and normal scars. Biochim Biophys Acta. 1975;405(2):412–21.
20. Hayakawa T, Hashimoto Y, Myokei Y, Aoyama H, Izawa Y. Changes in type of collagen during the development of human post-burn hypertrophic scars. Clin Chim Acta. 1979;93(1):119–25.
21. Ulrich D, Ulrich F, Unglaub F, Piatkowski A, Pallua N. Matrix metalloproteinases and tissue inhibitors of metalloproteinases in patients with different types of scars and keloids. J Plast Reconstr Aesthet Surg. 2010;63(6):1015–21.
22. Simon F, Bergeron D, Larochelle S, Lopez-Valle CA, Genest H, Armour A, et al. Enhanced secretion of TIMP-1 by human hypertrophic scar keratinocytes could contribute to fibrosis. Burns. 2012;38(3):421–7.
23. Dasu MR, Hawkins HK, Barrow RE, Xue H, Herndon DN. Gene expression profiles from hypertrophic scar fibroblasts before and after IL-6 stimulation. J Pathol. 2004;202(4):476–85.
24. Ghahary A, Shen YJ, Nedelec B, Wang R, Scott PG, Tredget EE. Collagenase production is lower in post-burn hypertrophic scar fibroblasts than in normal fibroblasts and is reduced by insulin-like growth factor-1. J Invest Dermatol. 1996;106(3):476–81.
25. Ghahary A, Shen YJ, Nedelec B, Scott PG, Tredget EE. Enhanced expression of mRNA for insulin-like growth factor-1 in post-burn hypertrophic scar tissue and its fibrogenic role by dermal fibroblasts. Mol Cell Biochem. 1995;148(1):25–32.
26. Amadeu TP, Braune AS, Porto LC, Desmouliere A, Costa AM. Fibrillin-1 and elastin are differentially expressed in hypertrophic scars and keloids. Wound Repair Regen. 2004;12(2):169–74.
27. Bhangoo KS, Quinlivan JK, Connelly JR. Elastin fibers in scar tissue. Plast Reconstr Surg. 1976;57(3):308–13.
28. Schilling JA. Wound healing. Surg Clin North Am. 1976;56(4):859–74.
29. Papakonstantinou E, Roth M, Karakiulakis G. Hyaluronic acid: a key molecule in skin aging. Dermatoendocrinol. 2012;4(3):253–8.
30. Honardoust D, Varkey M, Hori K, Ding J, Shankowsky HA, Tredget EE. Small leucine-rich proteoglycans, decorin and fibromodulin, are reduced in postburn hypertrophic scar. Wound Repair Regen. 2011;19(3):368–78.
31. Scott PG, Dodd CM, Ghahary A, Shen YJ, Tredget EE. Fibroblasts from post-burn hypertrophic scar tissue synthesize less decorin than normal dermal fibroblasts. Clin Sci (Lond). 1998;94(5):541–7.
32. Sayani K, Dodd CM, Nedelec B, Shen YJ, Ghahary A, Tredget EE, et al. Delayed appearance of decorin in healing burn scars. Histopathology. 2000;36(3):262–72.
33. Wang J, Dodd C, Shankowsky HA, Scott PG, Tredget EE, Wound Healing Research Group. Deep dermal fibroblasts contribute to hypertrophic scarring. Lab Invest. 2008;88(12):1278–90.
34. Honardoust D, Ding J, Varkey M, Shankowsky HA, Tredget EE. Deep dermal fibroblasts refractory to migration and decorin-induced apoptosis contribute to hypertrophic scarring. J Burn Care Res. 2012;33(5):668–77.
35. Kwan PO, Ding J, Tredget EE. Serum decorin, IL-1beta, and TGF-beta predict hypertrophic scarring postburn. J Burn Care Res. 2015;37:356–66.
36. Ding J, Hori K, Zhang R, Marcoux Y, Honardoust D, Shankowsky HA, et al. Stromal cell-derived factor 1 (SDF-1) and its receptor CXCR4 in the formation of postburn hypertrophic scar (HTS). Wound Repair Regen. 2011;19(5):568–78.
37. Ding J, Ma Z, Liu H, Kwan P, Iwashina T, Shankowsky HA, et al. The therapeutic potential of a C-X-C chemokine receptor type 4 (CXCR-4) antagonist on hypertrophic scarring in vivo. Wound Repair Regen. 2014;22(5):622–30.
38. Liu H, Ding J, Ma Z, Zhu Z, Shankowsky HA, Tredget EE. A novel subpopulation of peripheral blood mononuclear cells presents in major burn patients. Burns. 2015;41(5):998–1007.
39. Deshmane SL, Kremlev S, Amini S, Sawaya BE. Monocyte chemoattractant protein-1 (MCP-1): an overview. J Interferon Cytokine Res. 2009;29(6):313–26.
40. Nakazawa D, Shida H, Kusunoki Y, Miyoshi A, Nishio S, Tomaru U, et al. The responses of macrophages in interaction with neutrophils that undergo NETosis. J Autoimmun. 2016;67:19–28.
41. Selders GS, Fetz AE, Radic MZ, Bowlin GL. An overview of the role of neutrophils in innate immunity, inflammation and host-biomaterial integration. Regen Biomater. 2017;4(1):55–68.
42. Zhang J, Zhou Q, Yuan G, Dong M, Shi W. Notch signaling regulates M2 type macrophage polarization during the development of proliferative vitreoretinopathy. Cell Immunol. 2015;298(1–2):77–82.
43. Ferrante CJ, Pinhal-Enfield G, Elson G, Cronstein BN, Hasko G, Outram S, et al. The adenosine-dependent angiogenic switch of macrophages to an M2-like phenotype is independent of interleukin-4 receptor alpha (IL-4Ralpha) signaling. Inflammation. 2013;36(4):921–31.
44. Ferrante CJ, Leibovich SJ. Regulation of macrophage polarization and wound healing. Adv Wound Care (New Rochelle). 2012;1(1):10–6.
45. Braga TT, Agudelo JS, Camara NO. Macrophages during the fibrotic process: M2 as friend and foe. Front Immunol. 2015;6:602.
46. Zhu Z, Ding J, Ma Z, Iwashina T, Tredget EE. The natural behavior of mononuclear phagocytes in HTS formation. Wound Repair Regen. 2016;24(1):14–25.
47. Zhu Z, Ding J, Ma Z, Iwashina T, Tredget EE. Systemic depletion of macrophages in the subacute phase of wound healing reduces hypertrophic scar formation. Wound Repair Regen. 2016;24(4):644–56.
48. Zhu Z, Ding J, Ma Z, Iwashina T, Tredget EE. Alternatively activated macrophages derived from THP-1 cells promote the fibrogenic activities of human dermal fibroblasts. Wound Repair Regen. 2017;25:377–88.
49. Kryczka J, Boncela J. Leukocytes: the double-edged sword in fibrosis. Mediators Inflamm. 2015;2015:652035.
50. Castagnoli C, Trombotto C, Ondei S, Stella M, Calcagni M, Magliacani G, et al. Characterization of T-cell subsets infiltrating post-burn hypertrophic scar tissues. Burns. 1997;23(7):565–72.
51. Bernabei P, Rigamonti L, Ariotti S, Stella M, Castagnoli C, Novelli F. Functional analysis of T lymphocytes infiltrating the dermis and epidermis of post-burn hypertrophic scar tissues. Burns. 1999;25(1):43–8.
52. Wang J, Jiao H, Stewart TL, Shankowsky HA, Scott PG, Tredget EE. Increased TGF-beta-producing CD4+ T lymphocytes in post-burn patients and their potential interaction with dermal fibroblasts in hypertrophic scarring. Wound Repair Regen. 2007;15(4):530–9.
53. Wang JF, Jiao H, Stewart TL, Shankowsky HA, Scott PG, Tredget EE. Fibrocytes from burn patients regulate the activities of fibroblasts. Wound Repair Regen. 2007;15(1):113–21.
54. Yang L, Scott PG, Giuffre J, Shankowsky HA, Ghahary A, Tredget EE. Peripheral blood fibrocytes from burn patients: identification and quantification of fibrocytes in adherent cells cultured from peripheral blood mononuclear cells. Lab Invest. 2002;82(9):1183–92.

55. Yang L, Scott PG, Dodd C, Medina A, Jiao H, Shankowsky HA, et al. Identification of fibrocytes in postburn hypertrophic scar. Wound Repair Regen. 2005;13(4):398–404.
56. Linge C, Richardson J, Vigor C, Clayton E, Hardas B, Rolfe KJ. Hypertrophic scar cells fail to undergo a form of apoptosis specific to contractile collagen—the role of tissue transglutaminase. J Invest Dermatol. 2005;125(1):72–82.
57. Lian N, Li T. Growth factor pathways in hypertrophic scars: molecular pathogenesis and therapeutic implications. Biomed Pharmacother. 2016;84:42–50.
58. Kirfel G, Rigort A, Borm B, Schulte C, Herzog V. Structural and compositional analysis of the keratinocyte migration track. Cell Motil Cytoskeleton. 2003;55(1):1–13.
59. Clark RA, Lin F, Greiling D, An J, Couchman JR. Fibroblast invasive migration into fibronectin/fibrin gels requires a previously uncharacterized dermatan sulfate-CD44 proteoglycan. J Invest Dermatol. 2004;122(2):266–77.
60. Ding J, Ma Z, Shankowsky HA, Medina A, Tredget EE. Deep dermal fibroblast profibrotic characteristics are enhanced by bone marrow-derived mesenchymal stem cells. Wound Repair Regen. 2013;21(3):448–55.
61. Ding J, Tredget EE. The role of chemokines in fibrotic wound healing. Adv Wound Care (New Rochelle). 2015;4(11):673–86.
62. Geissmann F, Jung S, Littman DR. Blood monocytes consist of two principal subsets with distinct migratory properties. Immunity. 2003;19(1):71–82.
63. Willenborg S, Lucas T, van Loo G, Knipper JA, Krieg T, Haase I, et al. CCR2 recruits an inflammatory macrophage subpopulation critical for angiogenesis in tissue repair. Blood. 2012;120(3):613–25.
64. Low QEH, Drugea IA, Duffner LA, Quinn DG, Cook DN, Rollins BJ, et al. Wound Healing in MIP-1α−/− and MCP-1−/− Mice. Am J Pathol. 2001;159(2):457–63.
65. Ferreira AM, Takagawa S, Fresco R, Zhu X, Varga J, DiPietro LA. Diminished induction of skin fibrosis in mice with MCP-1 deficiency. Journal of Investigative Dermatology. 2006;126(8):1900–8.
66. Ekert JE, Murray LA, Das AM, Sheng H, Giles-Komar J, Rycyzyn MA. Chemokine (C-C motif) ligand 2 mediates direct and indirect fibrotic responses in human and murine cultured fibrocytes. Fibrogenesis Tissue Repair. 2011;4(1):23. -1536-4-23.
67. Liao WT, Yu HS, Arbiser JL, Hong CH, Govindarajan B, Chai CY, et al. Enhanced MCP-1 release by keloid CD14+ cells augments fibroblast proliferation: role of MCP-1 and Akt pathway in keloids. Exp Dermatol. 2010;19(8):e142–50.
68. Bodnar RJ, Yates CC, Wells A. IP-10 blocks vascular endothelial growth factor-induced endothelial cell motility and tube formation via inhibition of calpain. Circ Res. 2006;98(5):617–25.
69. Yates CC, Krishna P, Whaley D, Bodnar R, Turner T, Wells A. Lack of CXC chemokine receptor 3 signaling leads to hypertrophic and hypercellular scarring. Am J Pathol. 2010;176(4):1743–55.
70. Satish L, Blair HC, Glading A, Wells A. Interferon-inducible protein 9 (CXCL11)-induced cell motility in keratinocytes requires calcium flux-dependent activation of mu-calpain. Mol Cell Biol. 2005;25(5):1922–41.
71. Yates CC, Whaley D, Kulasekeran P, Hancock WW, Lu B, Bodnar R, et al. Delayed and deficient dermal maturation in mice lacking the CXCR3 ELR-negative CXC chemokine receptor. Am J Pathol. 2007;171(2):484–95.
72. Ishida Y, Gao JL, Murphy PM. Chemokine receptor CX3CR1 mediates skin wound healing by promoting macrophage and fibroblast accumulation and function. J Immunol. 2008;180(1):569–79.
73. Clover AJ, Kumar AH, Caplice NM. Deficiency of CX3CR1 delays burn wound healing and is associated with reduced myeloid cell recruitment and decreased sub-dermal angiogenesis. Burns. 2011;37(8):1386–93.
74. Robertson FM, Pellegrini AE, Ross MS, Oberyszyn AS, Boros LG, Bijur GN, et al. Interleukin-1alpha gene expression during wound healing. Wound Repair Regen. 1995;3(4):473–84.
75. Shephard P, Martin G, Smola-Hess S, Brunner G, Krieg T, Smola H. Myofibroblast differentiation is induced in keratinocyte-fibroblast co-cultures and is antagonistically regulated by endogenous transforming growth factor-β and interleukin-1. Am J Pathol. 2004;164(6):2055–66.
76. Lu T, Tian L, Han Y, Vogelbaum M, Stark GR. Dose-dependent cross-talk between the transforming growth factor-beta and interleukin-1 signaling pathways. Proc Natl Acad Sci U S A. 2007;104(11):4365–70.
77. Salgado RM, Alcantara L, Mendoza-Rodriguez CA, Cerbon M, Hidalgo-Gonzalez C, Mercadillo P, et al. Post-burn hypertrophic scars are characterized by high levels of IL-1beta mRNA and protein and TNF-alpha type I receptors. Burns. 2012;38(5):668–76.
78. Niessen FB, Andriessen MP, Schalkwijk J, Visser L, Timens W. Keratinocyte-derived growth factors play a role in the formation of hypertrophic scars. J Pathol. 2001;194(2):207–16.
79. Barrow RE, Dasu MR. Oxidative and heat stress gene changes in hypertrophic scar fibroblasts stimulated with interleukin-1beta. J Surg Res. 2005;126(1):59–65.
80. Chaudhuri V, Zhou L, Karasek M. Inflammatory cytokines induce the transformation of human dermal microvascular endothelial cells into myofibroblasts: a potential role in skin fibrogenesis. J Cutan Pathol. 2007;34(2):146–53.
81. Mia MM, Boersema M, Bank RA. Interleukin-1beta attenuates myofibroblast formation and extracellular matrix production in dermal and lung fibroblasts exposed to transforming growth factor-beta1. PLoS One. 2014;9(3):e91559.
82. Bhogal RK, Bona CA. Regulatory effect of extracellular signal-regulated kinases (ERK) on type I collagen synthesis in human dermal fibroblasts stimulated by IL-4 and IL-13. Int Rev Immunol. 2008;27(6):472–96.
83. Kilani RT, Delehanty M, Shankowsky HA, Ghahary A, Scott P, Tredget EE. Fluorescent-activated cell-sorting analysis of intracellular interferon-gamma and interleukin-4 in fresh and frozen human peripheral blood T-helper cells. Wound Repair Regen. 2005;13(4):441–9.
84. Tredget EE, Yang L, Delehanty M, Shankowsky H, Scott PG. Polarized Th2 cytokine production in patients with hypertrophic scar following thermal injury. J Interferon Cytokine Res. 2006;26(3):179–89.
85. Ray S, Ju X, Sun H, Finnerty CC, Herndon DN, Brasier AR. The IL-6 trans-signaling-STAT3 pathway mediates ECM and cellular proliferation in fibroblasts from hypertrophic scar. J Invest Dermatol. 2013;133(5):1212–20.
86. Peranteau WH, Zhang L, Muvarak N, Badillo AT, Radu A, Zoltick PW, et al. IL-10 overexpression decreases inflammatory mediators and promotes regenerative healing in an adult model of scar formation. J Invest Dermatol. 2008;128(7):1852–60.
87. Shi J, Li J, Guan H, Cai W, Bai X, Fang X, et al. Anti-fibrotic actions of interleukin-10 against hypertrophic scarring by activation of PI3K/AKT and STAT3 signaling pathways in scar-forming fibroblasts. PLoS One. 2014;9(5):e98228.
88. Elliott CG, Forbes TL, Leask A, Hamilton DW. Inflammatory microenvironment and tumor necrosis factor alpha as modulators of periostin and CCN2 expression in human non-healing skin wounds and dermal fibroblasts. Matrix Biol. 2015;43:71–84.
89. Goldberg MT, Han YP, Yan C, Shaw MC, Garner WL. TNF-alpha suppresses alpha-smooth muscle actin expression in human dermal fibroblasts: an implication for abnormal wound healing. J Invest Dermatol. 2007;127(11):2645–55.
90. Harrop AR, Ghahary A, Scott PG, Forsyth N, Uji-Friedland RTA, Tredget EE. Regulation of collagen synthesis and mRNA

expression in normal and hypertrophic scar fibroblasts in vitro by interferon-γ. J Surg Res. 1995;58(5):471–7.

91. Tredget EE, Shen YJ, Liu G, Forsyth N, Smith C, Robertson Harrop A, et al. Regulation of collagen synthesis and messenger RNA levels in normal and hypertrophic scar fibroblasts in vitro by interferon alfa-2b. Wound Repair Regen. 1993;1(3):156–65.
92. Ghahary A, Shen YJ, Nedelec B, Scott PG, Tredget EE. Interferons gamma and alpha-2b differentially regulate the expression of collagenase and tissue inhibitor of metalloproteinase-1 messenger RNA in human hypertrophic and normal dermal fibroblasts. Wound Repair Regen. 1995;3(2):176–84.
93. Wang J, Jiao H, Stewart TL, Shankowsky HA, Scott PG, Tredget EE. Improvement in postburn hypertrophic scar after treatment with IFN-alpha2b is associated with decreased fibrocytes. J Interferon Cytokine Res. 2007;27(11):921–30.
94. Wang J, Chen H, Shankowsky HA, Scott PG, Tredget EE. Improved scar in postburn patients following interferon-alpha2b treatment is associated with decreased angiogenesis mediated by vascular endothelial cell growth factor. J Interferon Cytokine Res. 2008;28(7):423–34.
95. Nedelec B, Shankowsky H, Scott PG, Ghahary A, Tredget EE. Myofibroblasts and apoptosis in human hypertrophic scars: the effect of interferon-α2b. Surgery. 2001;130(5):798–808.
96. Bi S, Chai L, Yuan X, Cao C, Li S. MicroRNA-98 inhibits the cell proliferation of human hypertrophic scar fibroblasts via targeting Col1A1. Biol Res. 2017;50(1):22-017-0127-6.
97. Gras C, Ratuszny D, Hadamitzky C, Zhang H, Blasczyk R, Figueiredo C. miR-145 Contributes to Hypertrophic Scarring of the Skin by Inducing Myofibroblast Activity. Mol Med. 2015;21:296–304.
98. Xiao K, Luo X, Wang X, Gao Z. MicroRNA185 regulates transforming growth factorbeta1 and collagen1 in hypertrophic scar fibroblasts. Mol Med Rep. 2017;15(4):1489–96.
99. Guo J, Lin Q, Shao Y, Rong L, Zhang D. miR-29b promotes skin wound healing and reduces excessive scar formation by inhibition of the TGF-beta1/Smad/CTGF signaling pathway. Can J Physiol Pharmacol. 2017;95(4):437–42.
100. Kwan P, Ding J, Tredget EE. MicroRNA 181b regulates decorin production by dermal fibroblasts and may be a potential therapy for hypertrophic scar. PLoS One. 2015;10(4):e0123054.
101. Rang Z, Wang ZY, Pang QY, Wang YW, Yang G, Cui F. MiR-181a Targets PHLPP2 to Augment AKT Signaling and Regulate Proliferation and Apoptosis in Human Keloid Fibroblasts. Cell Physiol Biochem. 2016;40(3–4):796–806.
102. Guo L, Xu K, Yan H, Feng H, Wang T, Chai L, et al. MicroRNA expression signature and the therapeutic effect of the microRNA21 antagomir in hypertrophic scarring. Mol Med Rep. 2017;15(3):1211–21.
103. Zhu HY, Li C, Bai WD, Su LL, Liu JQ, Li Y, et al. MicroRNA-21 regulates hTERT via PTEN in hypertrophic scar fibroblasts. PLoS One. 2014;9(5):e97114.
104. Zhou R, Zhang Q, Zhang Y, Fu S, Wang C. Aberrant miR-21 and miR-200b expression and its pro-fibrotic potential in hypertrophic scars. Exp Cell Res. 2015;339(2):360–6.
105. Liu Y, Li Y, Li N, Teng W, Wang M, Zhang Y, et al. TGF-beta1 promotes scar fibroblasts proliferation and transdifferentiation via up-regulating MicroRNA-21. Sci Rep. 2016;6:32,231.
106. Li G, Zhou R, Zhang Q, Jiang B, Wu Q, Wang C. Fibroproliferative effect of microRNA-21 in hypertrophic scar derived fibroblasts. Exp Cell Res. 2016;345(1):93–9.
107. Li P, He QY, Luo CQ. Overexpression of miR-200b inhibits the cell proliferation and promotes apoptosis of human hypertrophic scar fibroblasts in vitro. J Dermatol. 2014;41(10):903–11.
108. Cheng J, Wang Y, Wang D, Wu Y. Identification of collagen 1 as a post-transcriptional target of miR-29b in skin fibroblasts: therapeutic implication for scar reduction. Am J Med Sci. 2013;346(2):98–103.
109. Zhu Y, Li Z, Wang Y, Li L, Wang D, Zhang W, et al. Overexpression of miR-29b reduces collagen biosynthesis by inhibiting heat shock protein 47 during skin wound healing. Transl Res. 2016;178: 38–53.e6.
110. Nagata K. Expression and function of heat shock protein 47: a collagen-specific molecular chaperone in the endoplasmic reticulum. Matrix Biol. 1998;16(7):379–86.
111. Penn JW, Grobbelaar AO, Rolfe KJ. The role of the TGF-beta family in wound healing, burns and scarring: a review. Int J Burns Trauma. 2012;2(1):18–28.
112. Yu Q, Stamenkovic I. Cell surface-localized matrix metalloproteinase-9 proteolytically activates TGF-beta and promotes tumor invasion and angiogenesis. Genes Dev. 2000;14(2):163–76.
113. Wang R, Ghahary A, Shen Q, Scott PG, Roy K, Tredget EE. Hypertrophic scar tissues and fibroblasts produce more transforming growth factor-beta1 mRNA and protein than normal skin and cells. Wound Repair Regen. 2000;8(2):128–37.
114. Schmid P, Itin P, Cherry G, Bi C, Cox DA. Enhanced expression of transforming growth factor-beta type I and type II receptors in wound granulation tissue and hypertrophic scar. Am J Pathol. 1998;152(2):485–93.
115. Liu Y, Liu H, Meyer C, Li J, Nadalin S, Konigsrainer A, et al. Transforming growth factor-beta (TGF-beta)-mediated connective tissue growth factor (CTGF) expression in hepatic stellate cells requires Stat3 signaling activation. J Biol Chem. 2013;288(42):30,708–19.
116. Tang LY, Heller M, Meng Z, Yu LR, Tang Y, Zhou M, et al. Transforming growth factor-beta (TGF-beta) directly activates the JAK1-STAT3 axis to induce hepatic fibrosis in coordination with the SMAD pathway. J Biol Chem. 2017;292(10):4302–12.
117. Tao L, Liu J, Li Z, Dai X, Li S. Role of the JAK-STAT pathway in proliferation and differentiation of human hypertrophic scar fibroblasts induced by connective tissue growth factor. Mol Med Rep. 2010;3(6):941–5.
118. Kim JS, Choi IG, Lee BC, Park JB, Kim JH, Jeong JH, et al. Neuregulin induces CTGF expression in hypertrophic scarring fibroblasts. Mol Cell Biochem. 2012;365(1-2):181–9.
119. Colwell AS, Phan TT, Kong W, Longaker MT, Lorenz PH. Hypertrophic scar fibroblasts have increased connective tissue growth factor expression after transforming growth factor-beta stimulation. Plast Reconstr Surg. 2005;116(5):1387–90. discussion 1391-2.
120. Hu X, Li N, Tao K, Fang X, Liu J, Wang Y, et al. Effects of integrin alphanubeta3 on differentiation and collagen synthesis induced by connective tissue growth factor in human hypertrophic scar fibroblasts. Int J Mol Med. 2014;34(5):1323–34.
121. Bai X, He T, Liu J, Wang Y, Fan L, Tao K, et al. Loureirin B inhibits fibroblast proliferation and extracellular matrix deposition in hypertrophic scar via TGF-beta/Smad pathway. Exp Dermatol. 2015;24(5):355–60.
122. Wang Y, Liou N, Cherng J, Chang S, Ma K, Fu E, et al. siRNA-targeting transforming growth factor-β type I receptor reduces wound scarring and extracellular matrix deposition of scar tissue. Journal of Investigative Dermatology. 2014;134(7):2016–25.
123. Sisco M, Kryger ZB, O'Shaughnessy KD, Kim PS, Schultz GS, Ding XZ, et al. Antisense inhibition of connective tissue growth factor (CTGF/CCN2) mRNA limits hypertrophic scarring without affecting wound healing in vivo. Wound Repair Regen. 2008;16(5):661–73.
124. Bates DO. Vascular endothelial growth factors and vascular permeability. Cardiovasc Res. 2010;87(2):262–71.
125. Detmar M, Brown LF, Schon MP, Elicker BM, Velasco P, Richard L, et al. Increased microvascular density and enhanced leukocyte

rolling and adhesion in the skin of VEGF transgenic mice. J Invest Dermatol. 1998;111(1):1–6.
126. Kwak DH, Bae TH, Kim WS, Kim HK. Anti-vascular endothelial growth factor (bevacizumab) therapy reduces hypertrophic scar formation in a rabbit ear wounding model. Arch Plast Surg. 2016;43(6):491–7.
127. Wilgus TA, Ferreira AM, Oberyszyn TM, Bergdall VK, Dipietro LA. Regulation of scar formation by vascular endothelial growth factor. Lab Invest. 2008;88(6):579–90.
128. Lund SA, Giachelli CM, Scatena M. The role of osteopontin in inflammatory processes. J Cell Commun Signal. 2009;3(3-4):311–22.
129. Park CH, Chung JH. Epidermal growth factor-induced matrix metalloproteinase-1 expression is negatively regulated by p38 MAPK in human skin fibroblasts. J Dermatol Sci. 2011;64(2):134–41.
130. Song R, Bian HN, Lai W, Chen HD, Zhao KS. Normal skin and hypertrophic scar fibroblasts differentially regulate collagen and fibronectin expression as well as mitochondrial membrane potential in response to basic fibroblast growth factor. Braz J Med Biol Res. 2011;44(5):402–10.
131. Shi HX, Lin C, Lin BB, Wang ZG, Zhang HY, Wu FZ, et al. The anti-scar effects of basic fibroblast growth factor on the wound repair in vitro and in vivo. PLoS One. 2013;8(4):e59966.
132. Eto H, Suga H, Aoi N, Kato H, Doi K, Kuno S, et al. Therapeutic potential of fibroblast growth factor-2 for hypertrophic scars: upregulation of MMP-1 and HGF expression. Lab Invest. 2012;92(2):214–23.
133. Wang J, Ding J, Jiao H, Honardoust D, Momtazi M, Shankowsky HA, et al. Human hypertrophic scar-like nude mouse model: characterization of the molecular and cellular biology of the scar process. Wound Repair Regen. 2011;19(2):274–85.
134. Yang DY, Li SR, Wu JL, Chen YQ, Li G, Bi S, et al. Establishment of a hypertrophic scar model by transplanting full-thickness human skin grafts onto the backs of nude mice. Plast Reconstr Surg. 2007;119(1):104–9. discussion 110-1.
135. Ding J, Tredget EE. Transplanting Human skin grafts onto nude mice to model skin scars. Methods Mol Biol. 2017;1627:65–80.
136. Momtazi M, Kwan P, Ding J, Anderson CC, Honardoust D, Goekjian S, et al. A nude mouse model of hypertrophic scar shows morphologic and histologic characteristics of human hypertrophic scar. Wound Repair Regen. 2013;21(1):77–87.
137. Alrobaiea SM, Ding J, Ma Z, Tredget EE. A novel nude mouse model of hypertrophic scarring using scratched full thickness human skin grafts. Adv Wound Care (New Rochelle). 2016;5(7):299–313.
138. Momtazi M, Ding J, Kwan P, Anderson CC, Honardoust D, Goekjian S, et al. Morphologic and histologic comparison of hypertrophic scar in nude mice, T-cell receptor, and recombination activating gene knockout mice. Plast Reconstr Surg. 2015;136(6):1192–204.

Genetics of Scars and Keloids

4

Chao-Kai Hsu, Hsing-San Yang, and John A. McGrath

A keloid is an aggressively raised dermal lesion resulting from an abnormal wound healing process. Unlike hypertrophic scars, in which the raised dermal lesion stays within the confines of the initial wound, keloid scars grow beyond the original wound margins [1]. Histopathologically, keloids are characterized by keloidal collagen (thick hyalinized eosinophilic collagen fibers) with a horizontal, tongue-like advancing edge in the dermis [2]. Keloids often begin months, perhaps up to 1 year, after a skin injury or inflammatory process, such as acne vulgaris, folliculitis, chickenpox, or vaccinations [3, 4]. Normal wound healing processes involve expression of numerous genes and complex signaling pathways, where the interplay of these genes, molecules, and pathways means that any change in the gene expression can result in an abnormal wound healing response, including the formation of keloids [5].

The pathogenesis of keloids is very complex. Accumulating data implicates both local factors in the skin (tissue tension, cytokine and growth factors/receptors and their signaling pathways) and a genetic predisposition/contribution, including epigenetic influences [6–14]. In sum, the proposed mechanisms of keloid formation include: (1) mechanical force, (2) genetic susceptibility, (3) dysregulation of various cytokines/growth factors, and (4) aberrant collagen turnover. However, there is no single unifying hypothesis that can adequately explain the formation of keloids. In this chapter, we will focus on the genetic contributions to keloid pathogenesis.

4.1 Evidence/Phenomena for the Genetic Basis of Keloid Scarring

There is a strong body of evidence or phenomena that suggests a genetic element to keloid. Fundamentally, differences in the prevalence of keloids between populations of differing ancestries provide the first clue that keloid susceptibility may be heritable. Though keloids can occur in all populations, it is well known that dark-pigmented ethnicities, such as Asians and African people, are more susceptible (up to 15 times) to keloid formation [7, 15–17]. This is also reflected in the incidence of keloids as being the fifth most common skin disease in adult black patients in the UK [18].

Secondly, there have been numerous studies conducted on so-called "keloid pedigrees," in which susceptibility to keloids is shown to run among family lineages [19]. Omodare et al. first reported keloids with an autosomal recessive pattern of inheritance among 34 families from a Nigerian population [20]. Marneros et al. observed autosomal dominant inheritance with incomplete clinical penetrance and variable expression among 14 keloid families, mostly African-American ($n = 10$), but also including white ($n = 1$), Japanese ($n = 2$), and African-Caribbean ($n = 1$). The autosomal dominant pattern of inheritance is further supported by several studies of Han Chinese [21], Afro-Caribbean, African-American, and Asian-American origin [22]. In a cohort of 750 Taiwanese keloid patients, more than half reported a positive family history, with most having autosomal dominant inheritance with incomplete penetrance (unpublished data, Hsu CK) (Fig. 4.1). Overall, a single mode of inheritance for the keloid phenotype appears unlikely, but autosomal dominant inheritance with incomplete penetrance and variable expressivity seems most prob-

C.-K. Hsu
Department of Dermatology, National Cheng Kung University Hospital, College of Medicine, National Cheng Kung University, Tainan, Taiwan

International Center for Wound Repair and Regeneration (iWRR), National Cheng Kung University, Tainan, Taiwan

H.-S. Yang
Department of Dermatology, National Cheng Kung University Hospital, College of Medicine, National Cheng Kung University, Tainan, Taiwan

J. A. McGrath (✉)
St John's Institute of Dermatology, School of Basic and Medical Biosciences, King's College London, Guy's Hospital, London, UK
e-mail: john.mcgrath@kcl.ac.uk

© Springer Nature Singapore Pte Ltd. 2020
R. Ogawa (ed.), *Total Scar Management*, https://doi.org/10.1007/978-981-32-9791-3_4

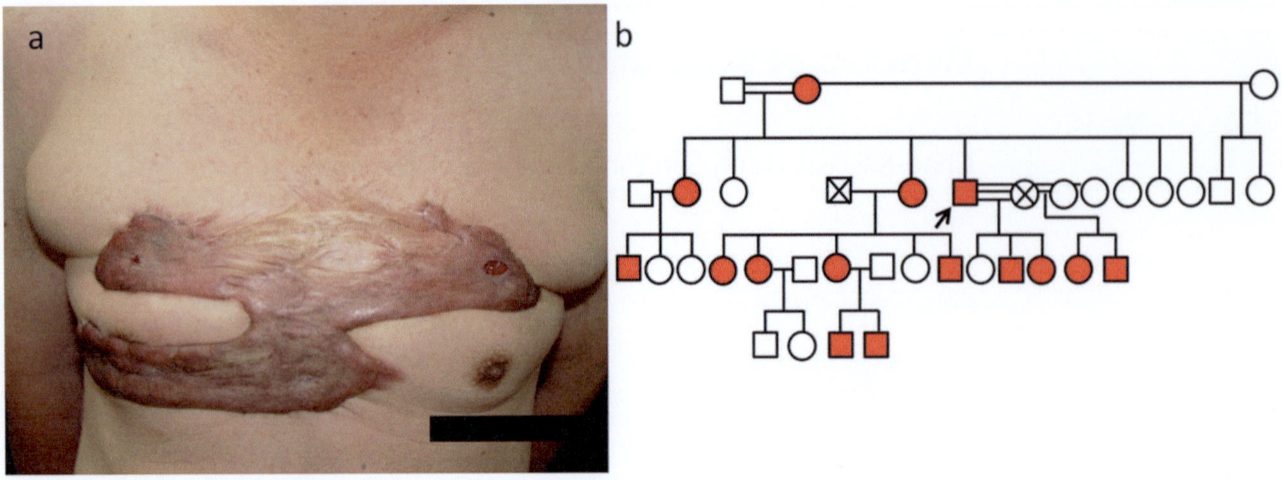

Fig. 4.1 An example of familial keloid. (**a**) A 58-year-old male manifests a large indurated plaque on the anterior chest. Some fistulas are noted within the keloid scar. (**b**) The pedigree indicates autosomal dominant inheritance with incomplete clinical penetrance

able based on reports from a number of independent groups in different ethnic populations.

Twin studies are also powerful tools to investigate the extent to which shared genetics contribute to a complex disease [23]. While monozygotic twins share 100% of their segregating genes, dizygotic twins share 50% on average. It is not difficult to understand the significance of the genetic factor in keloid pathogenesis while diseases with high concordance rates between monozygotic twins [19, 24].

4.2 Keloid-Associated Syndromes

A number of rare congenital syndromes are reported to be associated with familial keloids. These syndromes are mostly Mendelian disorders with a known molecular basis, and provide great opportunities to study the pathogenesis of keloids and to search for etiological clues, possible treatments, or preventive measures.

Rubinstein–Taybi syndrome (RSTS1; OMIM 180849, RSTS2; 613684) is the most common keloid-associated syndrome. This disorder is characterized by mental retardation, growth deficiency, microcephaly, broad thumbs and halluces, and dysmorphic facial features. There are several distinct facial features, such as highly arched eyebrows, broad nasal bridge, beaked nose, grimacing smile, and an increased prevalence of keloids (Fig. 4.2) [25]. A retrospective study revealed that 15 of 62 Dutch individuals with RTS had keloids, either spontaneously or after minor trauma, usually starting during early puberty [26]. RTS is caused by *CREBBP* or *EP300* gene mutation with autosomal dominant inheritance [26]. *CREBBP* gene codes for CREB-binding protein, while *EP300* codes for histone acetyltransferase p300 protein. Both are co-activators in the SMAD-related proteins/transforming growth factor (TGF)-β signaling pathways [27]. Furthermore, the involvement of histone acetyltransferase indicates that epigenetic modification may play a role in the pathogenesis of keloids [28], which has been supported by several studies [9, 29–31].

Atwal et al. recently reported a novel X-linked syndrome of cardiac valvulopathy, reduced joint mobility, and keloid scarring due to a missense mutation in *FLNA* (c.4726G>A; p.G1576R) [32]. The encoded protein, filamin A, is a SMAD-associated protein that provides a scaffold for cross talk between TGF-β superfamily and other signal transduction pathways [33].

Ehlers–Danlos syndrome (EDS) is a clinically and genetically heterogeneous group of heritable connective tissue disorders characterized by joint hypermobility, skin hyperextensibility, and tissue fragility. The 2017 classification describes 13 types of EDS [34]. Among these, keloidal plaques of the lower extremities have been reported in EDS type IV, which is caused by a heterozygous mutation in the gene for type III collagen (*COL3A1*) [35].

Collectively, these three different Mendelian syndromic disorders provide evidence for single gene contributions to keloid biogenesis, notwithstanding the protean nature of the primary disease pathologies in these diverse conditions.

4.3 Linkage Analysis Identified Several Loci and Candidate Genes

For patients with non-syndromic keloids, although familial inheritance plays prominently into our understanding of genetic influence, the identification of predisposing genes has been difficult to ascertain. Genetic linkage analysis is a powerful tool to detect the chromosomal location of potentially pathogenic genes [36]: it is based on the observation that the genes that reside physically close on a chromosome remain linked during meiosis and thus is a suitable technique to study keloid-prone individuals.

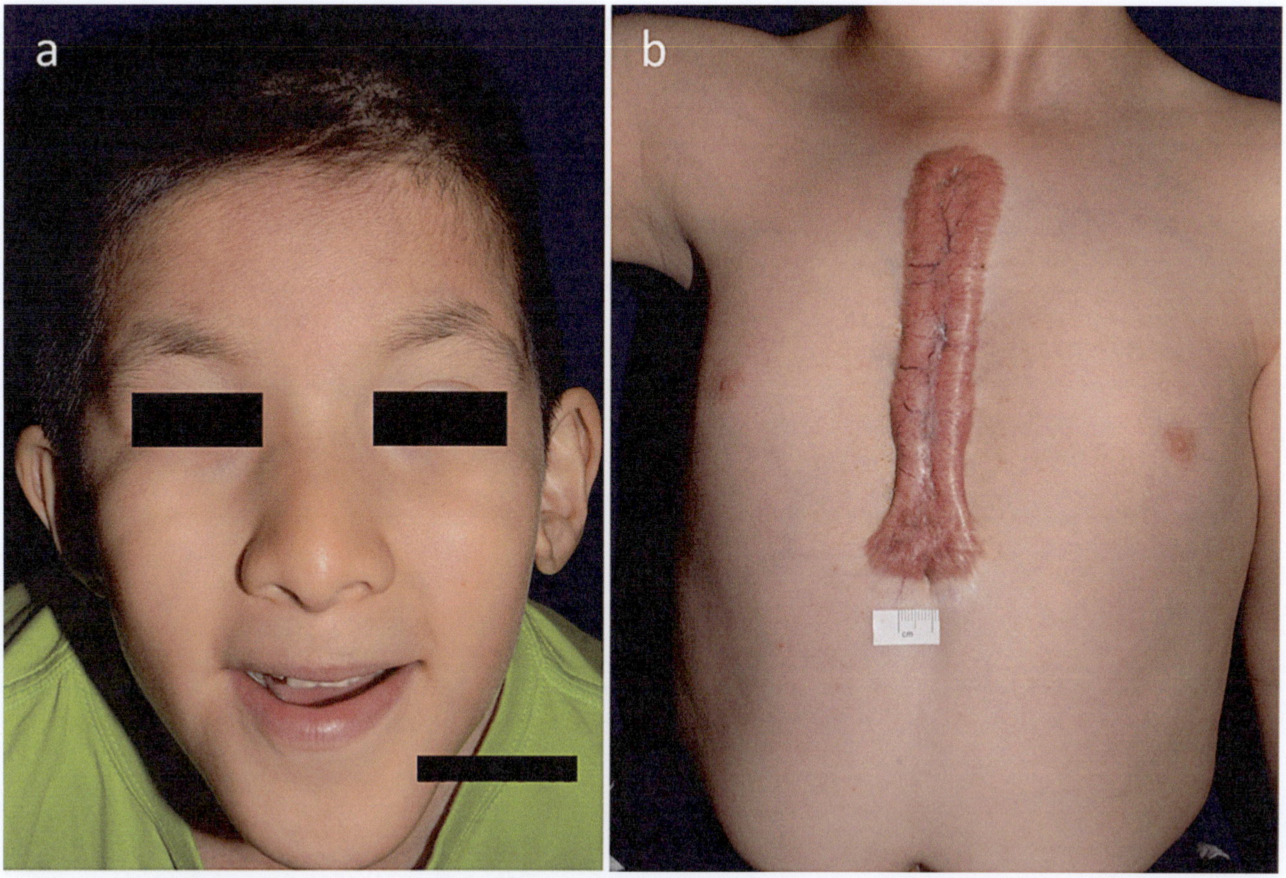

Fig. 4.2 (**a**) A 5-year-old boy with Rubinstein–Taybi syndrome. He presents with several features including distinct facies with highly arched eyebrows, broad nasal bridge, beaked nose, and grimacing smile. (**b**) A large keloid is noted on his anterior chest following cardiac surgery

Table 4.1 Summary of population studies on gene polymorphisms or mutations in selected genes

Gene name	Loci	Function	Ethnic	Methods	Reference
EGFR[a]	7p1w1	Cell migration Cell proliferation	African-American	Linkage analysis; Genome-wide association study	Marneros et al. (2004) [37]
TNFAIP6[a]	2q23	ECM synthesis	Japanese		
SMAD2 *SMAD4* *SMAD7*	18q21.1	ECM synthesis	Chinese	Linkage analysis	Yan et al. (2007) [38]
FOXL2[a]	1q41 3q22.3-23	GnRH/steroid hormones Signaling pathway	Japanese	Genome-wide association study	Nakashima et al. (2010) [40]
NEDD4	15q21.3	ECM synthesis			
HLA-DRB1[a]15	6p21.32	Immune responses	Caucasians of Northern European origin	Polymerase chain reaction sequence specific oligonucleotide probes (PCR-SSOP) typing system	Brown et al. (2008) [56]
CDC2L1	1p36	Cell-cycle control	Chinese	SNP sequencing	Zhang et al. (2012) [73]
TGF-β1	19q13.1	ECM synthesis	Malays	SNP genotyping	Emami et al. (2012) [59]
SMAD4	18q21.1	ECM synthesis	Malays		

[a]Close to the gene

Using linkage analysis on keloidal families with an autosomal dominant pattern of inheritance, susceptibility loci have been identified in a Japanese family to chromosome band 2q23 and in an African-American family to chromosome band 7p11, both with the logarithm of the odds (LOD) scores greater than 3 [37] (Table 4.1). The *TNFAIP6* gene at chromosome band 2q23 and the *EGFR* gene at chromosome band 7p11 were proposed as candidate genes within these respective loci. In a large Chinese family with keloids, linkage intervals were found at 15q22.31-q23, 18q21.1, and 10q23.31. The 18q21.1 region harbors the *SMAD2*, *SMAD7*, and *SMAD4* genes, which are involved in the regulation of TGF-β signaling pathways [38]. Sanger sequencing of these specific genes in the respective pedigrees, however, did not identify unique segregating variants.

4.4 Genome-Wide Association Study (GWAS)

Genome-wide association study (GWAS) is an observational study of a genome-wide set of single-nucleotide polymorphisms (SNP) in different individuals to determine if any SNP is associated with human disease [39]. Simply, the millions of genetic variants of each subject in both disease and control groups are read using SNP arrays. If the variant(s) is/are more frequent in the disease group, the variant(s) is/are said to be associated with the disease. The region marked by the identified SNPs is then considered as the "hot spot" of the human genome for the disease. As such, GWAS is a potentially useful investigative technique for ascertaining genomic susceptibility to keloids in a large number of affected and control individuals.

By performing a GWAS study in 824 individuals with keloid and 3205 unaffected controls in a Japanese population, Nakashima et al. identified four SNPs in three chromosomal regions: rs873549 at 1q41, rs940187 and rs1511412 at 3q22.3, and rs8032158 at 15p21.3 [40]. Among these, rs8032158 is found within the intron of the *NEDD4* gene. NEDD4 is known to upregulate expression of fibronectin and type 1 collagen that play a role in the accumulation of extracellular matrix [41]. In addition, NEDD4 participates in the ubiquitination and stability of the insulin-like growth factor (IGF)-1 receptor [42], and overexpression of IGF-1 receptor has been observed in keloidal lesions [43–45]. These loci (1q41 and 15q21.3) were further confirmed in 714 Chinese patients with keloids [46]. Ogawa et al. further determined rs8032158 at 15p21.3 as a biomarker of keloid severity among 204 Japanese patients [47].

4.5 Other Genome-Wide Studies on Keloid

Admixture mapping is a powerful method of gene mapping for diseases or traits that show differential risk by ancestry [48] and thus is also applicable to assessing genetic contributions to keloids. Admixture mapping has been applied most often to African-Americans with trace ancestry to Europeans and West Africans [48]. Velez Edwards et al. applied admixture mapping and identified a locus at 15q21.2-22.3 associated with keloid formation among 478 African-Americans [49]. Further analysis revealed a significant association at *MYO1E* (myosin 1E), and a genome scan also identified associations at *MYO7A* (myosin 7A). These two myosin genes suggest that an altered cytoskeleton may contribute to the enhanced migratory and invasive properties of keloid fibroblasts [50–52].

Shih and Bayat performed array-based comparative genomic hybridization on keloid tissue compared to an internal and external control tissue, and identified copy number variations in 6p21.32, 11q11, 17q12, 8p23.1, 22q13.1, 19p13.1, and 2q14.3 [53]. The association of keloid formation and *HLA-DRB5*, located at the region 6p21.32, was further confirmed by a validation qPCR study. Other HLA associations have been reported, including *HLA-DRB1∗15* in Caucasians and Chinese populations, as well as *HLA-DQA∗104*, *DQB1∗0501*, and *DQB1∗0503*, collectively implicating a significant immunogenetic contribution to keloid susceptibility [54–56].

Overall, however, no unique gene, collection of genes, or associate functional pathway can be directly implicated as the leading genomic susceptibility factor(s), and further research is needed to determine whether these putative genes or SNPs indeed contribute to keloid formation.

4.6 Other Genetic Studies of Keloids

4.6.1 TGF-β and SMADs

In terms of individual gene associations, there is plenty of evidence to implicate dysregulation of TGF-β and the downstream signaling molecules SMADs in keloid formation [11]. Therefore, several studies have focused on polymorphisms within these genes, including *TGF-β1*, *TGF-β2*, *TGF-β3*, *TGF-β receptor (TGF-βR)I*, *TGF-βRII*, *TGF-βRIII*, *SMAD3*, *SMAD6*, and *SMAD7*, and how these may contribute to the formation of keloids [57–63].

Nevertheless, several limitations may be present in these genetic studies. First, small population sizes and the lack of healthy control groups were included in these studies. Secondly, those genes selected for mutation or polymorphism studies were not chosen systemically and thus it may be difficult to draw conclusions about the genetic basis of keloid formation. Tu et al. conducted a meta-analysis of five case–control studies encompassing a total of 564 keloid cases and 620 healthy controls [64]. The results suggested that the TGF-β1 polymorphism (c.509C/T) is not associated with keloid susceptibility. The negative results of this analysis suggest that there is either an upstream gene or other genes that contribute to the expression of the TGFB genes in keloids. High-quality and large-scale studies are warranted to further validate these results.

4.6.2 TP53

The tumor suppressor p53 has been shown to play an important role in controlling cell proliferation and apoptosis, and so its potential dysregulation in keloid pathogenesis has been studied. Saed et al. reported *TP53* gene mutations in seven keloid tissue samples but none in healthy skin tissue or buccal swabs obtained from the same patients [65]. Their results were not confirmed, however, by another group [66].

4.6.3 ASAH1

Santos-Cortez et al. recently identified *ASAH1* as a susceptibility gene for familial keloids [67]. Through an analysis of whole-genome data, a locus on 8p23.3-p21.3 was mapped with an LOD score of 4.48. Whole-exome sequencing focusing on this locus then identified a missense mutation c.1202T>C (p.Leu401Pro) in the N-acylsphingosine amidohydrolase (ASAH1) gene in a large Yoruba family. The *ASAH1* gene encodes for the enzyme "acid ceramidase," which is responsible for the degradation of ceramide. Ceramide is related to tumorigenesis, and an increase in the intracellular ceramide may induce apoptotic signaling [68]. The ASAH1 protein is highly expressed in cancer cell lines and human alveolar macrophages, suggesting a role in proliferative lesions and inflammation [69]. Though the genotype of *ASAH1* co-segregates with the keloid phenotype in the large family, unfortunately, keloid tissue were not obtained from the carriers of the *ASAH1* variant. Therefore, the pathologic profile and the ceramide and ceramidase levels in keloids expressing the variant could be verified. Further functional studies are necessary to clarify the role of the *ASAH1* variant in keloid pathogenesis.

4.7 Future Perspectives

RNA-seq (RNA sequencing), also called whole transcriptome shotgun sequencing (WTSS), is a technology that also uses the capabilities of next-generation sequencing to reveal a snapshot of RNA presence and quantity from a genome at a given moment in time [70, 71]. RNA-seq data is therefore helpful in interpreting the "personalized transcriptome" and can be applied to improve understanding of the changes in transcriptomic profiles in keloid biogenesis. Onoufriadis et al. applied RNA-seq to explore transcriptomic alterations at an earlier time-point—during keloid formation [72]. A biopsy-rebiopsy procedure was performed on the buttock of eight keloid-prone subjects and six healthy controls after a 6-week interval. Comparing healthy controls before and after wounding identified 2215 differentially expressed genes, whereas the same analysis in the keloid-prone individuals identified 3161 differentially expressed genes. Of those genes, there were 513 genes specific to the healthy individuals and 1449 genes specific to the keloid phenotype. There were 22 pathways that were associated directly to the keloid-prone individuals. Of note, NOTCH signaling, MAPK signaling, and Toll-like receptor pathways were found to be altered in keloid-prone individuals after wounding. Gene association network analysis demonstrated a divergent average expression profile of cytokine signaling genes between keloid-prone and healthy individuals during wound healing. The study provided a comprehensive and integrative analysis of the keloid transcriptome and highlights biological pathways that feature during keloid formation. More importantly, the results may help to identify gene drivers.

4.8 Conclusion

Despite a strong body of evidence or phenomena suggesting a genetic component in keloid formation, there is still a significant amount of work that needs to be done to increase our current understanding of the genetic basis of keloid formation. Previous studies have suggested the possibility of polygenic inheritance pattern in keloid. Also, multiple genetic loci or genes have been identified in keloid pathogenesis. However, most of these findings require further functional studies to clarify potential pathogenicity. It is hoped that such work will help elucidate the molecular basis of keloid formation, and provide new strategies for prevention, diagnosis, and treatment.

References

1. Tuan TL, Nichter LS. The molecular basis of keloid and hypertrophic scar formation. Mol Med Today. 1998;4(1):19–24.
2. Lee JY, Yang CC, Chao SC, Wong TW. Histopathological differential diagnosis of keloid and hypertrophic scar. Am J Dermatopathol. 2004;26(5):379–84.
3. Brissett AE, Sherris DA. Scar contractures, hypertrophic scars, and keloids. Facial Plast Surg. 2001;17(4):263–72.
4. Robles DT, Moore E, Draznin M, Berg D. Keloids: pathophysiology and management. Dermatol Online J. 2007;13(3):9.
5. Gurtner GC, Werner S, Barrandon Y, Longaker MT. Wound repair and regeneration. Nature. 2008;453(7193):314–21.
6. Gauglitz GG, Korting HC, Pavicic T, Ruzicka T, Jeschke MG. Hypertrophic scarring and keloids: pathomechanisms and current and emerging treatment strategies. Mol Med. 2011;17(1–2):113–25.
7. Al-Attar A, Mess S, Thomassen JM, Kauffman CL, Davison SP. Keloid pathogenesis and treatment. Plast Reconstr Surg. 2006;117(1):286–300.
8. Butler PD, Longaker MT, Yang GP. Current progress in keloid research and treatment. J Am Coll Surg. 2008;206(4):731–41.
9. He Y, Deng Z, Alghamdi M, Lu L, Fear MW, He L. From genetics to epigenetics: new insights into keloid scarring. Cell Prolif. 2017;50:e12326.

10. Huang C, Murphy GF, Akaishi S, Ogawa R. Keloids and hypertrophic scars: update and future directions. Plast Reconstr Surg Glob Open. 2013;1(4):e25.
11. Berman B, Maderal A, Raphael B. Keloids and hypertrophic scars: pathophysiology, classification, and treatment. Dermatol Surg. 2017;43(Suppl 1):S3–S18.
12. Hsu CK, Lin HH, Harn HI, Hughes MW, Tang MJ, Yang CC. Mechanical forces in skin disorders. J Dermatol Sci. 2018;90(3):232–40.
13. Ogawa R, Hsu CK. Mechanobiological dysregulation of the epidermis and dermis in skin disorders and in degeneration. J Cell Mol Med. 2013;17(7):817–22.
14. Glass DA 2nd. current understanding of the genetic causes of keloid formation. J Investig Dermatol Symp Proc. 2017;18(2):S50–S3.
15. Kelly AP. Keloids. Dermatol Clin. 1988;6(3):413–24.
16. LeFlore IC. Misconceptions regarding elective plastic surgery in the black patient. J Natl Med Assoc. 1980;72(10):947–8.
17. Ud-Din S, Bayat A. Strategic management of keloid disease in ethnic skin: a structured approach supported by the emerging literature. Br J Dermatol. 2013;169(Suppl 3):71–81.
18. Child FJ, Fuller LC, Higgins EM, Du Vivier AW. A study of the spectrum of skin disease occurring in a black population in south-east London. Br J Dermatol. 1999;141(3):512–7.
19. Marneros AG, Norris JE, Olsen BR, Reichenberger E. Clinical genetics of familial keloids. Arch Dermatol. 2001;137(11):1429–34.
20. Omo-Dare P. Genetic studies on keloid. J Natl Med Assoc. 1975;67(6):428–32.
21. Chen Y, Gao JH, Liu XJ, Yan X, Song M. Characteristics of occurrence for Han Chinese familial keloids. Burns. 2006;32(8):1052–9.
22. Clark JA, Turner ML, Howard L, Stanescu H, Kleta R, Kopp JB. Description of familial keloids in five pedigrees: evidence for autosomal dominant inheritance and phenotypic heterogeneity. BMC Dermatol. 2009;9:8.
23. Phillips DI. Twin studies in medical research: can they tell us whether diseases are genetically determined? Lancet. 1993;341(8851):1008–9.
24. Bloom D. Multiple keloids in twin sisters. Arch Derm Syphilol. 1947;55(3):426.
25. Siraganian PA, Rubinstein JH, Miller RW. Keloids and neoplasms in the Rubinstein-Taybi syndrome. Med Pediatr Oncol. 1989;17(6):485–91.
26. van de Kar AL, Houge G, Shaw AC, de Jong D, van Belzen MJ, Peters DJ, et al. Keloids in Rubinstein-Taybi syndrome: a clinical study. Br J Dermatol. 2014;171(3):615–21.
27. Warner DR, Bhattacherjee V, Yin X, Singh S, Mukhopadhyay P, Pisano MM, et al. Functional interaction between Smad, CREB binding protein, and p68 RNA helicase. Biochem Biophys Res Commun. 2004;324(1):70–6.
28. Korzus E. Rubinstein-Taybi syndrome and epigenetic alterations. Adv Exp Med Biol. 2017;978:39–62.
29. Diao JS, Xia WS, Yi CG, Wang YM, Li B, Xia W, et al. Trichostatin A inhibits collagen synthesis and induces apoptosis in keloid fibroblasts. Arch Dermatol Res. 2011;303(8):573–80.
30. Fitzgerald O'Connor EJ, Badshah II, Addae LY, Kundasamy P, Thanabalasingam S, Abioye D, et al. Histone deacetylase 2 is upregulated in normal and keloid scars. J Invest Dermatol. 2012;132(4):1293–6.
31. Russell SB, Russell JD, Trupin KM, Gayden AE, Opalenik SR, Nanney LB, et al. Epigenetically altered wound healing in keloid fibroblasts. J Invest Dermatol. 2010;130(10):2489–96.
32. Atwal PS, Blease S, Braxton A, Graves J, He W, Person R, et al. Novel X-linked syndrome of cardiac valvulopathy, keloid scarring, and reduced joint mobility due to filamin A substitution G1576R. Am J Med Genet A. 2016;170a(4):891–5.
33. Sasaki A, Masuda Y, Ohta Y, Ikeda K, Watanabe K. Filamin associates with Smads and regulates transforming growth factor-beta signaling. J Biol Chem. 2001;276(21):17871–7.
34. Malfait F, Francomano C, Byers P, Belmont J, Berglund B, Black J, et al. The 2017 international classification of the Ehlers-Danlos syndromes. Am J Med Genet C Semin Med Genet. 2017;175(1):8–26.
35. Burk CJ, Aber C, Connelly EA. Ehlers-Danlos syndrome type IV: keloidal plaques of the lower extremities, amniotic band limb deformity, and a new mutation. J Am Acad Dermatol. 2007;56(2 Suppl):S53–4.
36. Lander E, Kruglyak L. Genetic dissection of complex traits: guidelines for interpreting and reporting linkage results. Nat Genet. 1995;11(3):241–7.
37. Marneros AG, Norris JE, Watanabe S, Reichenberger E, Olsen BR. Genome scans provide evidence for keloid susceptibility loci on chromosomes 2q23 and 7p11. J Invest Dermatol. 2004;122(5):1126–32.
38. Yan X, Gao JH, Chen Y, Song M, Liu XJ. Preliminary linkage analysis and mapping of keloid susceptibility locus in a Chinese pedigree. Zhonghua Zheng Xing Wai Ke Za Zhi. 2007;23(1):32–5.
39. Manolio TA. Genomewide association studies and assessment of the risk of disease. N Engl J Med. 2010;363(2):166–76.
40. Nakashima M, Chung S, Takahashi A, Kamatani N, Kawaguchi T, Tsunoda T, et al. A genome-wide association study identifies four susceptibility loci for keloid in the Japanese population. Nat Genet. 2010;42(9):768–71.
41. Chung S, Nakashima M, Zembutsu H, Nakamura Y. Possible involvement of NEDD4 in keloid formation; its critical role in fibroblast proliferation and collagen production. Proc Jpn Acad Ser B Phys Biol Sci. 2011;87(8):563–73.
42. Vecchione A, Marchese A, Henry P, Rotin D, Morrione A. The Grb10/Nedd4 complex regulates ligand-induced ubiquitination and stability of the insulin-like growth factor I receptor. Mol Cell Biol. 2003;23(9):3363–72.
43. Daian T, Ohtsuru A, Rogounovitch T, Ishihara H, Hirano A, Akiyama-Uchida Y, et al. Insulin-like growth factor-I enhances transforming growth factor beta induced extracellular matrix protein production through the P38/activating transcription factor-2 signaling pathway in keloid fibroblasts. J Invest Dermatol. 2003;120(6):956–62.
44. Ishihara H, Yoshimoto H, Fujioka M, Murakami R, Hirano A, Fujii T, et al. Keloid fibroblasts resist ceramide-induced apoptosis by overexpression of insulin-like growth factor I receptor. J Invest Dermatol. 2000;115(6):1065–71.
45. Yoshimoto H, Ishihara H, Ohtsuru A, Akino K, Murakami R, Kuroda H, et al. Overexpression of insulin-like growth factor-1 (IGF-I) receptor and the invasiveness of cultured keloid fibroblasts. Am J Pathol. 1999;154(3):883–9.
46. Zhu F, Wu B, Li P, Wang J, Tang H, Liu Y, et al. Association study confirmed susceptibility loci with keloid in the Chinese Han population. PLoS One. 2013;8(5):e62377.
47. Ogawa R, Watanabe A, Than Naing B, Sasaki M, Fujita A, Akaishi S, et al. Associations between keloid severity and single-nucleotide polymorphisms: importance of rs8032158 as a biomarker of keloid severity. J Invest Dermatol. 2014;134(7):2041–3.
48. Shriner D. Overview of admixture mapping. Curr Protoc Hum Genet. 2013;Chapter 1:Unit 1.23.
49. Velez Edwards DR, Tsosie KS, Williams SM, Edwards TL, Russell SB. Admixture mapping identifies a locus at 15q21.2-22.3 associated with keloid formation in African Americans. Hum Genet. 2014;133(12):1513–23.
50. Hsu CK, Lin HH, Harn HI, Ogawa R, Wang YK, Ho YT, et al. Caveolin-1 controls hyperresponsiveness to mechanical stimuli and

fibrogenesis-associated RUNX2 activation in keloid fibroblasts. J Invest Dermatol. 2018;138(1):208–18.
51. Harn HI, Hsu CK, Wang YK, Huang YW, Chiu WT, Lin HH, et al. Spatial distribution of filament elasticity determines the migratory behaviors of a cell. Cell Adh Migr. 2016;10(4):368–77.
52. Harn HI, Wang YK, Hsu CK, Ho YT, Huang YW, Chiu WT, et al. Mechanical coupling of cytoskeletal elasticity and force generation is crucial for understanding the migrating nature of keloid fibroblasts. Exp Dermatol. 2015;24(8):579–84.
53. Shih B, Bayat A. Comparative genomic hybridisation analysis of keloid tissue in Caucasians suggests possible involvement of HLA-DRB5 in disease pathogenesis. Arch Dermatol Res. 2012;304(3):241–9.
54. Shih B, Bayat A. Genetics of keloid scarring. Arch Dermatol Res. 2010;302(5):319–39.
55. Brown JJ, Bayat A. Genetic susceptibility to raised dermal scarring. Br J Dermatol. 2009;161(1):8–18.
56. Brown JJ, Ollier WE, Thomson W, Bayat A. Positive association of HLA-DRB1*15 with keloid disease in Caucasians. Int J Immunogenet. 2008;35(4-5):303–7.
57. Brown JJ, Ollier W, Arscott G, Ke X, Lamb J, Day P, et al. Genetic susceptibility to keloid scarring: SMAD gene SNP frequencies in Afro-Caribbeans. Exp Dermatol. 2008;17(7):610–3.
58. He S, Liu X, Yang Y, Huang W, Xu S, Yang S, et al. Mechanisms of transforming growth factor beta(1)/Smad signalling mediated by mitogen-activated protein kinase pathways in keloid fibroblasts. Br J Dermatol. 2010;162(3):538–46.
59. Emami A, Halim AS, Salahshourifar I, Yussof SJ, Khoo TL, Kannan TP. Association of TGFbeta1 and SMAD4 variants in the etiology of keloid scar in the Malay population. Arch Dermatol Res. 2012;304(7):541–7.
60. Bayat A, Bock O, Mrowietz U, Ollier WE, Ferguson MW. Genetic susceptibility to keloid disease and transforming growth factor beta 2 polymorphisms. Br J Plast Surg. 2002;55(4):283–6.
61. Bayat A, Bock O, Mrowietz U, Ollier WE, Ferguson MW. Genetic susceptibility to keloid disease and hypertrophic scarring: transforming growth factor beta1 common polymorphisms and plasma levels. Plast Reconstr Surg. 2003;111(2):535–43. discussion 44-6.
62. Bayat A, Bock O, Mrowietz U, Ollier WE, Ferguson MW. Genetic susceptibility to keloid disease: transforming growth factor beta receptor gene polymorphisms are not associated with keloid disease. Exp Dermatol. 2004;13(2):120–4.
63. Bayat A, Walter JM, Bock O, Mrowietz U, Ollier WE, Ferguson MW. Genetic susceptibility to keloid disease: mutation screening of the TGFbeta3 gene. Br J Plast Surg. 2005;58(7):914–21.
64. Tu Y, Lineaweaver WC, Zhang F. TGF-beta1-509C/T polymorphism and susceptibility to keloid disease: a systematic review and meta-analysis. Scars Burn Heal. 2017;3:2059513117709943.
65. Saed GM, Ladin D, Olson J, Han X, Hou Z, Fivenson D. Analysis of p53 gene mutations in keloids using polymerase chain reaction-based single-strand conformational polymorphism and DNA sequencing. Arch Dermatol. 1998;134(8):963–7.
66. Yan L, Lu XY, Wang CM, Cao R, Yin YH, Jia CS, et al. Association between p53 gene codon 72 polymorphism and keloid in Chinese population. Zhonghua Zheng Xing Wai Ke Za Zhi. 2007;23(5):428–30.
67. Santos-Cortez RLP, Hu Y, Sun F, Benahmed-Miniuk F, Tao J, Kanaujiya JK, et al. Identification of ASAH1 as a susceptibility gene for familial keloids. Eur J Hum Genet. 2017;25(10):1155–61.
68. Huang WC, Chen CL, Lin YS, Lin CF. Apoptotic sphingolipid ceramide in cancer therapy. J Lipids. 2011;2011:565316.
69. Coant N, Sakamoto W, Mao C, Hannun YA. Ceramidases, roles in sphingolipid metabolism and in health and disease. Adv Biol Regul. 2017;63:122–31.
70. Chu Y, Corey DR. RNA sequencing: platform selection, experimental design, and data interpretation. Nucleic Acid Ther. 2012;22(4):271–4.
71. Wang Z, Gerstein M, Snyder M. RNA-Seq: a revolutionary tool for transcriptomics. Nat Rev Genet. 2009;10(1):57–63.
72. Onoufriadis A, Hsu CK, Ainali C, Ung CY, Rashidghamat E, Yang HS, et al. Time series integrative analysis of RNA sequencing and microRNA expression data reveals key biologic wound healing pathways in keloid-prone individuals. J Invest Dermatol. 2018;138:2690–3.
73. Zhang G, Jiang J, Luo S, Tang S, Liang J, Yao P. Analyses of CDC2L1 gene mutations in keloid tissue. Clin Exp Dermatol. 2012;37(3):277–83.

Local, Systemic, and Genetic Risk Factors for Keloids and Hypertrophic Scars and the Reset Concept of Pathological Scar Therapy

5

Rei Ogawa

5.1 Introduction

Keloids and hypertrophic scars are red and elevated pathological inflammatory scars that are caused by aberrant wound healing after injury and irritation to the reticular dermis. These injuries include trauma, insect bite, burn, surgery, vaccination, skin piercing, acne, folliculitis, chicken pox, and herpes zoster. The importance of the reticular dermis in this pathology is demonstrated by the fact that superficial injury that does not reach the reticular dermis never causes keloid and hypertrophic scarring. The aberrant wound healing of these pathological scars is characterized by continuous inflammation that is mainly found in the reticular dermis. Specifically, the reticular layer of these scars is populated by large numbers of inflammatory cells that emit copious inflammatory signals, collagen-producing fibroblasts, proliferating endothelial cells, newly formed blood vessels, and vast accumulations of collagen [1].

In many classical textbooks, keloids and hypertrophic scars are defined as completely different scar types. Clinicians define hypertrophic scars as pathological scars that do not grow beyond the boundaries of the original wound, whereas keloids are defined as scars that spread into the surrounding normal skin. Pathologists also make a histological distinction between keloids and hypertrophic scars: keloids bear thick eosinophilic (hyalinizing) collagen bundles called "keloidal collagen," whereas hypertrophic scars lack these bundles and instead have distinctive dermal nodules [2]. However, there are many cases of scars that bear the growth and histological features of both hypertrophic scars and keloids (Fig. 5.1). These findings suggest that hypertrophic scars and keloids are actually manifestations of the same fibroproliferative skin disorder that merely differ in the intensity and duration of inflammation [3]. These features may in turn be shaped by genetic, systemic, and local risk factors for pathological scarring [1].

In general, it only becomes obvious that a scar has become pathological about 3 months after injury: at this point, the heavy ongoing inflammation and neovascularization in the reticular dermis start to manifest clinically as erythema, pruritis, pain, and scar tissue growth. Both patients and physicians often erroneously assume that, 7–14 days after surgery, the sutured surgical wounds have healed almost completely: at that stage the epidermis has regenerated, the wound is closed and dried, and the sutures can be removed. However, at that point, the inflammatory phase of normal wound healing is actually still ongoing (in normal wound healing, this phase only ends about 3–4 weeks after surgery). If the reticular dermis is subjected continuously or repetitively to one or more external and/or internal stimuli during this inflammation phase, this phase will become prolonged and the inflammation will strengthen, eventually leading to pathological scar growth.

The external and internal stimuli that are known to influence the characteristics and quantity of keloids and hypertrophic scars include multiple local, systemic, and genetic factors [1].

5.2 Local Risk Factors that Increase Dermal Inflammation

Multiple local factors can stimulate aberrant inflammation in the reticular dermis [1]. They include repeated injury and infection, such as that caused by piercings in the earlobe: the frequent attaching and detaching of the jewelry and rubbing of the jewelry-bearing lobe on the pillow at night repeatedly injure the pierced skin, which can get infected. This significantly increases the risk of developing ball-like earlobe

There are no financial disclosures to be made.

R. Ogawa (✉)
Department of Plastic, Reconstructive and Aesthetic Surgery, Nippon Medical School, Tokyo, Japan
e-mail: r.ogawa@nms.ac.jp

© Springer Nature Singapore Pte Ltd. 2020

R. Ogawa (ed.), *Total Scar Management*, https://doi.org/10.1007/978-981-32-9791-3_5

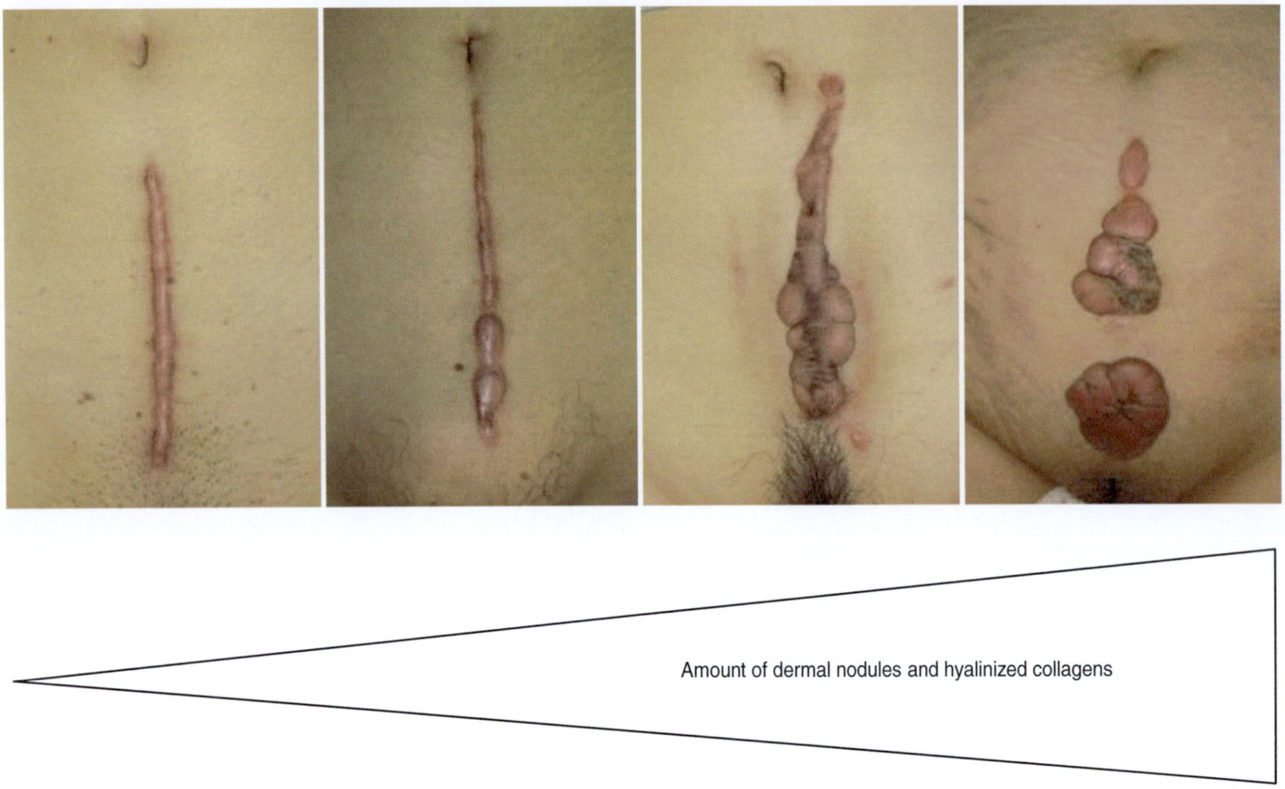

Fig. 5.1 Pathological scars on the abdomen of different patients: severity associates with the amount of characteristic histological features. Many pathological scars bear the growth and histological features of both hypertrophic scars and keloids. These four scars on the abdomen of four different patients bear both dermal nodules (originally considered to be a pathognomonic feature of hypertrophic scars) and hyalinized collagens (originally considered to be pathognomonic for keloids). Both features became more predominant as the clinical appearance of the scar became more severe. The severity of these clinical and histopathological features is likely to be determined by duration and intensity of the reticular dermal inflammation that is generated by local, systemic, and/or genetic risk factors. (This figure is part of a figure in reference [5]. It is reproduced here with the approval of the publisher)

keloids. The infectious agents that generate acne and folliculitis also associate with prolonged dermal inflammation. In addition, scratching of infected lesions, such as those generated by chickenpox, can increase the risk of pathological scarring.

Of the many local factors that contribute to pathological scar development, however, we believe that local mechanical forces play a particularly important role [4–6]. Several lines of evidence support this notion. First, keloids commonly adopt distinct site-specific shapes, namely, the typical butterfly, crab's claw, and dumbbell shapes on the shoulder, anterior chest, and upper arm, respectively (Fig. 5.2). This, together with our visual analysis using the finite element method, suggests that keloids are largely determined by the direction of the tension that is applied to the skin around the wound site (Fig. 5.3) [7]. For example, the direction of tension on the anterior chest wall is horizontal because of the contraction of the pectoralis major muscles. Consequently, keloids on the chest wall generally grow from left to right or vice versa (or both), depending on which side of the chest they are located (Fig. 5.4). In the case of keloids on the abdomen, the growth is in the cranial–caudal direction due to the contraction of the rectus abdominal muscle (Fig. 5.4). Similarly, the dumbbell-shaped keloids seen on the upper arm are often found to have started in childhood, which is when routine vaccinations occur. Their alignment along the long axis of the arm may reflect the strong growth of the arm during childhood.

Second, keloids show a marked preference for particular locations on the body: they usually occur at sites that are constantly or frequently subjected to tension (such as the anterior chest and scapular regions) but seldom in areas where stretching/contraction of the skin is rare (such as the parietal region or anterior lower leg). This is true even for patients with multiple/large keloids. Moreover, keloids on the upper eyelid are rare. This reflects the fact that eyelid skin is always relaxed regardless of whether the eyes are open or closed [8].

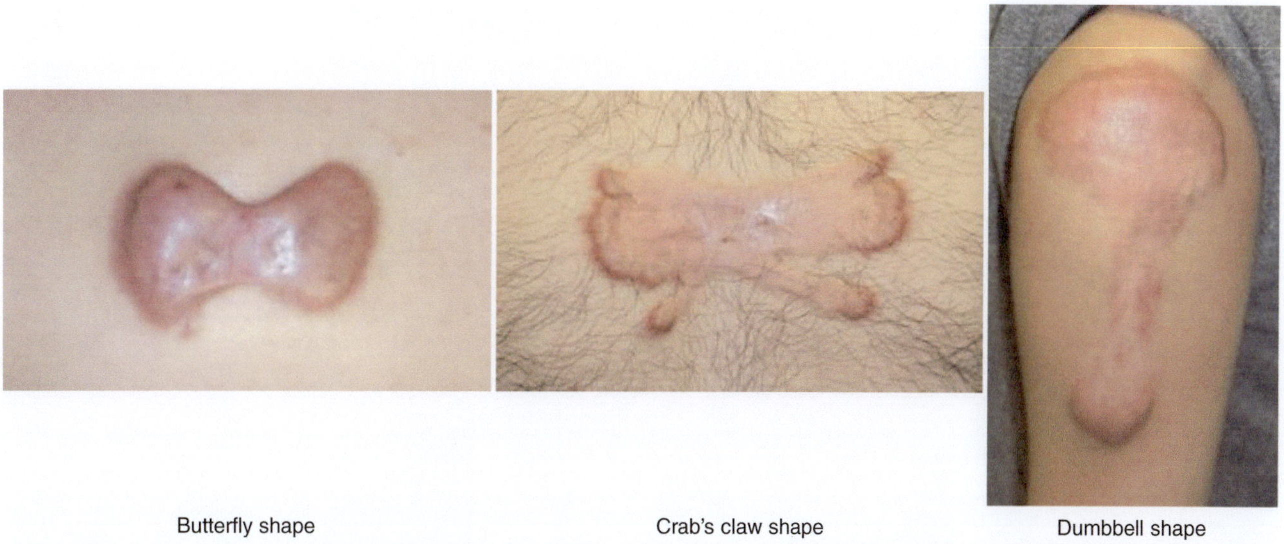

Fig. 5.2 Typical clinical appearance of keloids on different parts of the body. Keloids commonly adopt distinct site-specific shapes. In particular, keloids on the shoulder, anterior chest, and upper arm often take butterfly, crab's claw, and dumbbell shapes, respectively. This reflects the predominant directions of the skin tension that is placed on the edges of the wound/scar by the daily movements of the body region

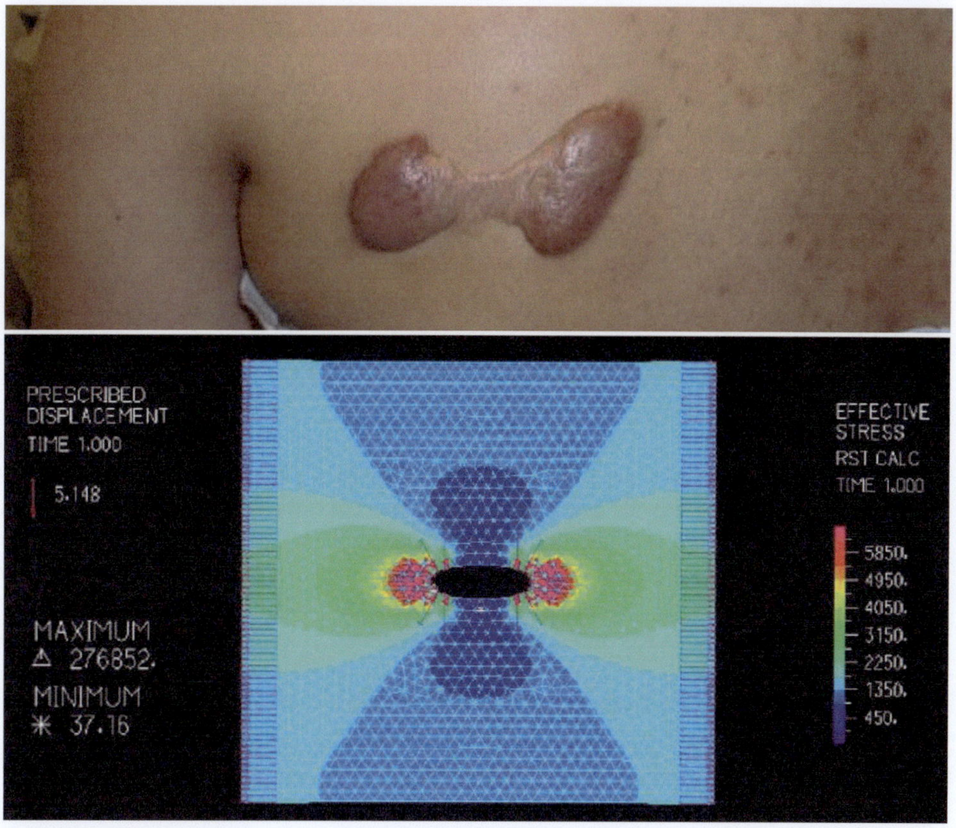

Fig. 5.3 Finite element analysis of the skin tension around a butterfly-shaped keloid on the shoulder. Keloid shape is largely determined by the directions of the tension that is applied to the skin around the wound site. (This figure is from reference [7]. It is reproduced here with the approval of the publisher)

Third, wounds on joints are particularly prone to hypertrophic scarring. This is also likely to reflect the strong repetitive tension placed on the wounds/scars during daily body movements.

In the case of earlobe keloids, mechanical force in the form of friction from the pillow and the weight of the keloid itself may also play a role once these keloids have formed.

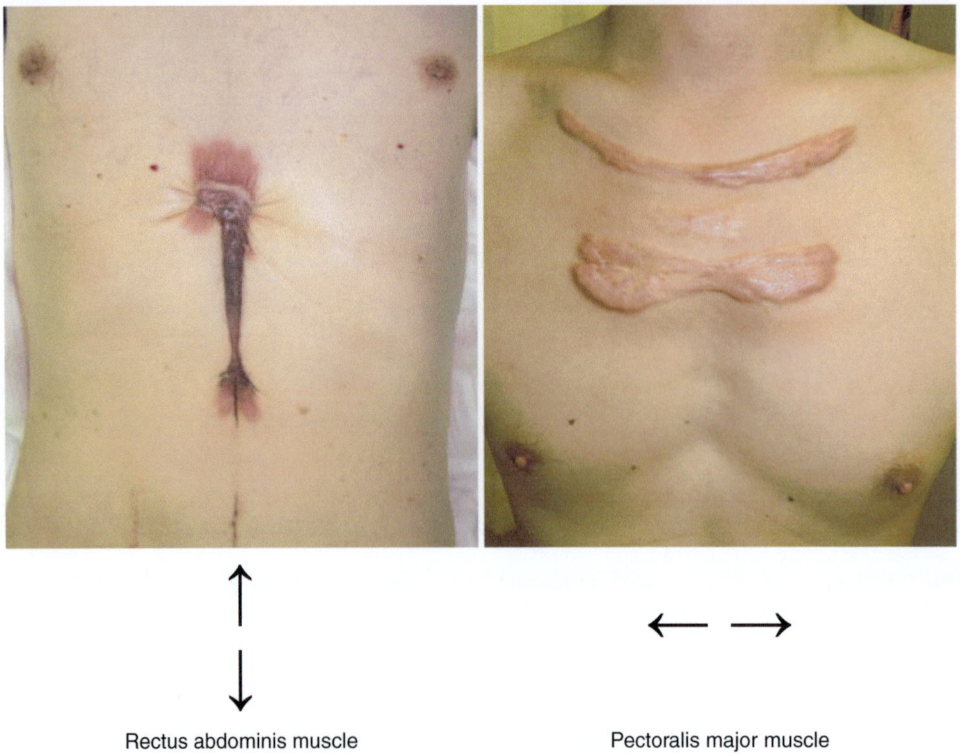

Fig. 5.4 Typical growth pattern of keloids on the abdomen and chest. Keloids on the abdomen always grow vertically, and the strongest inflammation is at their cranial and caudal ends. Keloids on the chest wall always grow horizontally, and the strongest inflammation is at the left and right ends

5.3 Systemic Risk Factors that Increase Dermal Inflammation

Adolescence and pregnancy associate with a higher risk of pathological scar development [9, 10]. This may reflect the fact that sex hormones such as estrogens and progesterones have vasodilatory and hyperpermeability effects, which may intensify inflammation and thereby promote the formation of and aggravate keloids and hypertrophic scars. This is supported by our unpublished data, which indicate that the incidence of keloids that are not caused by trauma suddenly increases at around 10 years of age. This suggests that the increases in sex steroid levels at the start of adolescence, not a higher likelihood of trauma, are responsible for the greater risk of pathological scar development in adolescents. Moreover, during pregnancy, the blood volume increases by 30–50%. This may also increase the risk of local tissue inflammation. In addition, pseudo-menopausal treatment for endometriosis or uterine myoma improves keloids markedly.

In the case of burn wounds, large and deep wounds are at a high risk of prolonged inflammation because the burn causes a prolonged proinflammatory cytokine storm. This increases the risk of pathological scarring. Indeed, it has been shown that, if a burn wound heals in less than 10 days, it has a 4% risk of developing into a hypertrophic scar, whereas a burn wound that takes 21 days or more to heal has a 70% or greater risk [11].

Our recent epidemiological study showed that another circulating factor, namely, hypertension, associates with the development of severe keloids [12]. This study assessed whether hypertension influences local keloid severity. Ordinal logistic regression analyses of 304 consecutive patients with keloids showed that blood pressure associated positively and significantly with both keloid size and number (both $p < 0.0001$). Thus, hypertension may aggravate keloids. This association may reflect the fact that hypertension associates with arteriosclerosis, which increases vascular resistance [6, 13]. This in turn accelerates the blood flow, which damages the blood vessels and induces local tissue inflammation.

The effect of hypertension on pathological scarring may be mediated, at least in part, by endothelial dysfunction, where the gaps between the endothelial cells are wide and therefore readily permit the influx of inflammatory cells into local tissues. Notably, endothelial dysfunction may also help mediate the proinflammatory and keloidogenic effects of skin stretching. Endothelial dysfunction may not only be secondary to factors such as hypertension and skin stretching, it may also have a primary cause such as a mutation. This possibility is supported by the fact that many young-onset keloid patients lack hypertension and other known keloidogenic factors [5, 14].

Conditions that induce systemic inflammation also promote pathological scarring. An example is Castleman's disease [15]. This rare lymphoproliferative disorder is characterized by the unregulated overproduction of interleukin-6, which leads to systemic lymphadenopathy and constitutional inflammatory symptoms. We experienced the case of an adult woman whose small auricular keloids developed at the age of 18 years but then became strongly aggravated after the onset of Castleman's disease 11 years later. Another example of systemic inflammatory conditions that promote pathological scarring is extensive burning: when patients with extensive burns undergo reconstructive surgery, they often develop hypertrophic scars. It is thought that this is due to the cytokine storm that is caused by the initial burn injury, which prevails for at least 1 year.

5.4 Genetic Risk Factors that Increase Dermal Inflammation

The fact that some patients with keloids and hypertrophic scars have a family history suggests that genetic factors associate with pathological scar development. This is supported by the fact that patients with darker skin are 15 times more likely than people with paler skin to develop pathological scars, primarily keloids [16], and that these scars are absent in albinos [17]. The genetic causes of pathological scar development may involve single nucleotide polymorphisms (SNPs): a genome-wide association study showed that four SNP loci in three chromosomal regions associate significantly with keloid development in the Japanese population [18]. Moreover, our study showed that the rs8032158 SNP associates with the clinical severity of keloids [19]. This SNP is located in intron 5 of the neuronal precursor cell-expressed developmentally down-regulated 4 (NEDD4) gene on chromosome 15 and may play a role in the aberrant cell proliferation seen in keloids, although further studies are needed to test this notion. There are probably many other genetic factors that have not yet been identified.

Chromosomal changes that relate to familial keloidogenesis have also been reported. To date, potential keloid-associated loci in Japanese, African-American, and Han Chinese families have been identified on chromosomes 2q23, 7p11 [20], and 10q23.31 [21], respectively, although the responsible genes have not yet been identified.

5.5 Pathological Scar Onset Model

Thus, it seems that keloids and hypertrophic scars are multifactorial disorders that are generated by genetic predisposition, systemic conditions, and/or local wound conditions (Fig. 5.5). These observations led us to propose the pathological scar onset model shown in Fig. 5.6. This model shows that it is the balance between the genetic and systemic risk factors (on the horizontal axis) and the local factors (on the vertical axis) that determines whether a wound becomes a

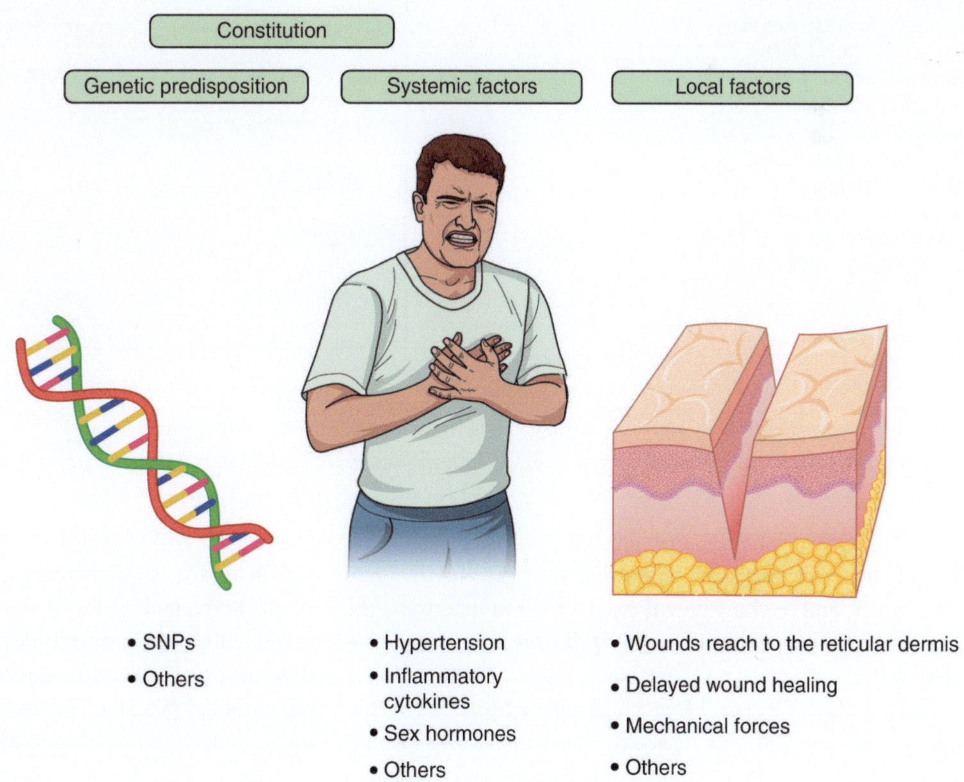

Fig. 5.5 Keloids and hypertrophic scars are multifactorial disorders. The inflammation in keloids and hypertrophic scars is driven by multiple factors, namely, genetic predisposition, systemic conditions, and local wound conditions

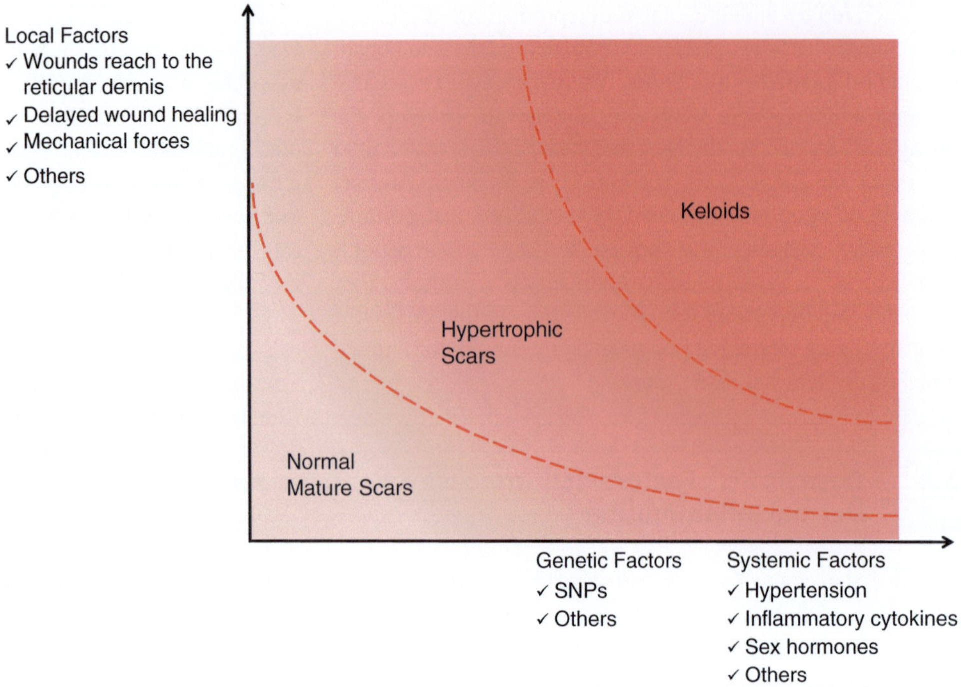

Fig. 5.6 Pathological scar onset model. The balance between genetic predisposition, systemic conditions, and local wound conditions may determine whether a wound becomes a keloid, a hypertrophic scar, or a normal scar. Genetic and systemic risk factors were put on the horizontal axis, and local factors were put on the vertical axis (This figure is from reference [7]. It is reproduced here with the approval of the publisher)

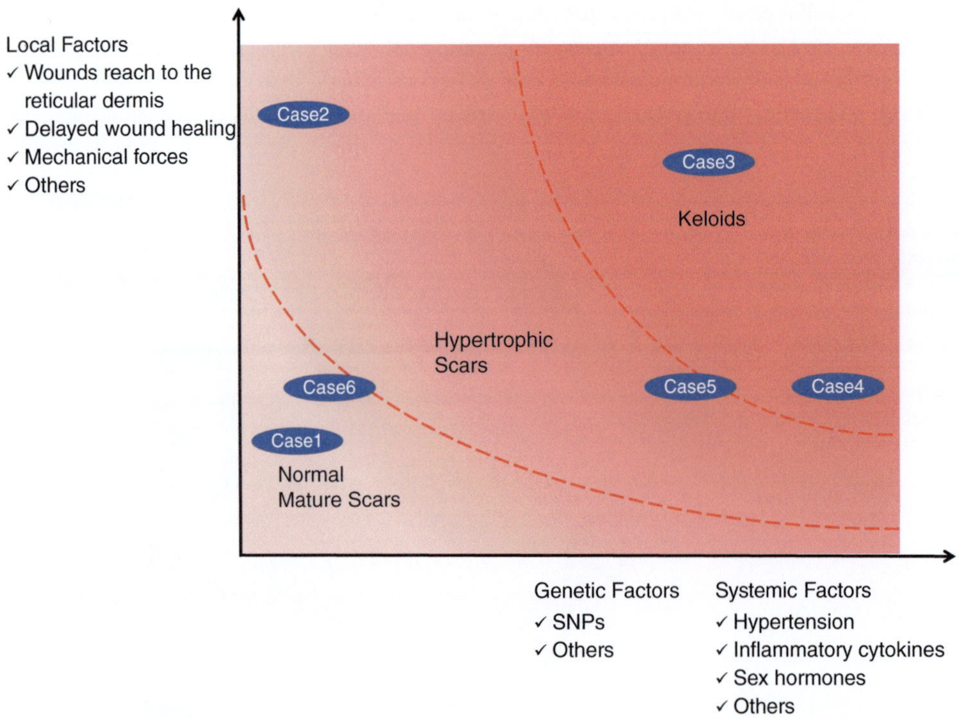

Fig. 5.7 Location of Cases 1–6 on the pathological scar onset model. The six cases are described in Figs. 5.8, 5.9, 5.10, 5.11, 5.12, and 5.13. Their location in the scar onset model is based on their degree of local risk factors (location on chest wall, major joints, or earlobe), their degree of genetic factors (as indicated by the number of other pathological scars), and their degree of systemic factors (presence of hypertension, pregnancy, adolescence, and/or inflammatory conditions)

keloid, hypertrophic scar, or normal scar [5]. To illustrate this model, and to show how it can be used to determine the best therapeutic approach, we will describe six cases (Fig. 5.7).

Case 1 (Fig. 5.8) is a 77-year-old male who had skin cancer on his face that was resected. The wounds healed normally and had matured completely before the end of the first postoperative year. This patient lacked any obvious systemic risk factors such as hypertension and did not have any keloids on his body, and his facial skin around the wounds was quite relaxed. Keloids also rarely develop on the face. Consequently, this case was placed in the bottom left corner of our scar onset model (i.e., the “normal mature scar” area), where the local, genetic, and systemic factors are all low (Fig. 5.7).

Case 2 (Fig. 5.9) is a 12-year-old girl who had a burn on her ankle joint that developed into a hypertrophic scar. Scar

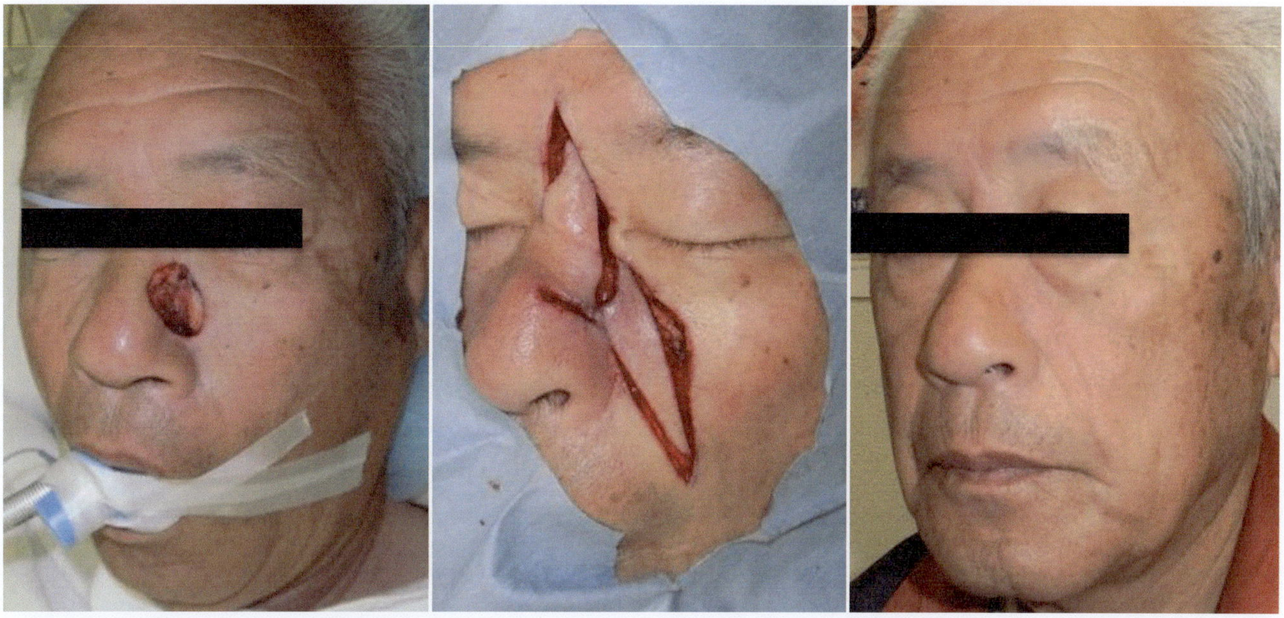

Fig. 5.8 Case 1 lacks risk factors and has a normal mature scar. This 77-year-old male developed a normal mature scar after excision of skin cancer: the right-hand panel shows his face 18 months after surgery. The normal scarring may reflect his lack of pathological scars and hypertension and the relaxed state of the skin around the wound. Thus, this case was placed at the bottom left of the scar onset model (Fig. 5.7)

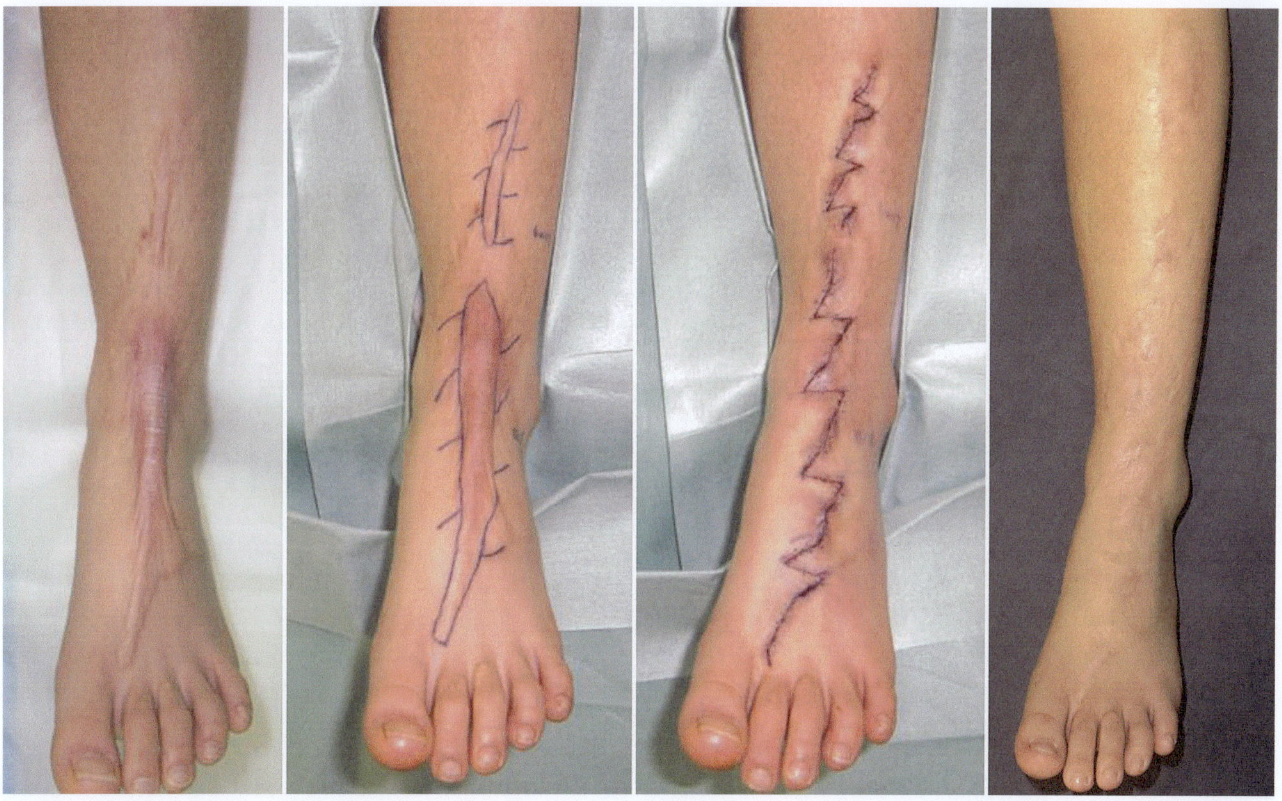

Fig. 5.9 Case 2 walked long distances: she has a hypertrophic scar on a joint. A 12-year-old girl developed a hypertrophic scar on her ankle after a burn injury. She lacked other pathological scars but had to walk long distances to school. Thus, the local risk factors are high while the genetic/systemic factors are low and this case was placed in the top left corner of the scar onset model (Fig. 5.7). After multiple z-plasties were performed, the scars matured readily and were almost invisible 18 months after surgery

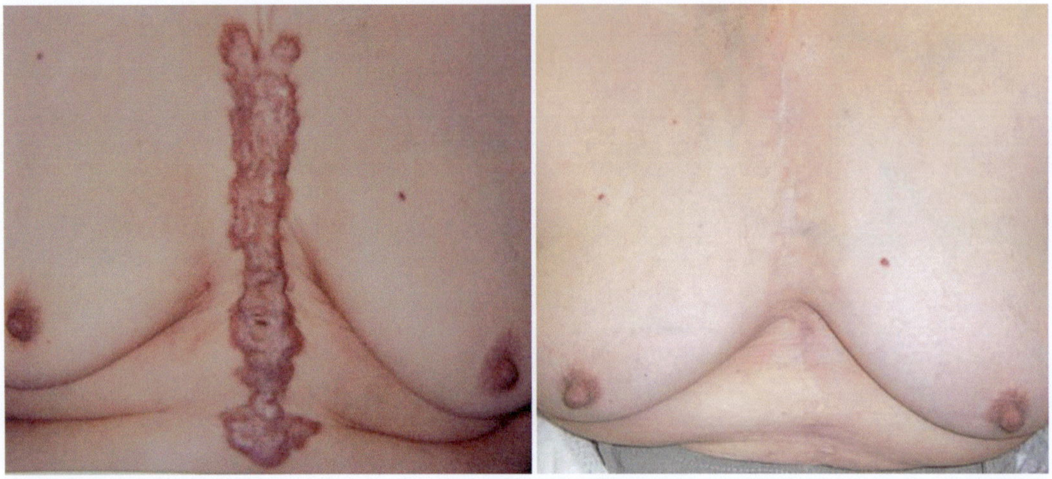

Fig. 5.10 Case 3 has hypertension: she developed chest keloids after cardiovascular surgery. A 68-year-old female developed keloids on her chest after cardiovascular surgery. While she had no other pathological scars, she had hypertension and arteriosclerosis and the scar was on an area that shows a strong predilection for keloidal growth. Thus, the local and systemic risk factors were high and this case was placed towards the top right corner of the scar onset model (Fig. 5.7). Resection and radiotherapy resulted in completely mature scars 18 months after the treatment

contracture followed. The patient did not have any obvious systemic risk factors, nor did she have any pathological scars on her body. However, she had to walk to school every day, and the ankle joint is a particularly mobile part of the body. This suggests that the cyclic tension imposed on her wound during these walks led to the development of the hypertrophic scar. Thus, this patient was placed in the upper left corner of our scar onset model (i.e., in the "hypertrophic scar" area), where the genetic/systemic factors are low but the local factors are high (Fig. 5.7). Thus, the treatment strategy should focus on releasing tension. Indeed, when multiple z-plasties were performed, the scars matured readily and were almost invisible 18 months after surgery.

Case 3 (Fig. 5.10) is a 68-year-old female who underwent cardiovascular surgery and then developed a keloid on the midline of her chest. She had hypertension and arteriosclerosis but no other keloids on her body. It seems that this case lacked genetic factors but that aging had increased the systemic factors; this combined with the injury on the high-tension anterior chest wall area is what caused the keloid to develop. Consequently, this patient was placed towards the top right corner of our scar onset model (i.e., the "keloid" area), where the genetic/systemic factors are middling but the local factors are high (Fig. 5.7). Thus, the treatment strategy should focus on releasing tension and strongly dampening the inflammation. Indeed, when the keloid was resected and radiotherapy was performed, the scars were completely mature 18 months after the treatment.

Case 4 (Fig. 5.11) is a 23-year-old male who developed a huge keloid on his earlobe after piercing his ears as a teenager. He had familial hypertension and many other hypertrophic scars and keloids on his body. However, the earlobe is not subjected to significant tension. It seems that this case had very high systemic factors but no local factors that would explain the onset of the keloid. Consequently, this patient was placed towards the bottom right corner of our scar onset model (i.e., in the "keloid" area), where the genetic/systemic factors are high and the local factors are low (Fig. 5.7). Surgery and radiotherapy were performed, and the scars were completely mature 18 months after the treatment.

Case 5 (Fig. 5.12) is a 32-year-old female who developed a mild keloid on her earlobe after piercing. She did not have any obvious systemic factors (although her estrogen level was not examined) and had no other pathological scars. Given the mildness of the keloid, the apparent absence of systemic/keloid factors, and the fact that the injury was on the low-tension earlobe, this patient was placed low down at the junction between the "keloid" and "hypertrophic scar" areas in our scar onset model (Fig. 5.7). Surgery and radiotherapy were performed, and the scars were completely mature 18 months after the treatment.

Case 6 (Fig. 5.13) is a 22-year-old female who developed a nodule just under the skin after piercing on the earlobe. The patient lacked any obvious systemic factors (although her estrogen level was not examined) and had no other pathological scars. Since the lesion was very minor, the patient lacked apparent systemic/genetic factors, and the injury was on the low-tension earlobe, this patient was placed low down at the junction between the "normal mature scar" and "hypertrophic scar" areas in our scar onset model (Fig. 5.7). Surgery and radiotherapy were performed, and the scars were completely mature 18 months after the treatment.

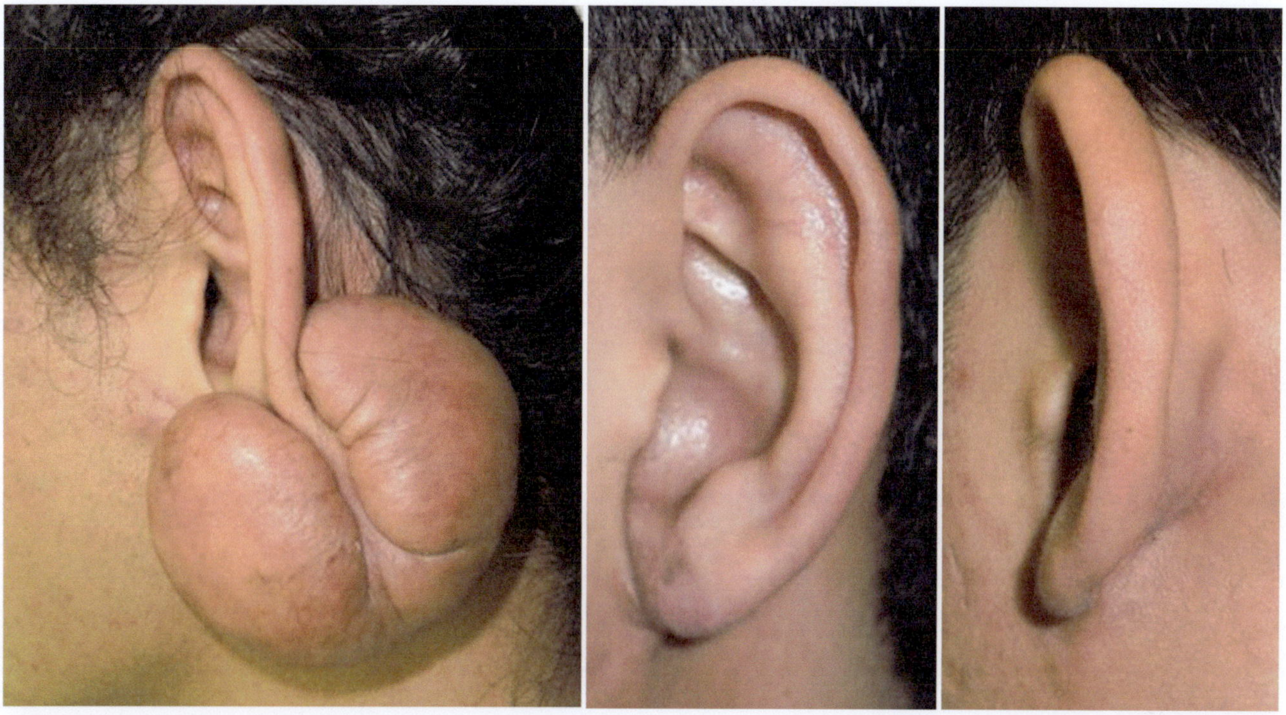

Fig. 5.11 Case 4 has familial hypertension and developed an earlobe keloid in adolescence. A 23-year-old male developed an earlobe keloid after piercing his ear as a teenager. He had familial hypertension and multiple pathological scars on his body. The earlobe is not a site of high tension, but the patient had very high genetic and systemic factors. Thus, this case was placed near the right perimeter of the scar onset model (Fig. 5.7). Surgery and radiotherapy were performed, and the scars were completely mature 18 months after the treatment. (This figure is part of a figure in reference#. It was reproduced with the approval of the publisher)

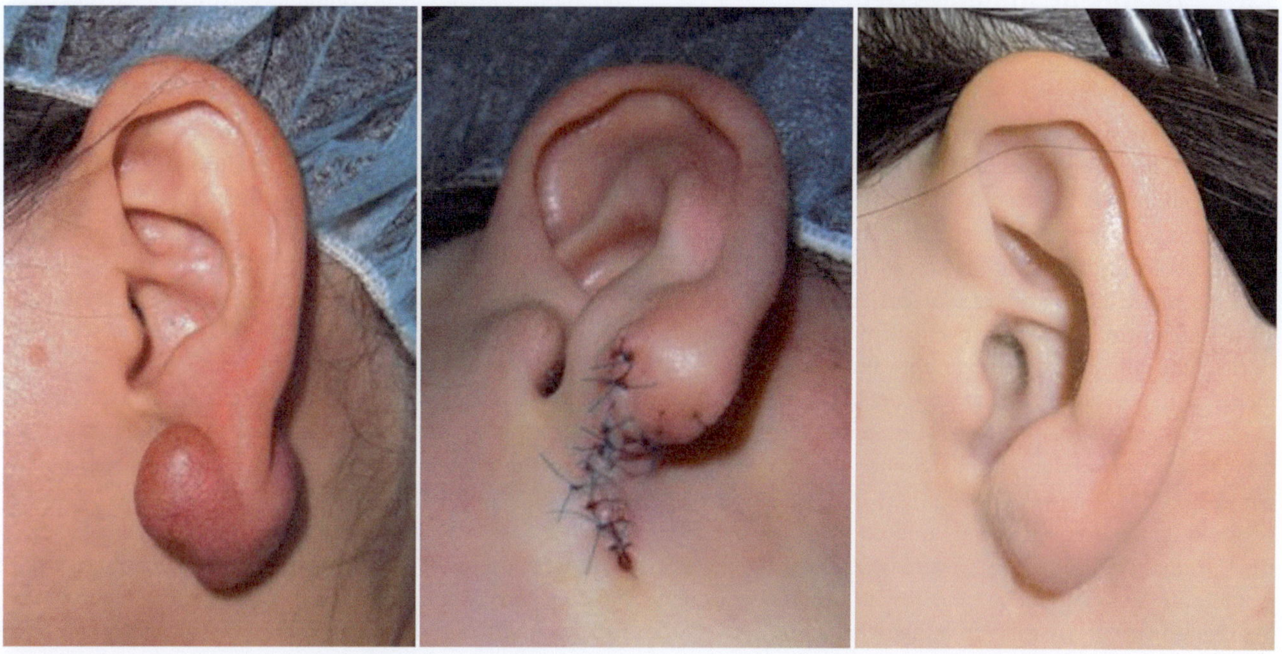

Fig. 5.12 Case 5 is a young woman without risk factors who developed a small earlobe keloid. A 32-year-old female developed a mild keloid on her earlobe after piercing. The keloid was on an area that is not subjected to skin tension, she did not have any obvious systemic factors, and had no other pathological scars. Thus, this case was placed at the junction between the "hypertrophic scar" and "keloid" areas in the scar onset model (Fig. 5.7). Surgery and radiotherapy were performed, and the scars were completely mature 18 months after the treatment. (This figure is part of a figure in reference#. It was reproduced with the approval of the publisher)

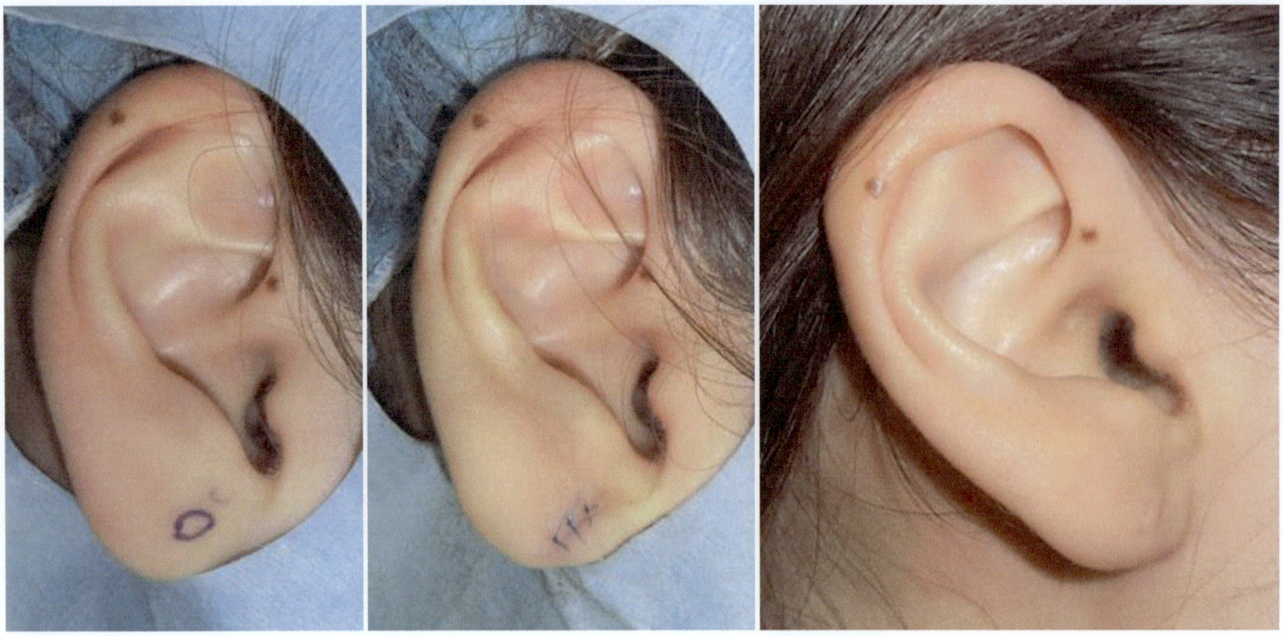

Fig. 5.13 Case 6 is a young woman without risk factors who developed a nodule after earlobe skin piercing. A 22-year-old female developed a nodule just under the skin after earlobe piercing. Since the lesion was very minor, the patient lacked apparent systemic/genetic factors, and the injury was on the low-tension earlobe, this patient was placed low down at the junction between the "keloid" and "hypertrophic scar" areas in our scar onset model. Surgery and radiotherapy were performed, and the scars were completely mature 18 months after the treatment

5.6 Treatment Strategies Depend on Inflammation Severity: The "Reset Concept"

Keloids and hypertrophic scars can be likened to a burning house on a hill, where the initial flame (a cutaneous injury) is fed continuously by strong wind drafts (daily body movements that place stretching tension on the wound/scar) and/or poor housing materials (systemic and genetic factors) until the whole house is ablaze (extensive inflammation). In such a situation, several (or even many) buckets of water (weak anti-inflammatory treatments such as steroid ointment) will not work. Depending on the ferocity of the flames (inflammation), a water cannon truck (radiation) may be able to subdue the fire. Sometimes, however, the whole house will have to be removed by a bulldozer (surgery) and the burning remnants doused by a water cannon truck (radiation) (Fig. 5.14). Thereafter, small flames and smoldering areas should be treated with watering cans and buckets of water (conservative therapies) until the fire (inflammation) has been completely extinguished and there is no risk of a new fire breaking out (recurrence) (Fig. 5.15). At that point, the ground (normal mature scar) can undergo reconstruction (surgery, fractional laser therapy, and/or makeup therapy) (Fig. 5.16). This analogy indicates that the key to successfully treating pathological scars is to carefully select the treatment modalities on the basis of the severity of the scar, its inflammation, and the factors that drive it.

This analogy also shows that removing the pathological scar by surgery serves to "reset" the skin back to when the inflammation had not gotten out of hand. I have called this the "Reset Concept" [22]. Once the strong and prolonged inflammation is removed, we can turn to therapies that control the proinflammatory factors that promoted the pathological scar in the first place (especially mechanical stress, which is easier to control than systemic and genetic factors); thus the approach is now preventive rather than therapeutic. Notably, the advantage of cutaneous scars is that they can be removed surgically, unlike the fibrosis of internal organs.

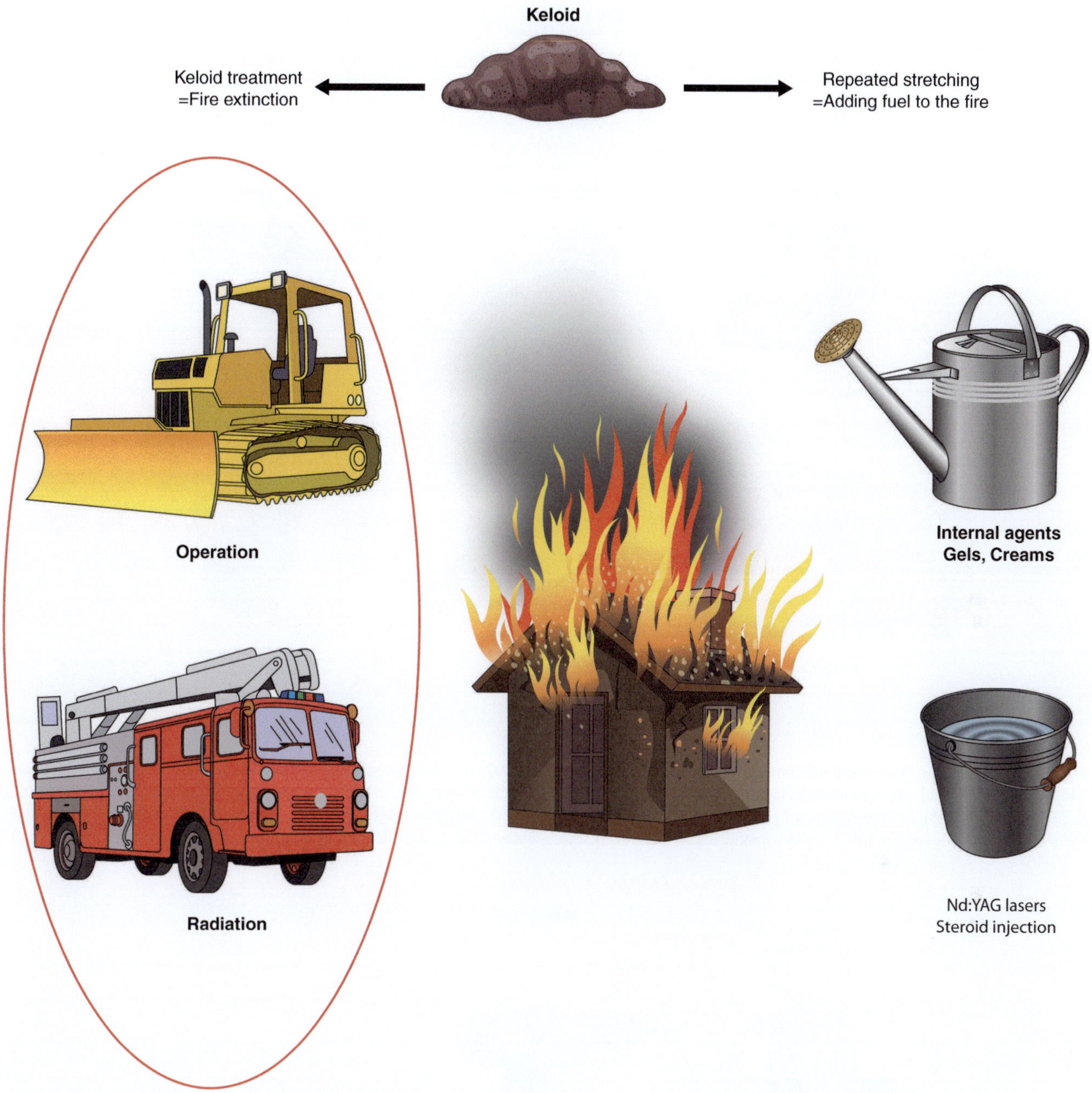

Fig. 5.14 Treatment strategy for keloids and hypertrophic scars when inflammation is severe. Keloids and hypertrophic scars can be likened to a burning house on a hill, where the initial flame (a cutaneous injury) has been continuously fanned by strong wind drafts (local mechanical tension). The poor housing materials (systemic and genetic factors) contribute to the spread of the flames (inflammation). Eventually, the whole house is blazing (very strong inflammation). Small doses of water from a watering can (internal agents, gels, and creams) or a bucket (Nd:YAG lasers and steroid injections) have little effect on the blaze. Sometimes, large amounts of water from a water cannon truck (radiation) can quell the fire (inflammation). However, sometimes, the whole house will have to be bulldozed (surgical removal) and the burning remnants doused with the water cannon truck (radiation)

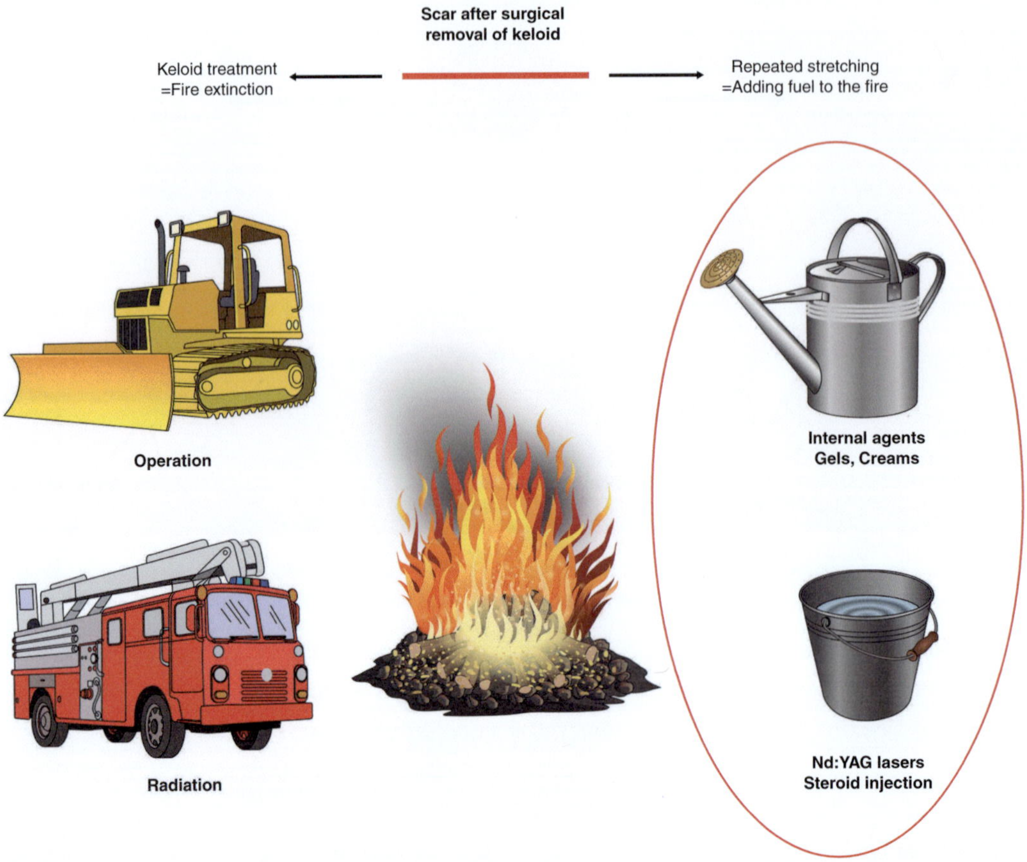

Fig. 5.15 Recurrence prevention strategy for patients whose keloids and hypertrophic scars are removed by surgery and/or radiation. After the burning house (the strongly inflamed pathological scar) is removed by a bulldozer (surgery) and/or a water cannon truck (radiation), the smoldering area should be treated with water from a watering can (internal agents, gels, or creams) or buckets (Nd:YAG laser treatment or steroid injection) until the fire (inflammation) has been extinguished completely and there is no risk of a new fire breaking out (recurrence)

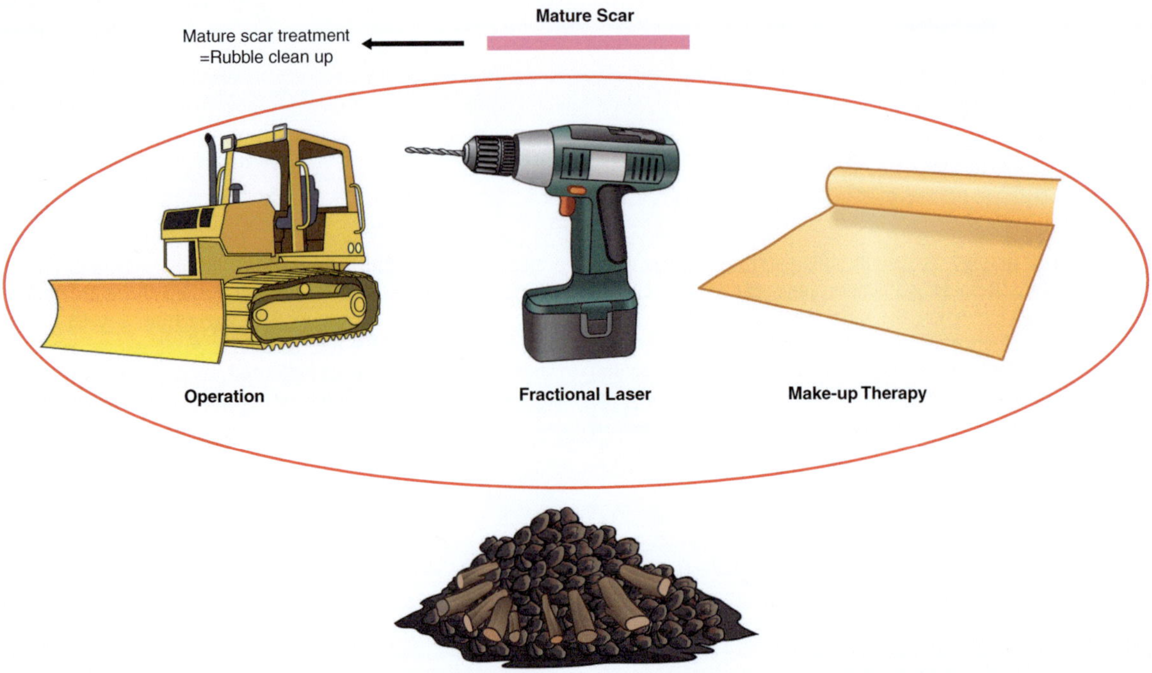

Fig. 5.16 Treatment strategy for patients with mature scars after their keloids and hypertrophic scars were removed by surgery and/or radiation. Once the fire (inflammation) has been eliminated, the ground (mature scar) can undergo reconstruction (further surgery, fractional laser therapy, and/or makeup therapy)

5.7 Conclusions

In recent years, our understanding of the pathological mechanisms that drive the development and progression of keloids and hypertrophic scars has grown rapidly. These scars are essentially lesions with chronic inflammation of the reticular dermis. The degree of inflammation is shaped by local, systemic, and genetic factors. Therefore, the treatment strategies should focus on assessing the degree of inflammation, and choosing the anti-inflammatory therapy that will adequately relieve it, and thereafter control the tension on the scars.

References

1. Ogawa R. Keloid and hypertrophic scars are the result of chronic inflammation in the reticular dermis. Int J Mol Sci. 2017;18(3):E606.
2. Huang C, Murphy GF, Akaishi S, Ogawa R. Keloids and hypertrophic scars: update and future directions. Plast Reconstr Surg Glob Open. 2013;1(4):e25.
3. Huang C, Akaishi S, Hyakusoku H, Ogawa R. Are keloid and hypertrophic scar different forms of the same disorder? A fibroproliferative skin disorder hypothesis based on keloid findings. Int Wound J. 2014;11(5):517–22.
4. Ogawa R. Mechanobiology of scarring. Wound Repair Regen. 2011;19(Suppl 1):s2–9.
5. Ogawa R, Akaishi S. Endothelial dysfunction may play a key role in keloid and hypertrophic scar pathogenesis: keloids and hypertrophic scars may be vascular disorders. Med Hypotheses. 2016;96:51–60.
6. Huang C, Liu L, You Z, Zhao Y, Dong J, Du Y, Ogawa R. Endothelial dysfunction and mechanobiology in pathological cutaneous scarring: lessons learned from soft tissue fibrosis. Br J Dermatol. 2017;177:1248–55.
7. Akaishi S, Akimoto M, Ogawa R, Hyakusoku H. The relationship between keloid growth pattern and stretching tension: visual analysis using the finite element method. Ann Plast Surg. 2008;60(4):445–51.
8. Ogawa R, Okai K, Tokumura F, Mori K, Ohmori Y, Huang C, Hyakusoku H, Akaishi S. The relationship between skin stretching/contraction and pathologic scarring: the important role of mechanical forces in keloid generation. Wound Repair Regen. 2012;20(2):149–57.
9. Moustafa MF, Abdel-Fattah MA, Abdel-Fattah DC. Presumptive evidence of the effect of pregnancy estrogens on keloid growth. Case report. Plast Reconstr Surg. 1975;56(4):450–3.
10. Mendelsohn ME, Karas RH. Estrogen and the blood vessel wall. Curr Opin Cardiol. 1994;9(5):619–26.
11. Deitch EA, Wheelahan TM, Rose MP, Clothier J, Cotter J. Hypertrophic burn scars: analysis of variables. J Trauma. 1983;23(10):895–8.
12. Arima J, Huang C, Rosner B, Akaishi S, Ogawa R. Hypertension: a systemic key to understanding local keloid severity. Wound Repair Regen. 2015;23(2):213–21.
13. Huang C, Ogawa R. The link between hypertension and pathological scarring: does hypertension cause or promote keloid and hypertrophic scar pathogenesis? Wound Repair Regen. 2014;22(4):462–6.
14. Noishiki C, Takagi G, Kubota Y, Ogawa R. Endothelial dysfunction may promote keloid growth. Wound Repair Regen. 2017;25:976–83.
15. Quong WL, Kozai Y, Ogawa R. A case of keloids complicated by Castleman's disease: interleukin-6 as a keloid risk factor. Plast Reconstr Surg Glob Open. 2017;5(5):e1336.
16. Miller MC, Nanchahal J. Advances in the modulation of cutaneous wound healing and scarring. BioDrugs. 2005;19(6):363–81.
17. Baisch A, Riedel F. Hyperplastic scars and keloids. Part I: basics and prevention. HNO. 2006;54(11):893–904.
18. Nakashima M, Chung S, Takahashi A, Kamatani N, Kawaguchi T, Tsunoda T, Hosono N, Kubo M, Nakamura Y, Zembutsu H. A genome-wide association study identifies four susceptibility loci for keloid in the Japanese population. Nat Genet. 2010;42(9):768–71.
19. Ogawa R, Watanabe A, Than Naing B, Sasaki M, Fujita A, Akaishi S, Hyakusoku H, Shimada T. Associations between keloid severity and single-nucleotide polymorphisms: importance of rs8032158 as a biomarker of keloid severity. J Invest Dermatol. 2014;134(7):2041–3.
20. Marneros AG, Norris JE, Watanabe S, Reichenberger E, Olsen BR. Genome scans provide evidence for keloid susceptibility loci on chromosomes 2q23 and 7p11. J Invest Dermatol. 2004;122:1126–32.
21. Chen Y, Gao JH, Yan X, Song M, Liu XJ. Location of predisposing gene for one Han Chinese keloid pedigree. Zhonghua Zheng Xing Wai Ke Za Zhi. 2007;23:137–40.
22. Ogawa R. The latest in keloid and hypertrophic scar pathophysiology and treatment strategies: keloids can be treated by employing up-to-date surgical management. Plastic surgery pulse news 5. Quality Medical Publishing, Inc.: St Louis; 2013.

Part II

Clinical Plactice of Scars

6 Scar Evaluation

Satoko Yamawaki

Scars induce cosmetic disfigurements, functional disorders, and psychological problems. The treatment of scars is challenging for plastic surgeons. Many treatment modalities are available for scars, including surgical excision, steroid injection, silicone gel sheeting, pressure treatment, and laser treatment. Thus, it is essential to robustly assess the outcomes of scar treatment. Assessment tools for scars fall into two categories, namely subjective assessment using scar rating scales and objective assessment using devices. We introduce the most common assessment methods in this chapter.

6.1 Subjective Assessment

6.1.1 Cosmetic Disfigurement Scale

Since the 1950s, many scar rating scales have been developed for burn scar assessment. Scars that form after burn injuries are typically red, stiff, stretched, and elevated from the surrounding skin. The scars sometimes develop hypertrophy, leading to contracture. Most of the patients have been children, and severe scars can lead to growth disorder owing to joint contracture as well as psychological problems. Smith et al. [1] reported a rating scale for burn scars that consists of five items, namely burn scar area, depth/thickness, skin color, and overall cosmetic disfigurement when fully clothed and when unclothed (Table 6.1). The authors evaluated the consistency of their scale and concluded that a dependable assessment requires input from more than four different raters.

S. Yamawaki (✉)
Department of Plastic and Reconstructive Surgery, Japanese Red Cross Fukui Hospital, Fukui-City, Fukui, Japan
e-mail: satokoy@kuhp.kyoto-u.ac.jp

Table 6.1 Cosmetic disfigurement scale reported by Smith et al. in 1988

1	Burn scar area is:				
	1: Smooth	2: Partly irregular	3: Mostly irregular		
2	Apparent depth or thickness of scarring:				
	1: Slight	2: Moderate	3: Severe		
3	Skin color of burn scar compared with normal skin:				
	1: No difference	2: Slightly darker	3: Darker	4: Very much darker	
4	Apparent overall cosmetic disfigurement if the patient were fully clothed:				
	1: None	2: Very slight	3: Slight	4: Moderate	5: Severe
5	Overall cosmetic disfigurement if the patient were not clothed:				
	1: Very slight	2: Slight	3: Moderate	4: Severe	5: Very severe

6.1.2 Hamilton Scale

Crowe et al. [2] further developed the scale that Smith et al. reported and described it as the Hamilton scale (Table 6.2). This scale assesses the thickness/height of the scar, the irregularity of the scar area, and the vascularity and color/pigmentation of the scar as compared with normal skin. The scale was designed with the aim of assessing the scar with a high reliability using input from only one rater.

6.1.3 Vancouver Scar Scale

The most commonly used scar assessment scale has been the Vancouver scar scale (VSS) [3]. The VSS is intended for use with outpatients, and it evaluates the typical features of scars, including their pigmentation, vascularity, pliability, and height (Table 6.3). The skin is blanched with a transparent plastic sheet to eliminate the effect of the vascularity when

© Springer Nature Singapore Pte Ltd. 2020

R. Ogawa (ed.), *Total Scar Management*, https://doi.org/10.1007/978-981-32-9791-3_6

assessing pigmentation. The assessment of vascularity is like a capillary refilling test, wherein the skin is pressed and then rated according to the return of the blood flow. The scar is picked with the fingers to assess its pliability. If the scar produces a deformity of distortion, it is rated as 5 points (i.e., the most severe rating). The consistency and reliability of the VSS have been confirmed; however, some problems have also been pointed out. Scars after burn injury sometimes show both hypo- and hyper-pigmentation after wound repair. Mixed pigmented scars are difficult to assess using the VSS. Moreover, this scale does not take each patient's symptoms into account.

Table 6.2 Hamilton scale reported by Crowe et al. in 1998

Total score 0–14					
1	Rate the thickness or height of the scar				
	0: No thickness or raising	1: Slight	2: Moderate	3: Severe	
2	Is it all the same height, or are there areas of irregularity?				
	0: All smooth	1: About 1/4 of the scar area	2: About 1/2	3: About 3/4	4: Majority
3	Rate the majority of the scar for vascularity, which describes how pink/red the scar is when compared with normal skin				
	0: Normal	1: Light to medium pink	2: Deep pink to light red	3: Medium to deep red	4: Purplish
4	Look at the color/pigmentation of the scar and compare it with normal skin				
	0: Normal or paler	1: Slightly darker	2: Darker	3: Much darker	

There have been some reports of modified versions of the VSS. Baryza and Baryza [4] reported that the VSS has a high interclass correlation coefficient and interrater reliability, but the κ values for its categories of pigmentation and height were only fair and moderate. Therefore, the authors amended the assessments of pigmentation and height and recommended to use a Plexiglas® sheet when assessing these subscales (Table 6.4).

Nedelec et al. [5] evaluated the change over time of each item and found that the scar height showed few changes with the progress of time. Therefore, they amended the height assessment. Moreover, they added each patient's self-reported symptoms of pain and itch (Table 6.5). Forbes-Duchart et al. [6] mentioned the difficulty of assessing differences in skin color between Caucasian and Australasian Aboriginal patients. A photograph of the typical skin color was shown in their article. They concluded that the total score of their modified VSS was meaningful for scar assessment.

6.1.4 Patient and Observer Scar Assessment Scale (POSAS)

The POSAS was invented by Draaijers et al. [7]. On this scale, the self-rated symptoms of the patients were adopted (Table 6.6) and the rating of each item used a 10-step score. The items rated by the observers consist of vascularization, pigmentation, thickness, relief, and pliability and those rated by the patients consist of pain, itching, color, stiffness, and thickness. All the items are assessed by the same numerical rating so that the individual scores can be summed to

Table 6.3 VSS reported by Sullivan et al. in 1990

Total score 0–12						
1	Pigmentation					
	0: Normal	1: Hypopigmentation	2: Hyperpigmentation			
2	Vascularity					
	0: Normal	1: Pink	2: Red	3: Purple		
3	Pliability					
	0: Normal	1: Supple	2: Yielding	3: Firm	4: Banding	5: Contracture
4	Height					
	0: Normal	1: Under 2 mm	2: Under 5 mm	3: Over 5 mm		

Table 6.4 Sections of the VSS amended by Baryza and Baryza (1995): pigmentation and height

Total score 0–15					
1	Pigmentation				
	0: Normal	1: Hypopigmentation	2: Mixed pigmentation	3: Hyperpigmentation	
4	Height				
	0: Normal	1: 0–1 mm	2: 1–2 mm	3: 2–4 mm	4: Over 4 mm

Table 6.5 Nedelec et al. [5] added each patient's opinion using a continuous scale

	Total score 0–14				
1	Pliability				
	0: Normal	1: Supple	2: Yielding	3: Firm	4: Adherent
2	Height				
	0: Normal	1: 1–2 mm	2: 3–4 mm	3: 5–6 mm	4: Over 6 mm
3	Vascularity				
	0: Normal	1: Pink	2: Red	3: Purple	
4	Pigmentation				
	0: Normal	1: Slight	2: Moderate	3: Severe	
	No pain			Worst pain ever experienced	
	No itchiness			Worst itchiness ever experienced	

Table 6.6 POSAS reported by Draaijers et al. in 2004

Observer scar assessment scale			Total score 5–50			
		Normal	1 2 3 4 5	6 7 8 9 10	Worst scar	
1	Vascularization					
2	Pigmentation					Hypo/mix/hyper
3	Thickness					
4	Relief					
5	Pliability					
Patient scar assessment scale			Total score 6–60			
		No complaints	1 2 3 4 5	6 7 8 9 10	Worst imaginable	
1	Is the scar painful?					
2	Is the scar itching?					
		Normal skin	1 2 3 4 5	6 7 8 9 10	Very different	
3	Is the color of the scar different?					
4	Is the scar more stiff?					
5	Is the thickness of the scar different?					
6	Is the scar irregular?					

produce a total score reliably and consistently. It is interesting that itching and height were found to have a greater influence on each patient's opinions about the scar than the other items. This scale has been proven to be useful for all types of scars.

6.1.5 Seattle Scale

Yeong et al. [8] introduced a scale that focuses on the differences between a scar and the adjacent normal skin. It consists of four items, namely surface irregularity, border height, thickness, and color differences. Each item is graded using a six-point scale from −1 to 4 (Table 6.7). This scale is known as the Seattle scale. Additionally, the authors recommended using photographs of the patients and the scar with the adjacent normal skin, which they called "teaching pictures." Such pictures can help raters to assess the scars simply, easily, and reliably.

6.1.6 Manchester Scar Scale

To obtain a quantitative assessment, Beausang et al. [9] proposed combining histological and clinical assessments of the scar. Their scale is called the Manchester scar scale (Table 6.8). They examined the epidermis and dermis using specimens obtained following scar excision at surgery. In addition, the papillary dermis and reticular dermis were examined separately. During the examination of the dermis, the orientation, density, and maturity of collagen fibers were assessed. This is because more mature scars exhibit thinner and more randomly oriented collagen fibers showing a basket-like weave pattern. The reticular dermis changed the most in the hypertrophic scars, but the findings of the epidermis and papillary dermis reflected the appearance of the scar according to their investigation. They commented on the reliability of the histological examination as follows: "In no case of a poor quality clinical scar was good histology found on microscopic examination." Other new items in the Manchester scar scale were the rating of how matte/shiny the scar is and the adoption of a

Table 6.7 Seattle scale reported by Yeong et al. in 1997

	Total score −4 to 16					
1	Burn scar surface					
	−1: Smooth	0: Normal	1: Rough	2: Rough	3: Rough	4: Rough
2	Burn scar border height					
	−1: Depressed	0: Normal	1: Raised	2: Raised	3: Raised	4: Raised
3	Burn scar thickness					
	−1: Thinner	0: Normal	1: Thicker	2: Thicker	3: Thicker	4: Thicker
4	Color differences between the scar and the adjacent normal skin					
	−1: Hypo-pigmented	0: Normal	1: Hyper	2: Hyper	3: Hyper	4: Hyper

Table 6.8 Manchester scar scale reported by Beausang et al. in 1998

Clinical assessment sheet						
Visual analogue scale						
	Excellent		________	Poor		
Total skin color	Lighter	Darker				
1	Color					
	1: Perfect	2: Slight mismatch	3: Obvious mismatch	4: Gross mismatch		
2	Matte/shiny					
	1: Matte	2: Shiny				
3	Contour					
	1: Flush with surrounding skin	2: Slightly proud/indented	3: Hypertrophic	4: Keloid		
4	Distortion					
	1: None	2: Mild	3: Moderate	4: Severe		
5	Texture					
	1: Normal	2: Just palpable	3: Firm	4: Hard		
Histological assessment scale		Total score 0–32				
1	Epidermis					
	0: Normal	1: Some restoration of rete ridges	2: No restoration			
2	Dermis					
	A	Collagen fiber orientation				
	0: Normal	1: Under 25% of fibers abnormal	2: 26–50%	3: 51–75%	4: 76–100%	5: Keloid-like
	B	Collagen fiber density				
	0: Normal	1: Under 25% of fibers abnormal	2: 26–50%	3: 51–75%	4: 76–100%	5: Keloid-like
	C	Collagen fiber maturity				
	0: Normal	1: Under 25% of fibers abnormal	2: 26–50%	3: 51–75%	4: 76–100%	5: Keloid-like

visual analogue scale (VAS) to capture each patient's opinion of their symptoms. They estimated that matte scars are better than shiny ones based on the layperson's common sense. The VAS was originally developed for measuring and assessing pain in the realm of pain research, and it has since been widely used in various clinical settings.

The first report of the VAS score being used for scar assessment was described by Quinn et al. [10]. Four plastic surgeons rated the scars in three categories, namely unacceptable, adequate, and excellent. Subsequently, the same observers rated the same scars using a VAS where their marks were measured as 0–100 mm as continuous data. They connected the categorical evaluation results to the VAS score and proposed the cutoff point of "poor" scars to be 35 mm on the VAS. The VAS is reproducible and reliable, but it is difficult to decide the cutoff points for all categories. This is because the VAS is conceptual and has no exact threshold value. After this report, Moiemen et al. [11] arranged the VAS to assess the efficacy of artificial skin for scar treatment. Their scale comprised seven items, namely range of movement, softness, appearance, itch, dryness, sweating, and sensation. Each item was assessed on a scale of −10 (worse) to +10 (better) by the patients. The VAS was used to rate the symptoms of the patients, such as pain and itchiness [12], and to quantify each patient's opinions. For example, to rate the patient's opinion regarding how their scars are perceived by other people, if the patient thinks that their scar is unattractive, he/she responds with a score of 0. By contrast, if he/she thinks that the scar is not noticed by other people, the patient responds with a score of 10 [13]. They also introduced a new scale called the Matching Assessment of Scars and Photographs. They arranged the scale that was reported by Yeong et al. [8] to include assessments of each patient's symptoms using the VAS, and proposed a scale that has a longer-term reliability.

6.1.7 Stony Brook Scar Evaluation Scale (SBSES)

Singer et al. [14] used the VAS score in combination with an observer-rated clinical assessment scale to create a new scale, which is termed the SBSES. This is one of several scales that combine the VAS score with clinical scar scales to assess the detailed characteristics of each scar. SBSES is composed of five categories, namely width, height, color, hatch marks/suture marks, and overall appearance, and each category is a dichotomous variable (Table 6.9). In this scale, a higher total score is associated with a better clinical outcome. They demonstrated not only high interrater and intrarater reliabilities but also a good correlation between the scar evaluation scale scores and VAS scores, unlike previous reports. The category of hatch/suture marks is included in the subscale, so this scale is appropriate for the short-term assessment of postoperative scars [15]. Furthermore, the use of this scale has been recommended by the U. S. Food and Drug Administration.

In VSS, a functional joint mobility disorder was assessed as a "contracture" on the subscale of pliability. Schneider et al. [16, 17] focused on the range of motion in joints affected by contractures caused by scars. They aimed to examine the incidence and severity of the joint contracture and to determine the main predictors of a contracture occurring after a burn injury. For instance, the active range of motion of the elbow is measured in all planes, namely flexion, extension, pronation, and supination, using a goniometer and inclinometer. According to the disturbance of the range of motion, the severity of each contracture was classified into mild, moderate, and severe (Table 6.10). The most frequently affected joint was the shoulder, followed by the elbow and the knee. The length of the hospital stay and the total burn surface area (TBSA) burned and grafted were the main predictors of contracture development. The main predictors of the severity of the contracture were the TBSA grafted, amputation, and inhalation injury. The length of the hospital stay and the TBSA burned and grafted were also associated with the number of contractures. In conclusion, they proposed that an early intervention of rehabilitation in burn patients prevents the development of a contracture.

Table 6.9 SBSES reported by Singer et al. in 2007

Total score 0–5		
1	Width	
	0: Over 2 mm	1: Less than or equal to 2 mm
2	Height	
	0: Elevated or depressed in relation to the surrounding skin	1: Flat
3	Color	
	0: Darker including red, purple, brown, or black	1: Same
4	Hatch marks or suture marks	
	0: Present	1: Absent
5	Overall appearance	
	0: Poor	1: Good
VAS:	0–100 mm	

Table 6.10 Schneider et al. [16, 17] focused on the range of motion of each joint

	Joint	Muscle action	Contracture severity		
			Mild	Moderate	Severe
1	Shoulder	Flexion	120–180	60–119	<60
		Extension	32–50	16–31	<16
		Abduction	120–180	60–119	<60
		Adduction	32–50	16–31	<16
2	Elbow	Flexion	93–140	4–92	<46
		Extension	−140–93	−46–92	>−46
		Pronation	53–80	26–52	<26
		Supination	53–80	26–52	<26
3	Hip	Flexion	67–100	34–66	<34
		Extension	20–30	10–19	<10
		Abduction	26–40	13–25	<13
		Adduction	13–20	7–12	<7
4	Knee	Flexion	100–150	50–99	<50
		Extension	−150 to 100	−99 to 50	>−50

A few years later, Fearmonti et al. [18] quoted the concept that Schneider et al. reported and developed a new POSAS. He aimed to distinguish pathologic scars from nonpathologic scars, since it is important to identify pathologic scars so that they can be treated. We previously reported a scar assessment scale called the Kyoto scar scale [19]. It is composed of both objective and subjective symptoms. The objective symptoms assessed were redness, hardness, and elevation. The subjective symptoms assessed were pain and itch. We graded the scars into four categories, namely excellent, good, fair, and poor, according to the total score.

6.1.8 Japan Scar Workshop (JSW) Scar Scale

All the scales that we mentioned above assess the treatment outcomes of the scars, but the optimal treatment modality will differ depending on the type of scar. It is difficult to differentiate keloids from intractable hypertrophic scars, but those two types of scars require distinct treatment strategies.

JSW Scar (JSS) 2015 (Classification and Evaluation of Keloids and Hypertrophic Scars)

Classification (For grading and selection of appropriate treatment methods)

Risk factors		
1. Human race	Africans	2
	Others	1
	Caucasians	0
2. Familial tendency	Clearly exists	1
	Not clearly	0
3. Number	Multible	2
	Solitary	0
4. Region	Anterior chest, Scapular-Shoulder, Suprapubic	2
	Others	0
5. Age at onset	0—30 y/o	2
	31—60 y/o	1
	60— y/o	0
6. Causes	Unknown or minute	3
	Specific wound type such as surgery	0
Present symtoms		
7. Size (cm²)	Over 20cm²	1
	Under 20cm²	0
8. Vertical growth (Elevation) (Figure 1)	Clearly exists	2
	Not clearly	0
9. Horizontal growth (Figure 2)	Clearly exists	3
	Not clearly	0
10. Shape (Figure 3)	Characteristic shape	3
	Others	0
11. Erythema around scars (Figure 4)	Clearly present	2
	Not present	0
12. Subjective symptoms	Always exist	2
	Intermittent	1
	None	0
		Total 0—25

Remarks

0—5	Character like matured scars	(intractability : low risk)
6—15	Character like hypertrophic scars	(intractability : middle risk)
16—25	Character like keloids	(intractability : high risk)

Evaluation (For judging treatment results and for following-up)

1. Induration			
0 : None	1 : Weak	2 : Mild	3 : Strong
2. Elevation (Figure 5)			
0 : None	1 : Weak	2 : Mild	3 : Strong
3. Redness of scars (Figure 6)			
0 : None	1 : Weak	2 : Mild	3 : Strong
4. Erythema around scars (Figure 7)			
0 : None	1 : Weak	2 : Mild	3 : Strong
5. Spontaneous and pressing pain			
0 : None	1 : Weak	2 : Mild	3 : Strong
6. Itch			
0 : None	1 : Weak	2 : Mild	3 : Strong
			Total 0-18

Remarks

Weak: symptoms exist in less than 1/3 of the area, or are intermittently

Strong: symptoms exist in the entire region, or are continuous

Mild: between weak and strong

Ogawa R, Akaishi S, Akita S, Okabe K, Shimizu T, Sunaga A, Tosa Y, Nagao M, Yamawaki S. JSW Scar Scale Working Group. Japan Scar Workshop (JSW) Scar Scale 2015. Available online at; http://www.scar-keloid.com/en/index.html

Fig. 6.1 The JSW scar scale for the classification and evaluation of scars

Keloids sometimes need additional radiotherapy after their surgical excision. Therefore, it is important to accurately differentiate between keloids and hypertrophic scars before starting treatment. Following this perspective, the JSW invented the JSW scar scale [20], which classifies scars as mature scars, hypertrophic scars, and keloids and evaluates their characteristics (Fig. 6.1). In the classification, 12 items are assessed, namely ethnicity, familial tendency, number of lesions, whether the region is a common site of scarring, age at onset, causes, size, vertical growth, horizontal growth, shape, erythema around the scar, and the frequency of subjective symptoms. Standardized photographs are adopted to assess the subscales of vertical growth, horizontal growth, shape, and erythema around the scar. According to the total score of the scale, the scars are categorized as mature scars (0–5 points), hypertrophic scars (6–15 points), and keloids (16–25 points). We can decide the treatment strategy based on this result. The evaluation comprises six subscales, namely induration, elevation, redness of scars, erythema around scars, spontaneous/pressing pain, and itch. All the subscales are graded on a four-point scale as none, weak, mild, or strong. The raters can refer to the photographs of typical cases to assist in the evaluation. The JSW scar scale is used for the classification of scars before starting treatment as well as their evaluation after treatment. It is easy to use, helpful, and feasible for use in clinical settings.

There are many scar rating scales. VSS and POSAS have been used widely, because they assess the main features of scars and are simple, easy to use, noninvasive, fast, and inexpensive. Therefore, they are suitable for use in clinical practice. The recommended guidelines for using scar rating scales reliably are as follows. First, the site and the area to

Table 6.11 An overview of the devices available for the assessment of scar features

Color	Thickness	Pliability	Surface area	Volume
Chroma Meter®	Ultrasonography	Ultrasonography	Tracing	Molding
LabScan®	Biopsy	Tonometer	Image tool	3D camera
DermaSpectrometer®		Durometer	3D camera	
Mexameter®		Pneumatometer		
Laser Doppler flowmetry		Cutometer®		
		Elastometer®		

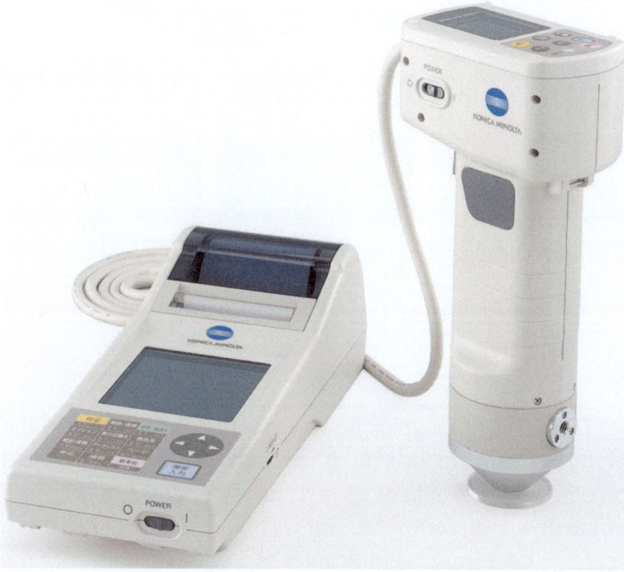

Fig. 6.2 The Chroma Meter® (CR-400, provided by Konica Minolta, Tokyo, Japan)

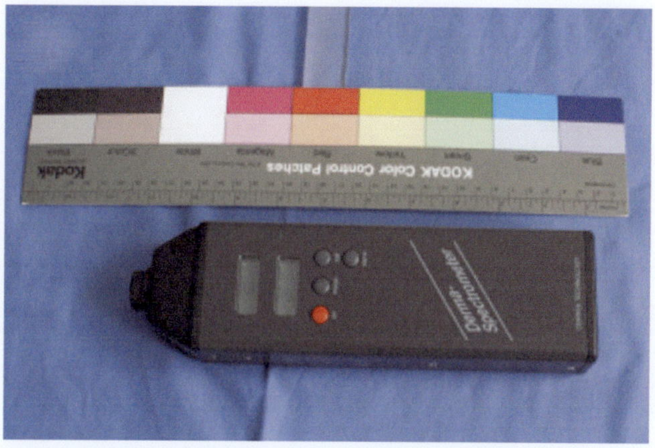

Fig. 6.3 The DermaSpectrometer® (Cortex Technology, publication permission given by Wolters Kluwer Health)

rate should be the same every time. Sullivan et al. [3] proposed that the area to rate should be 4 cm^2, while Tyack et al. [21] proposed that it should be 3 × 3 cm^2. Second, we should decide which area is rated and select an appropriate control area. Finally, scales with many items and a large total score tend to be capable of identifying smaller differences between scars than scales whose total score is small.

6.2 Objective Assessment

All scars have the common features of color, thickness, pliability, and surface area. Various devices are available for the assessment of those features of scars. We introduce an overview of the devices for the measurement of each scar feature in Table 6.11.

6.2.1 Color

Abnormal skin color is a major complaint of patients with scars. The color of a scar reflects the contents of hemoglobin and melanin in the skin. There are two categories of tools for the measurement of skin color.

First, tristimulus reflectance colorimetry illuminates the skin and collects the reflected light to measure three parameters: $L*$, lightness (brightness); $a*$, the amount of green and red (redness); and $b*$, the amount of yellow and blue (pigmentation). The Chroma Meter® (CR-400, Konica Minolta, Tokyo, Japan, Fig. 6.2) and LabScan® (HunterLab, Reston, VA) are widely used devices that employ this mechanism and measure both redness and pigmentation. The Chroma Meter® has been proven to be reliable and consistent for use with subjective scar assessment scales such as VSS and POSAS [22, 23]. The LabScan® measures the light wavelengths that human eyes recognize and shows an excellent reliability. This device is commonly used for research studies. We should be aware that a high vascularization sometimes masks the pigmentation when using these devices. The Chroma Meter® is easier to operate and cheaper than the LabScan®.

Second, narrow-band spectrophotometry calculates the erythema index and melanin index based on the differences between the absorption of red and green light by hemoglobin and melanin, respectively. The DermaSpectrometer® (Cortex Technology, Hadsund, Denmark, Fig. 6.3) has a proven validity and reliability as compared with the Chroma Meter® and subjective scar assessment scales [22, 23]. Oliveira et al. [23] showed that a blood flow index cutoff of 2.5 has a high sensitivity and specificity of 73% and 83.3%, respectively.

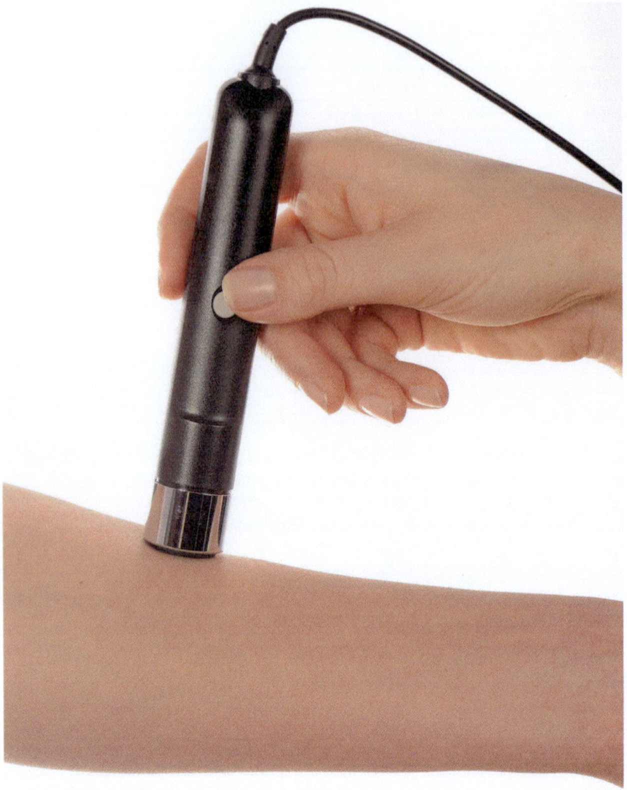

Fig. 6.4 The Mexameter® (Courage and Khazaka, provided by Integral Corporation)

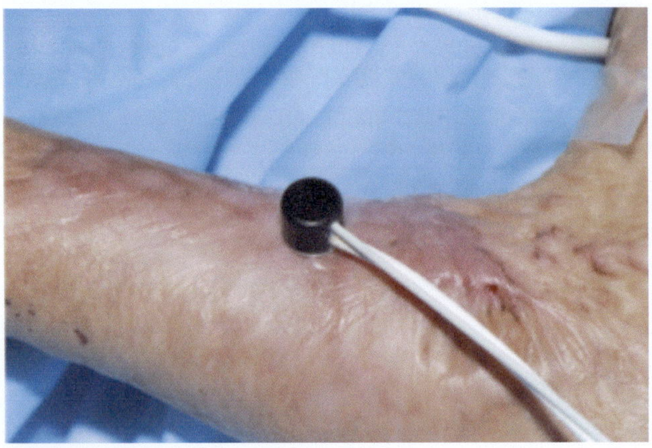

Fig. 6.5 Laser Doppler flowmetry (publication permission given by Wolters Kluwer Health)

The Mexameter® (Courage and Khazaka, Cologne, Germany, Fig. 6.4) illuminates the assessed area with three different light wavelengths of 568, 660, and 880 nm. Then, it measures the light reflected by the skin. Thus, it also assesses both erythema and pigmentation. The probe of the Mexameter® is small and easy to handle. Additionally, it has shown a high interobserver reliability and a strong correlation with VSS [24].

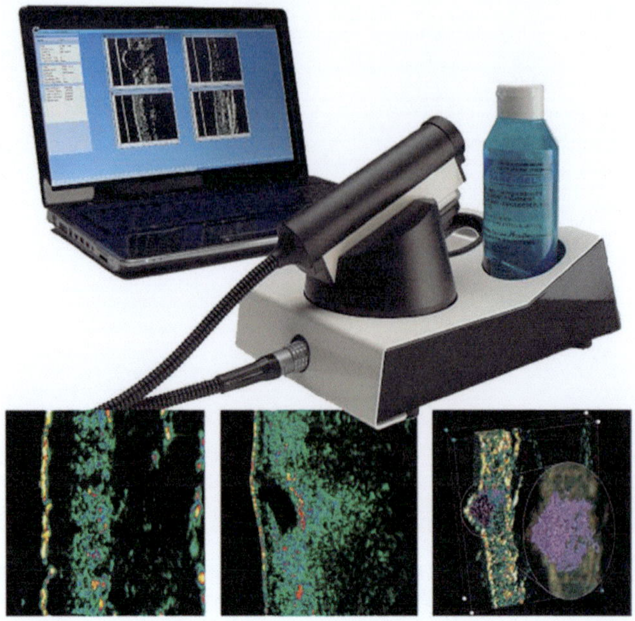

Fig. 6.6 The DermaScan® C (Cortex Technology, provided by Integral Corporation)

Third, Laser Doppler flowmetry (Fig. 6.5) evaluates the blood perfusion in the skin. It measures the movement of red blood cells in an area of approximately 1 mm^2 [25–27]. The blood flow in hypertrophic scars is higher than that in mature scars and decreases significantly at 18–24 months after the burn injury [23, 26]. That is, the data measured by Laser Doppler flowmetry can provide information about the characteristics and maturity of a scar. Ehrlich and Kelley [26] suggested that this technique can be useful for the prediction of hypertrophic scar formation. In addition, Laser Doppler flowmetry has been used to determine the depth of burn injuries. Merz et al. [28] concluded that wounds with Laser Doppler flowmetry readings of more than 100 AU will heal within 3 weeks.

6.2.2 Thickness

The thickness of a scar is measured by comparing it with the adjacent normal skin in clinical settings. Since scars are caused by the proliferation of collagen and fibroblasts in the dermis, we can measure the protrusion and depth of the lesions using appropriate devices or techniques. The biopsy of the skin is one solution for measuring these scar characteristics [9, 29]. However, this technique is invasive, and the skin shrinks after being fixed with paraformaldehyde. The skin biopsy technique is appropriate for the histological examination of the scars. Another solution for determining the scar thickness is ultrasonography (US) [30, 31]. Nedelec et al. [24, 32] used the DermaScan® C (Cortex Technology, Fig. 6.6), which is specialized for the measurement of skin characteristics via US. The authors suggested that sites with a thickness exceeding 2.034 mm should be categorized as hypertrophic scars. The examination of the skin using general US has recently become possible owing to the progress of US technology. US devices are commonly used in clinical settings and they offer a good reproducibility, low invasiveness, and high accuracy. Moreover, US has recently been applied to assess the stiffness of skin lesions [33, 34]. We will discuss the measurement of stiffness using US further in the next section.

6.2.3 Pliability

Scars commonly have a reduced pliability as compared with normal skin. The increased stiffness of scars sometimes induces pain and itching because of the difference in their flexibility as compared with the adjacent normal skin. In addition, their stiffness aggravates scar contractures and contributes to the limited range of joint motion. There are several devices based on different mechanisms for measuring the pliability of the scars. The tonometer was originally developed in the field of ophthalmology for the assessment of intraocular pressure [31, 35]. It provides an indentational load in the vertical direction. The pneumatometer and durometer (Fig. 6.7) are types of tonometer that measure pressure via an airflow system. These devices showed a high consistency with the VSS [23]. The durometer had a sensitivity of 87% and a specificity of 91.7% under the cutoff of 40. The pneumatometer showed a sensitivity of 87.5% and a specificity of 100% under the cutoff of 20. We should consider that the tonometer is influenced by the underlying hard tissue [36]. The Cutometer® (Courage and Khazaka, Fig. 6.8) measures the viscoelasticity of skin by analyzing the vertical deformation of the skin surface after applying a negative pressure of 500 mbar to the skin for a period of 1 s, followed by the application of a normal pressure for 1 s. The data is uploaded to a computer. The Cutometer® uses handheld probes of several different diameters ranging from 2 to 8 mm. The 6-mm probe is appropriate for the measurement of dermal elasticity [37]. The device obtains data for several parameters (Fig. 6.9). Among the measured parameters, Uf and Ue are speculated to be reliable measures of elasticity [22, 38–40]. The Cutometer® has been used widely and

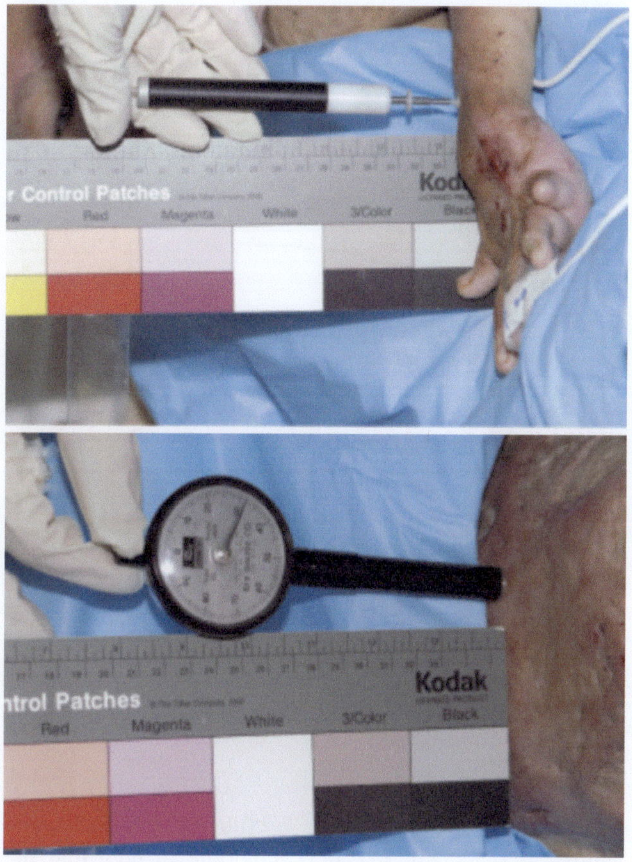

Fig. 6.7 The pneumatometer/durometer (publication permission given by Wolters Kluwer Health)

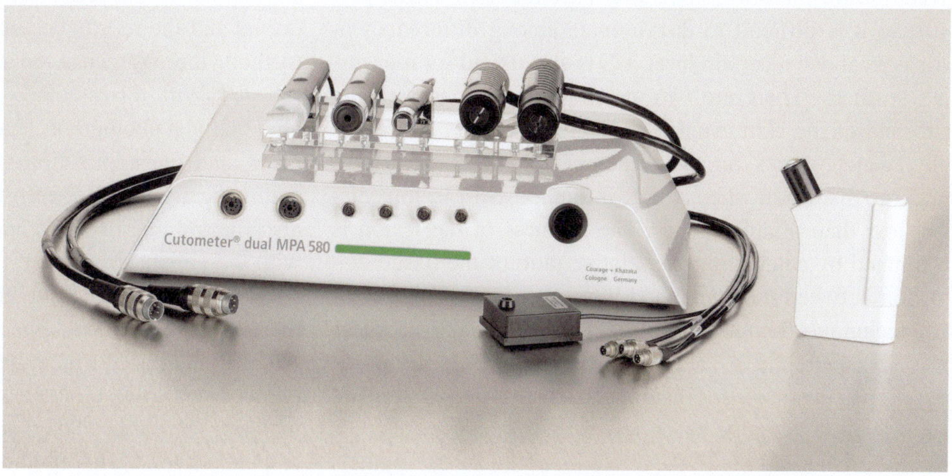

Fig. 6.8 The Cutometer® (Courage and Khazaka, provided by Integral Corporation)

Table 1. Definition of cutometer parameters

Ue	Immediate Distension
Uv	Delayed distension
Ur	Immediate retraction
Uf	Final deformation
Ua	Resilient distension
R	Residual deformation
Uv/Ue	Viscoelastic ratio
Ur/Uf	Gross elasticity or relative elastic recovery
Ur/Ue	Net elasticity or elastic function
Ua/Uf	Biological elasticity

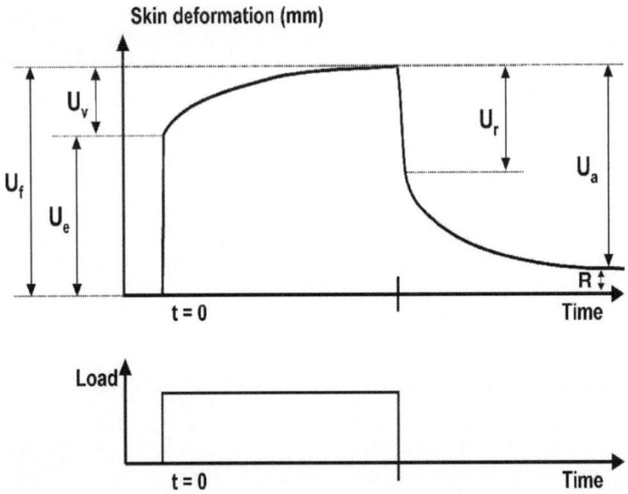

Fig. 6.9 An example of a Cutometer® plot and the definition of each parameter (publication permission given by Wolters Kluwer Health)

many articles have shown its usefulness, reliability, and validity [22, 32, 40, 41]. It is important to note that the Cutometer® is influenced by the humidity, temperature, and site of the body being assessed. We need to pay attention to the selection of the control subject. In addition, the devices available for measuring pliability have a ceiling effect [24, 40], so it is difficult to discriminate among differences in stiffness above a certain level. US is also useful for measuring stiffness. There are two techniques for measuring the stiffness of the skin using US. The first is strain elastography, which works on the principle that the lesions will undergo distortion when a force is applied. Stiff lesions distort less than pliable tissues. The stiffness of the lesion is estimated by calculating the relative ratio of the tissue distortion between the lesion and normal dermis. The second US technique for measuring the stiffness of skin is shear wave elastography. A shear wave elastography emits short-duration acoustic pulses that induce tissue compression and subsequently generate shear waves that propagate into the tissue perpendicularly to the direction of the acoustic pulse. We select the region of interest in the scar and the velocity is calculated automatically. Thus, the stiffness is revealed by the wave propagation velocity. In harder tissues, the waves propagate at a higher velocity, and the waves also propagate at a higher velocity in immature scars that show an abnormal accumulation of collagen by histopathological analysis than they do in mature scars [33, 34].

6.2.4 Surface Area

The surface area of scars relates to their severity, especially for burn injuries. Tracing the outline of scars has been performed as an evaluation method for a long time. Currently, it is common to combine photographs of the scars with the computational image analysis tools that are easily available. Although the tracing technique and photography combined with computational analysis are both reliable and reproducible, especially for areas smaller than 25 cm^2, the latter is easier to perform and obtain data from [42]. There are several drawbacks regarding the measurement of surface area. First, the surface area of the scar may change when it either expands or contracts; therefore, it is difficult to estimate the area of the original wound from the area of a scar. Second, the surface area increases in patients who underwent a skin graft after a burn injury. Finally, the curvature of the body disturbs the accuracy of surface area measurements, even if we use computational image analysis methods.

6.2.5 Volume

To measure the volume of scars, dental molds have been used in the past [5, 43, 44]. The use of this approach is cumbersome because several steps are needed to measure the volume, namely to make a negative impression, to make a positive impression, and to measure the volume. The molds are applied to the scars directly; thus, skin distortion often occurs and the results become inaccurate. As an alternative method, three-dimensional cameras have become popular [45–47]. With this method, we select three arbitrary points after taking a photograph. The system is connected to a computer, and the application software calculates the volume automatically. It can measure not only the surface area but also the volume of scars and requires no physical contact with the patient. Moreover, it can calculate the slope of the body surface, so the issue about the curvature of the body mentioned above can be resolved. Using this method, Ardehali et al. [45] found that steroid injections for 8 weeks reduced the volume of the scars by more than 50% in the majority of cases. They successfully identified the low responders for whom another treatment modality should be considered. The limitations of three-dimensional photography are the cost of the apparatus and the time-consuming analysis steps, which make it challenging to use this method daily in the clinical settings.

To determine the appropriate treatment modality, the assessment of the treatment outcome is very important. The objective assessment of scars is quantitative, accurate, reliable, reproducible, and valid. Each device is accurate; for instance, the VECTRA® three-dimensional imaging system (Canfield Scientific, Parsippany, NJ) can measure the scar volume with a measurement error of less than 1 mm^3. However, almost all the devices mentioned above can each assess only one feature of scars, even though scars have several features that reflect their severity such as their color, stiffness, surface area, and thickness. In addition, it is questionable whether the patients would appreciate small improvements in their scars that can only be measured using such devices. Another issue is that these devices are expensive and generally require time-consuming analysis steps. As a result, the assessment of scars using these devices is usually more appropriate for research than for daily clinical practice. At present, each rater should select the appropriate device depending on the purpose of a given research study or clinical evaluation procedure.

References

1. Smith GM, Tompkins DM, Bigelow ME, et al. Burn-induced cosmetic disfigurement: can it be measured reliably? J Burn Care Rehabil. 1988;9(4):371–5.
2. Crowe JM, Simpson K, Johnson W, et al. Reliability of photographic analysis in determining change in scar appearance. J Burn Care Rehabil. 1998;19(2):183–6.
3. Sullivan T, Smith J, Kermode J, et al. Rating the burn scar. J Burn Care Rehabil. 1990;11(3):256–60.
4. Baryza MJ, Baryza GA. The Vancouver Scar Scale: an administration tool and its interrater reliability. J Burn Care Rehabil. 1995;16(5):535–8.
5. Nedelec B, Shankowsky HA, Tredget EE. Rating the resolving hypertrophic scar: comparison of the Vancouver Scar Scale and scar volume. J Burn Care Rehabil. 2000;21(3):205–12.
6. Forbes-Duchart L, Mrashall S, Strock A, et al. Determination of inter-rater reliability in pediatric burn scar assessment using a modified version of the Vancouver Scar Scale. J Burn Care Res. 2007;28(3):460–7.
7. Draaijers LJ, Tempelman FR, Botman YA, et al. The patient and observer scar assessment scale: a reliable and feasible tool for scar evaluation. Plast Reconstr Surg. 2004b;113(7):1960–5. discussion 1966–1967.
8. Yeong EK, Mann R, Engrav LH, et al. Improved burn scar assessment with use of a new scar-rating scale. J Burn Care Rehabil. 1997;18(4):353–5. discussion 352.
9. Beausang E, Floyd H, Dunn KW, et al. A new quantitative scale for clinical scar assessment. Plast Reconstr Surg. 1998;102(6):1954–61.
10. Quinn JV, Drzewiecki AE, Stiell IG, et al. Appearance scales to measure cosmetic outcomes of healed lacerations. Am J Emerg Med. 1995;13(2):229–31. https://doi.org/10.1016/0735-6757(95)90100-0.
11. Moiemen NS, Staiano JJ, Ojeh NO, et al. Reconstructive surgery with a dermal regeneration template: clinical and histologic study. Plast Reconstr Surg. 2001;108(1):93–103.
12. Masters M, McMahon M, Svens B. Reliability testing of a new scar assessment tool, Matching Assessment of Scars and Photographs (MAPS). J Burn Care Rehabil. 2005;26(3):273–84.
13. Martin D, Umraw N, Gomez M, et al. Changes in subjective vs objective burn scar assessment over time: does the patient agree with what we think? J Burn Care Rehabil. 2003;24(4):239–44. discussion 238. https://doi.org/10.1097/01.BCR.0000075842.55039.03.
14. Singer AJ, Arora B, Dagum A, et al. Development and validation of a novel scar evaluation scale. Plast Reconstr Surg. 2007;120(7):1892–7. https://doi.org/10.1097/01.prs.0000287275.15511.10.
15. Bae SH, Bae YC. Analysis of frequency of use of different scar assessment scales based on the scar condition and treatment method. Arch Plast Surg. 2014;41(2):111–5. https://doi.org/10.5999/aps.2014.41.2.111.
16. Schneider JC, Holavanahalli R, Helm P, et al. Contractures in burn injury: defining the problem. J Burn Care Res. 2006;27(4):508–14. https://doi.org/10.1097/01.BCR.0000225994.75744.9D.
17. Schneider JC, Holavanahalli R, Helm P, et al. Contractures in burn injury part II: investigating joints of the hand. J Burn Care Res. 2008;29(4):606–13. https://doi.org/10.1097/BCR.0b013e31817db8e1.
18. Fearmonti R, Bond J, Erdmann D, et al. A review of scar scales and scar measuring devices. Eplasty. 2010;10:e43.
19. Yamawaki S, Naitoh M, Ishiko T, et al. Keloids can be forced into remission with surgical excision and radiation, followed by adjuvant therapy. Ann Plast Surg. 2011;67(4):402–6. https://doi.org/10.1097/SAP.0b013e31820d684d.
20. Ogawa R, Akaishi S. Endothelial dysfunction may play a key role in keloid and hypertrophic scar pathogenesis—keloids and hypertrophic scars may be vascular disorders. Med Hypotheses. 2016;96:51–60. https://doi.org/10.1016/j.mehy.2016.09.024.
21. Tyack Z, Simons M, Spinks A, et al. A systematic review of the quality of burn scar rating scales for clinical and research use. Burns. 2012;38(1):6–18. https://doi.org/10.1016/j.burns.2011.09.021.
22. Draaijers LJ, Botman YA, Tempelman FR, et al. Skin elasticity meter or subjective evaluation in scars: a reliability assessment. Burns. 2004a;30(2):109–14. https://doi.org/10.1016/j.burns.2003.09.003.
23. Oliveira GV, Chinkes D, Mitchell C, et al. Objective assessment of burn scar vascularity, erythema, pliability, thickness, and planimetry. Dermatol Surg. 2005;31(1):48–58.
24. Nedelec B, Correa JA, Rachelska G, et al. Quantitative measurement of hypertrophic scar: intrarater reliability, sensitivity, and specificity. J Burn Care Res. 2008b;29(3):489–500. https://doi.org/10.1097/BCR.0b013e3181710869.
25. Atiles L, Mileski W, Purdue G, et al. Laser Doppler flowmetry in burn wounds. J Burn Care Rehabil. 1995;16(4):388–93.
26. Ehrlich HP, Kelley SF. Hypertrophic scar: an interruption in the remodeling of repair—a laser Doppler blood flow study. Plast Reconstr Surg. 1992;90(6):993–8.
27. Perry DM, McGrouther DA, Bayat A. Current tools for noninvasive objective assessment of skin scars. Plast Reconstr Surg. 2010;126(3):912–23. https://doi.org/10.1097/PRS.0b013e3181e6046b.
28. Merz KM, Pfau M, Blumenstock G, et al. Cutaneous microcirculatory assessment of the burn wound is associated with depth of injury and predicts healing time. Burns. 2010;36(4):477–82. https://doi.org/10.1016/j.burns.2009.06.195.
29. Verhaegen PD, van der Wal MB, Middelkoop E, et al. Objective scar assessment tools: a clinimetric appraisal. Plast Reconstr Surg. 2011;127(4):1561–70. https://doi.org/10.1097/PRS.0b013e31820a641a.

30. Fong SS, Hung LK, Cheng JC. The cutometer and ultrasonography in the assessment of postburn hypertrophic scar—a preliminary study. Burns. 1997;23(Suppl 1):S12–8.
31. Katz SM, Frank DH, Leopold GR, et al. Objective measurement of hypertrophic burn scar: a preliminary study of tonometry and ultrasonography. Ann Plast Surg. 1985;14(2):121–7.
32. Nedelec B, Correa JA, Rachelska G, et al. Quantitative measurement of hypertrophic scar: interrater reliability and concurrent validity. J Burn Care Res. 2008a;29(3):501–11. https://doi.org/10.1097/BCR.0b013e3181710881.
33. Aya R, Yamawaki S, Muneuchi G, et al. Ultrasound elastography to evaluate keloids. Plast Reconstr Surg Glob Open. 2014;2(2):e106. https://doi.org/10.1097/GOX.0000000000000048.
34. Aya R, Yamawaki S, Yoshikawa K, et al. The shear wave velocity on elastography correlates with the clinical symptoms and histopathological features of keloids. Plast Reconstr Surg Glob Open. 2015;3(7):e464. https://doi.org/10.1097/GOX.0000000000000445.
35. Esposito G, Ziccardi P, Scioli M, et al. The use of a modified tonometer in burn scar therapy. J Burn Care Rehabil. 1990;11(1):86–90.
36. Falanga V, Bucalo B. Use of a durometer to assess skin hardness. J Am Acad Dermatol. 1993;29(1):47–51.
37. van Zuijlen PP, Angeles AP, Kreis RW, et al. Scar assessment tools: implications for current research. Plast Reconstr Surg. 2002;109(3):1108–22.
38. Lee KC, Dretzke J, Grover L, et al. A systematic review of objective burn scar measurements. Burns Trauma. 2016;4:14. https://doi.org/10.1186/s41038-016-0036-x.
39. Matsuzaki K, Kumagai N, Fukushi S, et al. Cultured epithelial autografting on meshed skin graft scars: evaluation of skin elasticity. J Burn Care Rehabil. 1995;16(5):496–502.
40. Rennekampff HO, Rabbels J, Reinhard V, et al. Comparing the Vancouver Scar Scale with the cutometer in the assessment of donor site wounds treated with various dressings in a randomized trial. J Burn Care Res. 2006;27(3):345–51. https://doi.org/10.1097/01.BCR.0000216311.61266.00.
41. van Zuijlen PP, Vloemans JF, van Trier AJ, et al. Dermal substitution in acute burns and reconstructive surgery: a subjective and objective long-term follow-up. Plast Reconstr Surg. 2001;108(7):1938–46.
42. van Zuijlen PP, Angeles AP, Suijker MH, et al. Reliability and accuracy of techniques for surface area measurements of wounds and scars. Int J Low Extrem Wounds. 2004;3(1):7–11. https://doi.org/10.1177/1534734604263200.
43. Ahn ST, Monafo WW, Mustoe TA. Topical silicone gel for the prevention and treatment of hypertrophic scar. Arch Surg. 1991;126(4):499–504.
44. Sawada Y. A method of recording and objective assessment of hypertrophic burn scars. Burns. 1994;20(1):76–8.
45. Ardehali B, Nouraei SA, Van Dam H, et al. Objective assessment of keloid scars with three-dimensional imaging: quantifying response to intralesional steroid therapy. Plast Reconstr Surg. 2007;119(2):556–61. https://doi.org/10.1097/01.prs.0000252505.52821.76.
46. Taylor B, McGrouther DA, Bayat A. Use of a non-contact 3D digitiser to measure the volume of keloid scars: a useful tool for scar assessment. J Plast Reconstr Aesthet Surg. 2007;60(1):87–94. https://doi.org/10.1016/j.bjps.2005.12.051.
47. van der Aa T, Verhiel SH, Erends M, et al. A simplified three-dimensional volume measurement technique in keloid scars: Validity and reliability. J Plast Reconstr Aesthet Surg. 2015;68(11):1574–80. https://doi.org/10.1016/j.bjps.2015.07.001.

Clinical and Pathological Diagnosis of Scars

7

Chenyu Huang, Longwei Liu, Zhifeng You, Zhaozhao Wu, Yanan Du, and Rei Ogawa

Cutaneous scars are often seen in dermatology clinics. They can be due to trauma or surgery. Occasionally, their cause is unknown. Until recently, most studies on the etiology of cutaneous scars examined the underlying genetic, endocrinological, immunological, and nutritional causes [1]. This focus changed recently when multiple lines of evidence from various fields showed that local mechanics [2, 3], endothelial dysfunction [4], and lipid metabolism [5] may also contribute to scarring. However, while efforts have been made to elucidate the molecular mechanisms by which the latter etiological factors promote scarring [6], these mechanisms are currently mainly supported by indirect theoretical evidence rather than hard data. These uncertainties regarding scar etiology mean that the choice between the various treatment modalities for individual scars today continues to depend on current scar diagnostics, which are based on the physician's clinical evaluations and the pathologist's findings under the microscope. This chapter will provide an overview of the various scar categories that exist currently. Specifically, the manifestations of these distinct scar types, how they are diagnosed and differentiated from each other, and their complications will be described in detail.

7.1 Classification of Cutaneous Scars

Cutaneous scars (also known as dermatological scars) are essentially the result of aberrant wound healing that causes excessive accumulation of cellular and extracellular components. Depending on the focus of the researcher, scars can be classified in various ways. Specifically, they can be categorized according to the original cause (e.g., trauma, burn, acne, vaccination, and incision), their shape and appearance (e.g., linear and webbed scars), the function-impairing deformities that they cause (e.g., adhesion and contracture), their general severity (e.g., degeneration and hypertrophy), and their potential complications (e.g., ulcer and malignancy). In this chapter, we will classify scars according to their clinical and pathological features into normal scars, atrophic scars, hypertrophic scars, keloids, and malignant ulcers of scars.

7.2 Scar Assessment Scales Used to Evaluate Scar Severity

Regardless of the scar classification system that is chosen, it is necessary to accurately assess the severity of the individual scar, as this will help the physician to choose the most appropriate therapeutic strategy. Smith et al. reported the first scar severity measurement technique in 1988: they reported that when panels of four or more hospital staff reviewed color slide photographs, they reliably rated scar severity variables such as cosmetic disfigurement in terms of irregularity, thickness, and discoloration [7]. Thereafter, various scar assessment scales were proposed and, in some cases, further modified. These scales include the Vancouver scar scale (VSS) [8], the Seattle scale [9], the Manchester scar scale [10], the Hamilton scale [11], the patient and observer scar assessment scale (POSAS) [12], the matching assessment of scars and photographs (MAPS) tool [13], the Stony Brook scar evaluation scale (SBSES) [14], and the University of North Carolina "4P" scar scale (UNC4P) [15, 16]. The relative advantages and disadvantages of each scale have been well discussed and are detailed in several specific reviews [17, 18]. The most widely used scales are the VSS and POSAS. VSS scores are based on semiquantitative estimation by therapists of scar pigmentation, vascularity, pliability, and

C. Huang (✉)
Department of Dermatology, Beijing Tsinghua Changgung Hospital, School of Clinical Medicine, Tsinghua University, Beijing, China

L. Liu · Z. You · Z. Wu · Y. Du
Department of Biomedical Engineering, School of Medicine, Tsinghua University, Beijing, China

R. Ogawa
Department of Plastic, Reconstructive and Aesthetic Surgery, Nippon Medical School, Tokyo, Japan

© Springer Nature Singapore Pte Ltd. 2020
R. Ogawa (ed.), *Total Scar Management*, https://doi.org/10.1007/978-981-32-9791-3_7

height/thickness. POSAS scores are based on estimations by both the patient and the observer. Thus, the patient scar assessment scale (P-SAS) is used to estimate the degree of pain and pruritus and the color, stiffness, thickness, and irregularity of the scar relative to the normal skin, while the observer scar assessment scale (O-SAS) is used to evaluate the extent of vascularization, pigmentation, thickness, relief, and pliability. In addition, in 2015, we developed a new scoring system in the Japanese Scar Workshop. This JSW scar scale is used to specifically diagnose pathological scars and is based on the notion that HSs and keloids represent successively worse stages of dermal inflammation [19, 20].

These various scar scales and our clinical experiences suggest that a number of key variables dictate scar severity. Along with the cause of the scar and its age and location, all of these variables should be assessed to the best, regardless of the type of scar. These variables relate to the objective appearance and functional impairment caused by the scars and the subjective effects of the scar, as experienced by the patient, on sensation and psychosocial aspects. The objective assessment involves primary visual and tactile variables, including color (pigmentation and vascularity), height or thickness, width, pliability, and surface roughness. The objective assessment also examines the effect of the scar on secondary hair growth (hypotrichosis or hypertrichosis) and distortion (e.g., contracture) and scar-related complications, including chronic wound, infection, lymphedema, and skin cancer. In the subjective assessment, the patient is asked whether there is pain, itchiness, or dysesthesia and whether the scar has had psychosocial consequences (Table 7.1). These variables can be measured in a qualitative manner (e.g., yes or no), graded in a semiquantitative fashion (e.g., mild, moderate, and severe), or estimated quantitatively (e.g., mm or mm^2).

Regardless of the scar scale or tool or approach that is chosen, scar severity should be assessed with the aim of identifying the most suitable therapy given the patient's expectations (as indicated by the subjective variables) and clinical feasibility (as determined by the doctor's objective evaluations).

7.3 Clinical and Pathological Diagnoses of Cutaneous Scars

In this chapter, dermatological scars will be classified as normal scars, atrophic scars, hypertrophic scars, keloids, and malignant ulcers of scars. Although individual patients may bear various types of scars (even within the same scar), these different scar types will be discussed here as independent lesions that can be differentially diagnosed on the basis of their clinical manifestations (e.g., history, symptoms, signs, and characteristics) and pathological features (e.g., cellular and extracellular matrix [ECM] changes). We will also discuss how keloids can be differentiated from hypertrophic scars, which resemble them, thereby assuring the most appropriate therapy for both types of scars.

7.3.1 Normal scars

Normal scars (also known as mature scars) usually present as superficial and mature scars that have a pliable texture and a flat or slightly elevated appearance. There may or may not be changes in pigmentation. The original injury generally occurred one or more years ago. Clinically, they can have a linear (Fig. 7.1a) or bridge (Fig. 7.1b) shape and do not provoke functional impairment or significant aesthetic concerns. The hypopigmentation of such normal scars can be so mild that it is difficult even for physicians to distinguish their exact boundaries from the neighboring normal skin. However, when compared to normal skin at the pathological level, there are clear changes. First, the epidermis of normal scars is thinner and has flattened rete ridges. Second, the dermal collagen bundles are broader and are more likely to be aligned parallel to the epidermis. Third, the collagens in the deep dermis exhibit obvious fragmentation that makes it difficult to distinguish the papillary/superficial dermis from the reticular/deep dermis. Fourth, the elastic fibers in the superficial dermis appear to be smaller in diameter than the elastic fibers in normal skin (0.54 vs. 1.08 μm); this is also observed in the deep dermis (1.16 vs. 1.99 μm) (both $p < 0.05$) [21].

Table 7.1 Clinical variables that are assessed during comprehensive assessment of cutaneous scar severity

Objective (appearance and function)	Primary	Visual	Color:	pigmentation, vascularity
			Height/thickness:	contour, irregularity
			Width	
		Tactile	Pliability	
			Roughness	
	Secondary	Hair	Hypotrichosis/hypertrichosis	
		Distortion	Contracture	
	Complication:	chronic wound, infection, lymphedema, skin cancer		
Subjective	Sensation			
	Psychosocial			

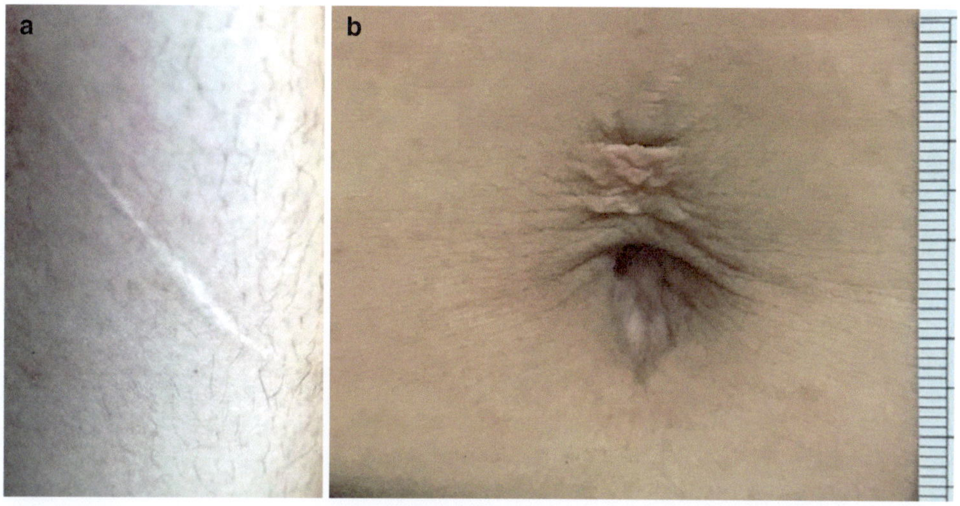

Fig. 7.1 The different shapes that can be taken by normal scars. (**a**) Linear scar on the left forearm. (**b**) Scar bridge above the umbilicus

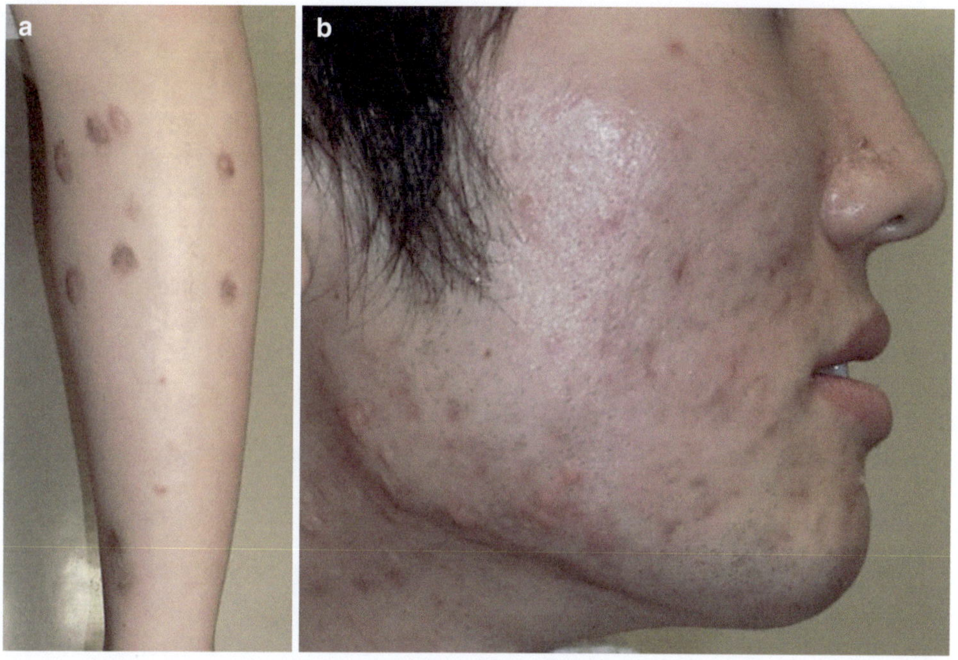

Fig. 7.2 Atrophic scars after external fixation of bone fracture or acne. (**a**) Atrophic scars after external fixation of bone fracture. Note the hypertrophic scars on the medial side. (**b**) Atrophic scars after acne on the face. Note that the scars on the lower jaw are hypertrophic

This is supported by stereological analysis that shows that the elastic system, which is composed of fibrillin-1 and elastin, is disrupted in normal scars. Specifically, in both the superficial and deep dermis, the fibrillin-1-containing fibers in normal scars occupy less volume (as shown by lower fibillin-1 volume densities) than those in normal skin. However, the dermal fibrillin-1 volume density in normal scars is higher than that in hypertrophic scars and keloids. This pattern was also observed for the elastin-containing fibers in the superficial dermis (i.e., elastin volume density: normal skin > normal scars > hypertrophic scars ≈ keloids). However, in the deep dermis, normal skin, normal scars, and hypertrophic scars have similar elastin fiber volumes, although all have lower elastin volume density in the deep dermis than keloids [22].

7.3.2 Atrophic Scars

Atrophic scars (also known as depressive scars) are scars that exhibit indentation or depression in the skin below the level of the surrounding tissues. Hyperpigmentation or hypopigmentation may be present. They are often caused by cystic acne, surgery, burns, and trauma.

Clinically, atrophic scars occur most commonly on the face and head and the skin lying above the tibia. The obviously sunken appearance of these scars associates somewhat with collagen damage or abnormalities in collagen production and injury, atrophy, or deficit of the underlying subcutaneous tissue. They are typically seen in acne scars on the face and scars above the tibia (Fig. 7.2). Goodman has proposed that postacne atrophic scars can be divided into three subtypes on the basis of the depth and extent of inflammation, namely, superficial macular scars, deeper dermal scars, and perifollicular scars. These subtypes are characterized by discolored macules, sharp-walled/ice pick/troughed scars, and hypopigmented papular scars, respectively [23]. Quite often, atrophic scars that lie close to the underlying bone (such as those overlying the tibia) tend to have thin and fragile skin that is susceptible to friction and wounding. This instability potentiates repeated ulcerations or secondary chronic ulceration. The latter may result in malignant transformation (see Sect. 7.4).

Pathologically, atrophic scars are characterized by drawing-in of the epithelium, an exaggeratedly atrophic dermis, and atrophy of the underlying fat. The collagen bundles are obviously atrophic under the microscope and the elastin fibers are thin, disrupted, and fragmented (Fig. 7.3) [24]. These pathological patterns may reflect the changes in gelatinolysis: ELISA and gelatin zymography analyses of the pro and active forms of matrix metalloproteinase (MMP)-2 in normal human skin and various scar types showed that atrophic scars have much lower MMP-2 levels (0.006 ng/mg protein) than normal skin (0.216 ng/mg protein), hypertrophic scars (0.407 ng/mg protein), and keloids (1.223 ng/mg protein). As a result, atrophic scars have lower active/pro-MMP-2 ratios (0.48) than normal skin (0.54), hypertrophic scars (0.69), and keloids (0.97) [25]. MMP-2 usually has baseline expression in various noninflammatory cells and plays a maintenance role in normal dermis. These findings suggest the involvement of deranged gelatinolytic activity in the remodeling phase in atrophic scars [26].

7.3.3 Hypertrophic Scars

Hypertrophic scars are pathological raised scars that develop either immediately or within months from obvious wounds that are caused by burn, trauma, or incision. The mass of these scars characteristically remains within the boundary of the original wound and may flatten spontaneously 1–2 years after they appear (Fig. 7.4a). These scars are aesthetically unappealing and can have psychological consequences when they are on exposed parts of the body. Moreover, if they are located over or near a joint, they can impair joint function due to their contracture (Fig. 7.4b). In such cases, surgery that releases the contracture and thereby restores joint function is needed.

At the pathological level, it has long been thought that hypertrophic scars are distinguished from other scar types, including keloids, by the presence of dermal nodules [27]. These well-demarcated nodules are composed of focal aggregates of fibroblasts and randomly oriented collagen fibers [28]. The pathological diagnosis of hypertrophic scars is further supported by the expression pattern of α-smooth muscle actin (α-SMA); it is thought that hypertrophic scars have diffuse expression of α-SMA while keloids display little or only focal expression of α-SMA [27]. Notably, compared to normal scars, the epidermis of hypertrophic scars exhibits enhanced expression of the keratins K6 and K16. This signifies keratinocyte activation, which may delay re-epithelization and prolong epidermal inflammation [29]. Indeed, hypertrophic scars exhibit elevated numbers of Langerhans cells, increased expression of epidermal interleukin-4, and reduced expression of epidermal interleukin-1α

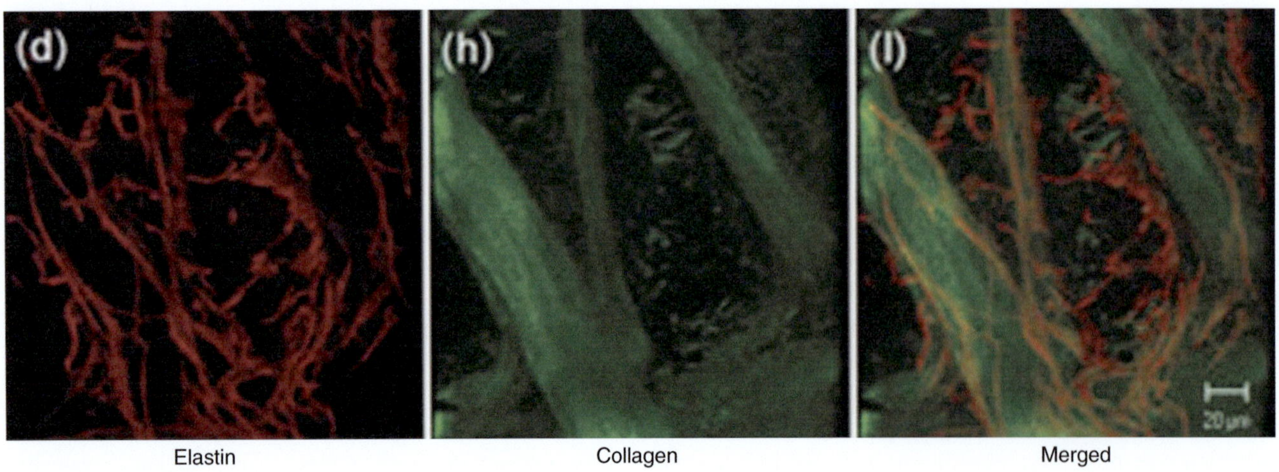

Fig. 7.3 Evaluation of elastin and collagen fibers in unstained atrophic scars without fixation and sectioning. Two-photon excited fluorescence (TPEF) was used to identify the elastin fibers (red, left panel), while the second harmonic generation (SHG) technique was used to indicate the collagen fibers (green, middle panel). The three-dimensional TPEF and SHG images are overlapped in the right panel. The images are from Zhu et al. with permission (Quantification of scar margin in keloid different from atrophic scar by multiphoton microscopic imaging. Scanning. 2011;33(4):195–200)

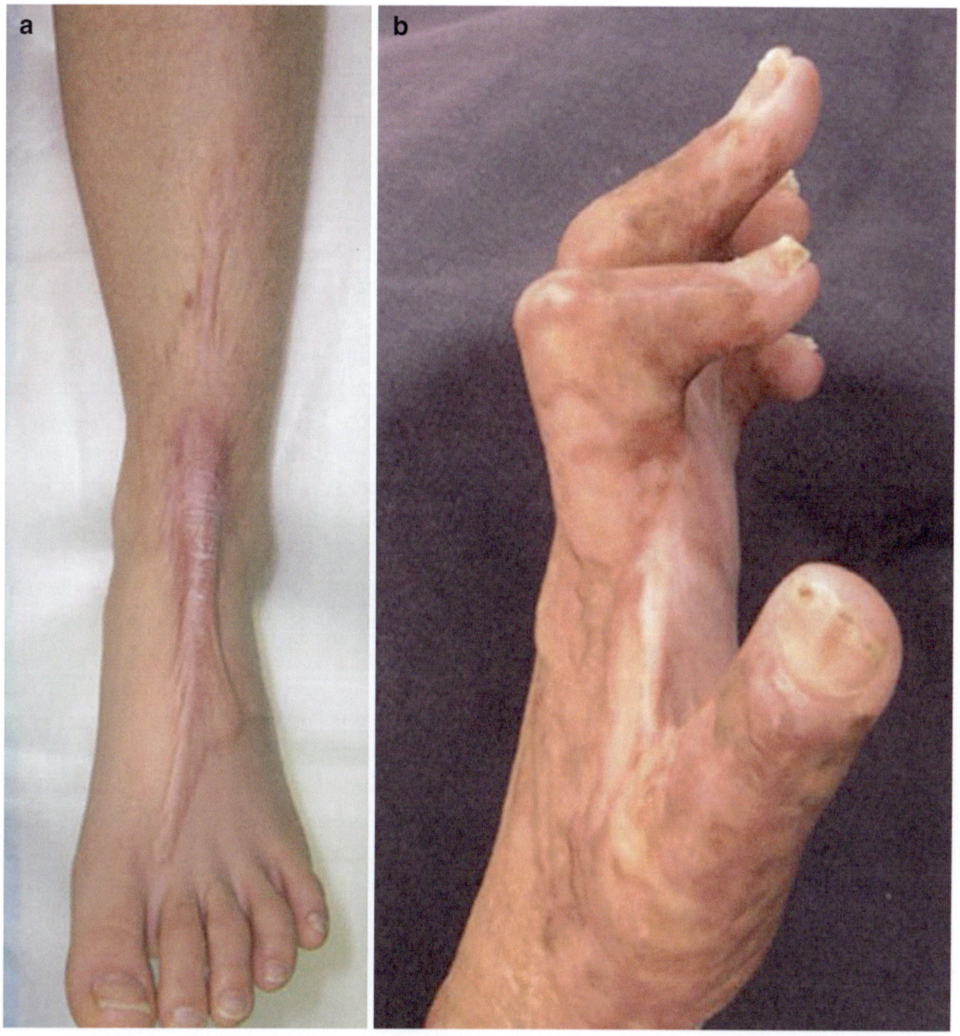

Fig. 7.4 Hypertrophic scars and the functional impairment caused by their contracture. (**a**) Thick hypertrophic scar without functional impairment. (**b**) Typical claw hand after burn

[30, 31]. Moreover, Rossiello et al. showed that the epidermis of hypertrophic scars expresses higher levels of cyclooxygenase-1 than the epidermis of normal skin and keloid specimens [32]. These findings support the notion that excessive, prolonged, and/or abnormal inflammatory/immunological signaling from the epidermis may promote aberrant dermal remodeling and thereby contribute to the formation of hypertrophic scars [33].

The dermis of hypertrophic scars is markedly expanded compared to the dermis of normal skin and the loosely arrayed wavy collagen bundles are flatter, less clearly demarcated, somewhat fragmented, and shortened compared to those in normal skin. However, the majority of the collagen bundles still run parallel to the epithelial surface [34] and Friedman et al. showed that the average type I/III collagen ratio is 7.73, which is similar to the ratio in normal skin (6.28) or normal scar (5.97) and much lower than the ratio in keloids (17.28) [35]. Hyaluronan, which is an ECM component that is distributed throughout the papillary dermis intensely in normal skin and thinner in mature scars, only occurs as a narrow strip in hypertrophic scars. Keloids display even less papillary dermis hyaluronan [36]. Fibronectin in the dermis, which decreases gradually in maturing scars, persists in hypertrophic scars as diffuse lines or curls [37]. However, hypertrophic scars do not exhibit more mast cells than normal scars [30].

7.3.4 Keloids

Keloids are pathological scars that are the result of excessive wound healing. The word "excessive" here is consistent with their striking clinical features. First, even minor traumas such as a 'mosquito bite' or minor local folliculitis can result in keloids. Second, keloids grow continuously due to massive and prolonged inflammation, especially on the advancing edge, which is often erythematous. Third, keloids grow beyond the confines of their original wound, thus causing them to project into the neighboring healthy skin. They never regress over time and surgical excision rarely stops their growth and indeed associates with high recurrence rates. However, since it takes time for these diagnostic temporal and spatial clinical symptoms of keloids to manifest themselves, it takes 3 months to 1 year after the wounding for the doctors to distinguish these scars from normal scars, which mature around this time.

The prevalence of keloids varies from 0.09% in the United Kingdom to 16% in the Congo [38, 39]. Our epidemiological data of 1500 anatomic regions in 483 Japanese patients show that keloids are mostly seen on the anterior chest (48.9%), scapular regions (26.9%), and lower jaw-neck regions (12.1%) [40] (Fig. 7.5). Notably, these areas are highly mobile and/or are exposed to high stretching tension; by contrast, keloids rarely develop on areas such as the parietal region or the anterior lower leg where skin stretching/contraction is rare [40]. Furthermore, keloids often take typical shapes on particular areas of the body. For example, chest keloids resemble a crab's claw, keloids on the scapular region have butterfly or dumbbell shape, and earlobe keloids take a ball shape. Local mechanics analyses show that these shapes are largely determined by the predominant directions and distribution of skin tension that characterize these different areas of the body [41] (Fig. 7.6). This notion is further supported by an in vitro study that showed that dermal fibroblasts, which are present in vast numbers in keloids, are highly sensitive to cyclic stretching simulation: when stimulated in this manner, they become resistant to apoptosis and rapidly migrate and reorient themselves perpendicular to the direction of stretch [42].

Pathologically, the most pathognomonic characteristic of keloids is the presence of hyalinized collagen in the reticular dermis. Moreover, compared to normal scars or normal skin, keloids exhibit pronounced infiltration of inflammatory cells, namely, T cells, B cells, and alternative macrophages (M_2). Notably, they have normal intraepidermal Langerhans cell numbers [43]. Keloids also exhibit mast cell activation, as indicated by the upregulated expression of the specific activation marker MC β-tryptase [44]. Several studies suggest that, like in hypertrophic scars, epithelial–mesenchymal interactions may contribute to keloid pathogenesis. First, in vitro studies suggest that the keratinocytes from keloid epidermis induce fibroblasts to secrete connective tissue growth factor in a paracrine fashion. This factor enhances fibrosis by either acting as a cofactor or a downstream mediator of transforming growth factor β [45]. Second, Rossiello et al. found that keloid epidermis expresses higher levels of cyclooxygenase-2 than the epidermis of normal skin and hypertrophic scars [32]. Proliferating cell nuclear antigen expression analyses of skin specimens show that the fibroblasts in the keloid dermis are more proliferative

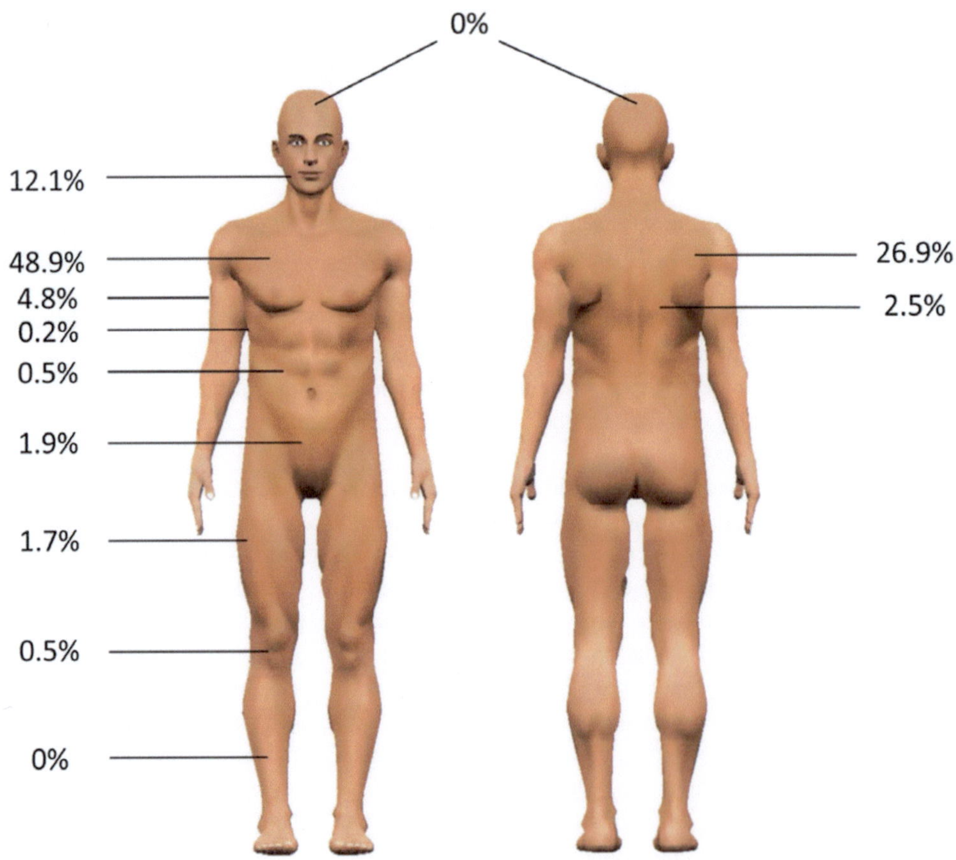

Fig. 7.5 Site-specific frequency of keloids. Pathological scarring associates with skin stretching/contraction: mechanical forces play a key role in keloid pathogenesis. From Ogawa et al. Wound Repair Regen. 2012;20(2):149–57

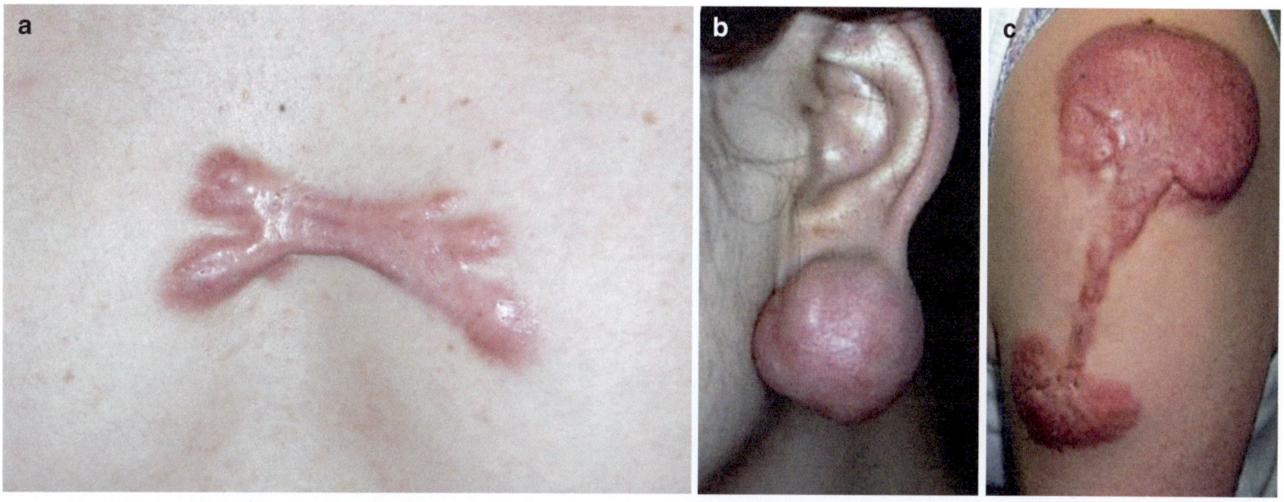

Fig. 7.6 The typical skin tension-dependent shapes of keloids on specific sites that are particularly prone to keloid formation. (**a**) Crab's claw on the chest. (**b**) Ball on the earlobe. (**c**) Dumbbell on the scapular region

(75.1% ± 8.1%) than those in hypertrophic scar (45.6% ± 10.6%, $p < 0.01$) and normal skin (38.8% ± 6.3%, $p < 0.01$) [46]. Moreover, as mentioned above, Friedman et al. showed that keloids have much higher type I/III collagen ratio than normal skin (17.28 vs. 6.28) [35]. Uitto et al. observed a greater type I/III procollagen mRNA ratios in keloid (22.1 ± 7.8) than in normal human skin (5.2 ± 2.1) cell cultures, due to elevated procollagen type I mRNA expression and unaltered procollagen III mRNA expression [47]. Keloids also exhibit higher fibronectin expression than normal skin [48], and hyaluronan is primarily detected in the thickened granular and spinous layers of the epidermis and the least in the papillary dermis [36].

It is generally not difficult to diagnose keloids if the patient has the typical clinical history, the lesion is on an area that is prone to keloid formation, and the lesion is itchy or painful. However, sometimes physicians mistake keloids for other diseases that have a similar appearance, such as chondroid syringoma [49]. This mistake is promoted by the fact that physicians rarely suggest that keloid-like lesions should be biopsied. Moreover, physicians sometimes do not realize that some keloidal response arise because the patient has an unsuspected inflammatory disease (e.g., nodular/keloidal scleroderma [50]). The most deleterious of these misdiagnoses is when the lesion is actually a malignant tumor (e.g., malignant dermatofibrosarcoma protuberans [DFSP]) or an infectious disease (e.g., lobomycosis). This is problematic because treating these lesions with steroid injection, which is the common therapeutic approach for keloids, not only delays the correct diagnosis, it may aggravate the disease.

In relation to these misdiagnosed diseases, DFSP is a spindle cell tumor in the dermis that resembles keloids, especially its sclerosing [51] or atrophic [52] types (Fig. 7.7). The differential diagnosis depends on the typical findings of DSFP, namely, monomorphous spindle-shaped cells that are arranged in a storiform pattern in a fibrous stroma [51], and on immunohistochemical staining for CD34 expression: keloids do not express CD34, whereas 75% of DFSP tumor cells do [53–55].

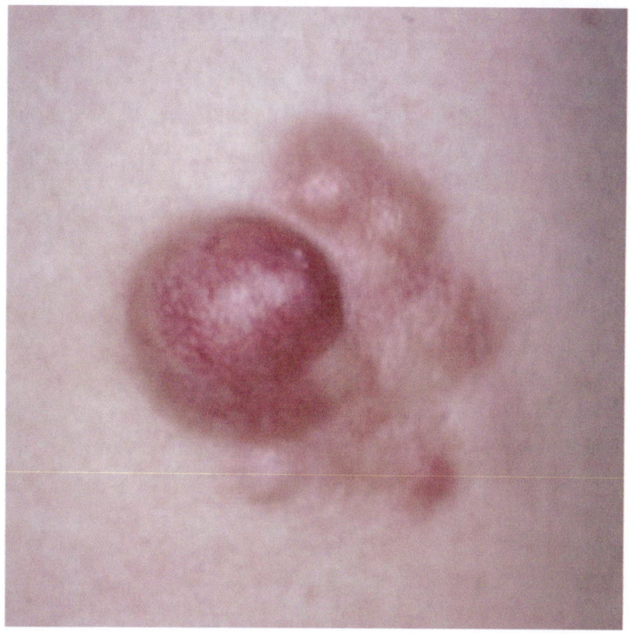

Fig. 7.7 DFSP on the abdomen

Lobomycosis (also called lacaziosis or keloidal blastomycosis) is a chronic fungal infection of the skin that is caused by *Lacazia loboi*, which is endemic in rural regions in south/central America (Fig. 7.8). The clinical presentation is post-traumatic cutaneous nodules [56] or keloidal-like lesions that initially present as single plaque, papule, or nodule [57] in the highly exposed areas several years after initial expo-

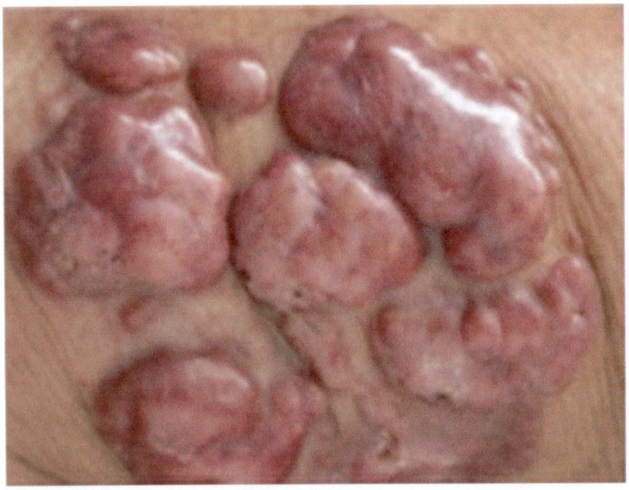

Fig. 7.8 Typical primary fibrous appearance of lobomycosis. These lesions present as nodular plaques that are covered by smooth and shiny skin and that have small exulcerated areas and visible telangiectasias. From Francesconi et al. Lobomycosis: epidemiology, clinical presentation, and management options. Therapeutics and Clinical Risk Management 2014;10:851–860

sure and incubation. Differentially diagnosing these lesions from keloids is further confused by the fact that fungal infection is suspected to be a contributing factor for keloid pathogenesis [58]. However, the diagnosis of lobomycosis can be readily established by scraping the lesion and determining whether the fungus and/or other fungal structures (e.g., catenular or Rosario bead distribution) can be directly visualized under a microscope [59].

7.3.5 Similarities and Differences Between Hypertrophic Scars and Keloids

Hypertrophic scars and keloids are both pathological scars. However, keloids differ from hypertrophic scars in that they never stop growing and exhibit high recurrence rates after treatment. This refractoriness of keloids to treatment in particular has caused clinicians and pathologists to expend considerable efforts on distinguishing between hypertrophic scars and keloids: the hope was that this would lead to orderly and effective guidelines for treating these two pathological scar entities. However, recent progress in this field has upended the paradigm that hypertrophic scars and keloids are disparate scar types: rather, there is increasing evidence that hypertrophic scars and keloids are actually different stages of the same fibroproliferative skin disorder.

There are indeed marked clinical differences between classical hypertrophic scars and keloids. Hypertrophic scars usually derive from a definite trauma, whereas keloids can develop from minute wounds such as a 'mosquito bite', vaccination, or hair folliculitis; in fact, they sometimes seem to arise without any skin injury. Hypertrophic scars do not favor particular sites of the body, although they are notorious for inducing transarticular contraction that impairs joint function and necessitates reconstructive surgery. By contrast, keloids occur on areas of the body that are exposed to marked local mechanics. Hypertrophic scars also confine their growth within the original wound, whereas keloids grow beyond the original wound. Moreover, hypertrophic scars tend to stop growth gradually and the rate of recurrence after surgery is low. By contrast, keloids never regress spontaneously and often recur after surgery (Table 7.2).

Table 7.2 Clinical differentiation between hypertrophic scars and keloids

Clinical feature	Hypertrophic scars	Keloids
Definite injury history	+	±
Prevalence	Varies, injury dependent	0.9–16%
Predilection site	Unspecific	Mechanic related (e.g., chest, deltoid, earlobe)
Specific shape	–	Tension related (e.g., butterfly, dumbbell, ball)
Contracture	+	–
Excessive growth	Within the original wound boundary	Beyond the original wound boundary
Spontaneous regression	±	–
Recurrence after excision	Low	High

Pathologists also proposed that several pathognomonic features distinguish hypertrophic scars from keloids, namely, α-SMA (diffuse in hypertrophic scars, little or focal in keloids), dermal nodules (present in hypertrophic scars, absent in keloids), and hyalinized collagen (present in keloids, absent in hypertrophic scars). However, multiple lines of evidence show that these pathological distinctions are not as clear-cut as was once believed. First, with regard to α-SMA, it was found that collagen nodules of some hypertrophic scars contained no α-SMA expressing myofibroblasts [60], whereas 45% of keloids do express it. The strongest and most diffuse staining is actually found in keloid but not HS lesions [61]. Moreover, pathological scars can show both α-SMA$^+$ staining within dermal nodules (characteristic of hypertrophic scars) and large amounts of hyalinized collagens (characteristic of keloids) [61]. These findings suggest that α-SMA staining cannot really be considered to be a pathognomonic marker of hypertrophic scars.

The notion that hyalinized collagens are pathognomonic for keloids has also been cast into doubt: Lee detected this diagnostic hallmark in only 55% of their keloid specimens [61]. Moreover, in many cases, the hyalinized keloidal fibers can exhibit quite different features within the same keloid

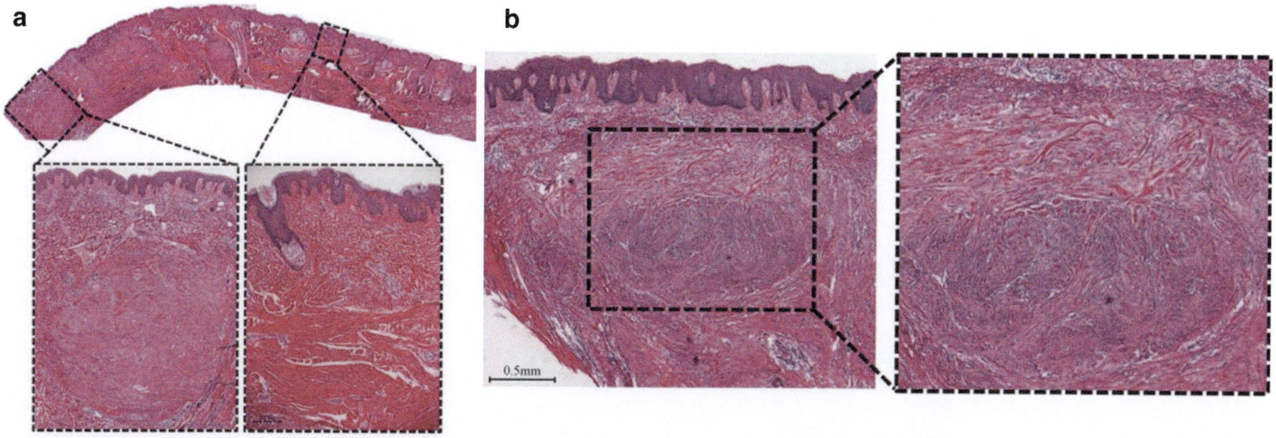

Fig. 7.9 A keloid sample that exhibits spatial transition from hypertrophic scar morphology to keloidal morphology. Samples such as this support the notion that hypertrophic scars and keloids are successive stages of the same fibroproliferative skin disorder. From: Huang et al. Are keloid and hypertrophic scar different forms of the same disorder? A fibroproliferative skin disorder hypothesis based on keloid findings. Int Wound J. 2014;11(5):517–22. (**a**) The same keloid sample can bear both keloidal collagen and dermal nodules. This HE staining slide shows a cross section of a resected lesion from a keloid patient. The center of the lesion is in the middle and to the right of the section, while the lesion periphery is to the left. The reticular dermis of this keloid is vastly expanded, as is usual for keloids. The hyalinized keloidal collagens predominate in the center of the lesion and become increasingly sparser towards the periphery of the lesion. By contrast, the dermal nodules demonstrate increased nodular size and cellularity, less well-defined nodular outlines, and decreased quantity and thickness of collagens to the periphery of the sample. (**b**) The dermal nodules, which are composed of focal fibroblast aggregates and randomly oriented collagen fibers, have hyalinized collagens scattered on their top. The nature of these hyalinized collagen fibers change with location: at the nodule base, the fibers are short, wavy, and have a random orientation in relation to the epidermis. They are also non-eosinophilic. By contrast, the fibers at the nodule top are long, straight, and lie parallel to the epidermis. They are also strongly eosinophilic

sample. Thus, in the keloid center, the fibers are often large and thick and show strong eosinophilic staining and parallel alignment to the epithelial surface. Moreover, the intercollagen fibers are thin and sparsely dispersed. By contrast, in the keloid periphery, the collagens are often not hyalinized and they are thin in diameter, low in density, and random in orientation. In addition, the intercollagen fibers are more normal than those in the center [62].

Of particular significance, the same keloid sample can also bear both keloidal hyalinized collagens and the dermal nodules that are considered to be pathognomonic for hypertrophic scars. An example is shown in Fig. 7.9a. Interestingly, we have observed on numerous occasions that these ambiguous lesions exhibit a spatial transition from hypertrophic scar features to keloidal features. First, as described above, the hyalinized collagen fibers predominate in the center of the lesion and become increasingly sparser towards the periphery of the lesion. By contrast, while the dermal nodules gradually increase in size towards the lesion periphery and become much less well demarcated until they become the predominant feature (Fig. 7.9a). Second, the dermal nodules themselves are typically comprised of focal fibroblast aggregates that contain randomly oriented collagen fibers. However, the nodules also contain hyalinized fibers whose appearance changes as we move from looking at the base of the nodule to its top. Thus, the hyalinized fibers at the nodule base are short, wavy, randomly oriented, and non-eosinophilic. By contrast, the hyalinized fibers at the nodule top are long, straight, oriented parallel to the epidermis, and strongly eosinophilic (Fig. 7.9b) [62].

These findings led us to hypothesize that hypertrophic scars and keloids are successive stages of the same fibroproliferative skin disorder (Fig. 7.9). It may be that the fate of a wound (i.e., hypertrophic scar or keloid) depends on how much inflammation is generated. This is supported by the fact that keloids have more activated inflammatory cells (e.g., macrophages) and higher CD4/CD8 ratios than normal skins [63]. This notion is also supported by the fact that pronounced inflammation also associates with a particularly pernicious feature of keloids, namely, their growth into surrounding normal tissue, since their leading edge often exhibits much greater inflammation (as well as erythema and pruritus) than their core [62].

7.4 Malignant Ulcer

Malignant ulcers that arise in preexisting scars are called Marjolin's ulcer. They are secondary to chronic ulceration in the scars (Fig. 7.10). Scar-related risk factors for post-scar malignant ulceration include scar fragility that increases susceptibility to trauma and an irregular shape that makes it difficult to clean the scar and increases the risk of ulcer and infection. The latency period between the original wounding

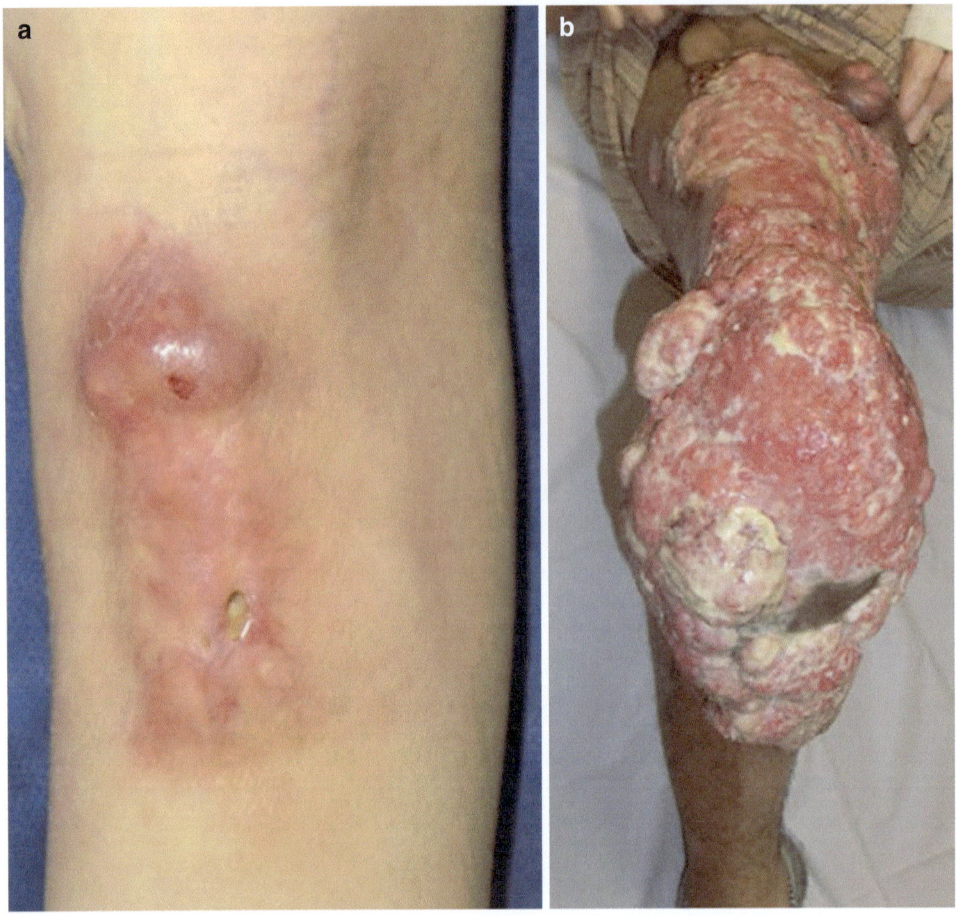

Fig. 7.10 Malignant ulceration secondary to burns scars. Biopsies confirmed that the scars had developed into squamous cell carcinoma. (**a**) Postburn Marjolin's ulcer, which developed from a scar on the right lower extremity. (**b**) Marjolin's ulcer, which developed from extensive burn scars on the right leg

and malignancy varies from as little as 6 weeks [64] to as long as 70 years [65]: the average latency period is about 35 years [66]. Such malignant transformation occurs in nearly 2% of the burn scars [67]. The lymphatic obstruction within scars may delay the dissemination of the tumor cells somewhat, thereby inhibiting local and systemic metastasis. However, if the malignant cells in Marjolin's ulcer reach the lymphatic vessels, the tumor will spread rapidly [65].

Chronic ulcers that arose more than 6 weeks previously should be biopsied to determine whether Marjolin's ulcer has developed. The diagnosis is dependent on the scar and ulcer history and the clinical and laboratory examinations [68], as follows:

- *History:* The patient has had a chronic ulcer within the margins of the scar for longer than 3 months.
- *Symptomatic triad:* Nodule formation, induration, and ulceration.
- *Clinical findings:* Exuberant/excessive granulation tissue, rolled/everted wound margins, bleeding on contact, foul-smelling purulence, crusting over, increased size, and pain.
- *Staging and grading:* Marjolin's ulcer can be graded on the basis of the frequency of differentiated cells. Grade I = >75%, Grade II = 75–25%, and Grade III = <25%. Higher grades associate with a greater risk of metastasis and a worse prognosis [69, 70].
- *Morphological forms:* The common form is the flat, indurated, infiltrative, ulcerative variant with poor differentiation. The less frequent form is the exophytic, papillary variety, which is well differentiated and associates with a better prognosis [65].
- *Pathological types:* The most frequently seen tumor in Marjolin's ulcer is squamous cell carcinoma (71%), followed by basal cell carcinoma (12%), melanoma (6%), sarcoma (5%), and other rare neoplasms such as fibrosarcoma, liposarcoma, and DFSP [71].

7.5 Summary

Given the stage of scar research at present, the commonly seen scars in the clinic can be divided into normal scars, atrophic scars, hypertrophic scars, and keloids. The objective and subjective clinical variables in various scar scales and tools can be used to diagnose the scars and thereby determine the treatment that will assure the best outcomes in terms of local appearance and function and avoidance of

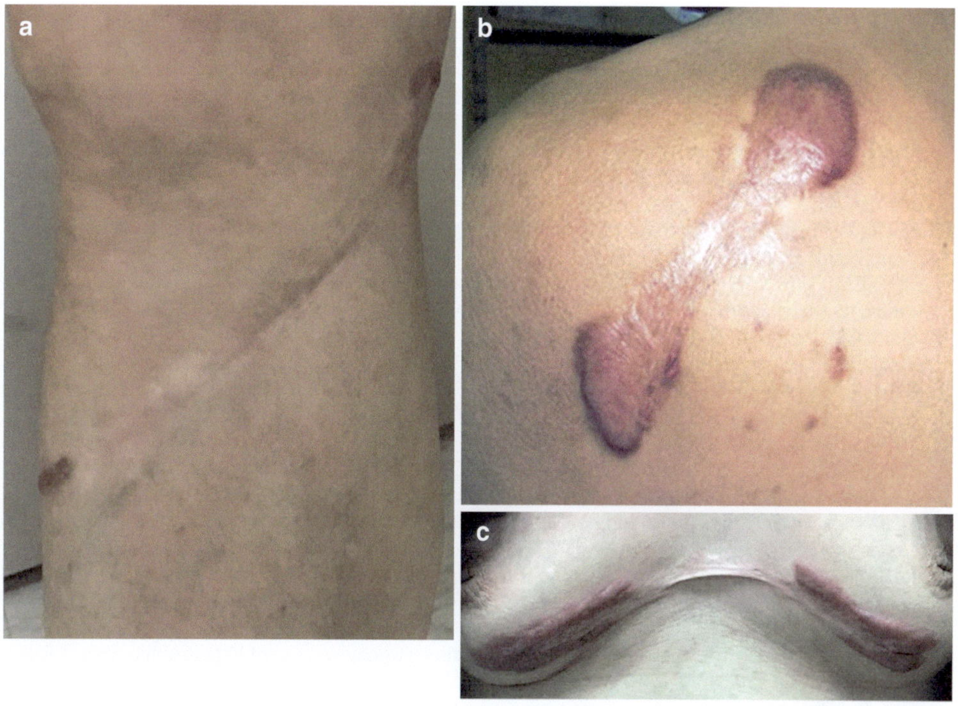

Fig. 7.11 Patients can have various types of scars within the same lesion. (**a**) Many years after the initial wounding on the anteromedial side of the right leg, this patient exhibits normal healing in the central part of the scar and the development of a keloid at both ends. Note that the normally healed part of the scar exhibits minute depigmentation. (**b**) The left scapular scar of this patient exhibits normal healing in its center and keloids on either end. Note the transition of different degrees of inflammation, as indicated by the erythema, from the center to the peripheries. (**c**) The scar of this patient exhibits normal scarring in the center and both hypertrophic scars and keloids at each end

complications such as malignant ulcer. However, biopsies are the best way to make a definite diagnosis. At the pathological level, the dermal event of collagen accumulation as a result of excessive wound healing is the shared characteristics in skin scarring. However, the scars can also differ in terms of their cellular and ECM constituents, which in turn lead to distinct pathological features. For example, hyalinized fibers are often seen in keloids, while dermal nodules are often seen in hypertrophic scars. However, while these features were once believed to be pathognomonic for keloids and hypertrophic scars, respectively, increasing lines of evidence suggest that this distinction is not as clear-cut as was once believed. In particular, the same pathological scar sample can bear both hyalinized collagen fibers and dermal nodules. Moreover, since such ambiguous samples often exhibit spatial transitions in these features, we propose that hypertrophic scars and keloids may be different stages in the same soft tissue fibroproliferative disease.

Currently, there are no clinical or pathological thresholds or other definitive markers that will allow physicians to distinguish between the various scar types with full confidence, especially at the early stages of wound healing. This situation can be further complicated by the fact that some patients have more than one scar type concomitantly, each of which exhibits distinct degrees of local inflammation (Fig. 7.11). We recommend performing a biopsy if there is any confusion. Moreover, we emphasize that scars, especially those with complications, should be diagnosed with the aim of identifying the therapy that best improves the functional and aesthetic impairments and thereby provides a better quality of life. Thus, scar diagnoses and therapeutics should be based on not only what is feasible from the point of view of the physician but also the patient's preferences.

To date, researchers have put significant effort into identifying clinical and pathological variables and markers that help to identify the best therapy for individual scars and patients. However, these variables and markers have diagnostic limitations. To improve this situation, further research that elucidates the molecular etiologies of the different scar types is needed. This research may reveal laboratory biomarkers that improve scar diagnosis and/or can serve as targets for therapeutic pharmaceuticals. One promising avenue in this field is the role of local mechanics in scar formation. Further progress in our understanding of the mechanobiological mechanism that drives soft tissue fibroproliferative disorders [72] could well potentiate the discovery of laboratory markers that aid scar diagnosis and/or could be targeted in novel mechanotherapeutic interventions [73] that act at the molecular, cellular, or tissue level to facilitate normal wounding and prevent, ameliorate, or reverse the formation or progression of pathological scars.

References

1. Huang C, Murphy GF, Akaishi S, Ogawa R. Keloids and hypertrophic scars: update and future directions. Plast Reconstr Surg Glob Open. 2013;1(4):e25.
2. Huang C, Ogawa R. The link between hypertension and pathological scarring: does hypertension cause or promote keloid

and hypertrophic scar pathogenesis? Wound Repair Regen. 2014;22(4):462–6.
3. Huang C, Liu L, You Z, Wang B, Du Y, Ogawa R. Keloid progression: a stiffness gap hypothesis. Int Wound J. 2017;14(5):764–71.
4. Huang C, Liu L, You Z, Zhao Y, Dong J, Du Y, Ogawa R. Endothelial Dysfunction and mechanobiology in pathological cutaneous scarring: lessons learned from soft tissue fibrosis. Br J Dermatol. 2017;177(5):1248–55.
5. Huang C, Ogawa R. Roles of lipid metabolism in keloid development. Lipids Health Dis. 2013;12:60.
6. Huang C, Akaishi S, Ogawa R. Mechanosignaling pathways in cutaneous scarring. Arch Dermatol Res. 2012;304(8):589–97.
7. Smith GM, Tompkins DM, Bigelow ME, Antoon AY. Burn-induced cosmetic disfigurement: can it be measured reliably? J Burn Care Rehabil. 1988;9(4):371–5.
8. Sullivan T, Smith J, Kermode J, McIver E, Courtemanche DJ. Rating the burn scar. J Burn Care Rehabil. 1990;11(3):256–60.
9. Yeong EK, Mann R, Engrav LH, Goldberg M, Cain V, Costa B, Moore M, Nakamura D, Lee J. Improved burn scar assessment with use of a new scar-rating scale. J Burn Care Rehabil. 1997;18(4):353–5.
10. Beausang E, Floyd H, Dunn KW, Orton CI, Ferguson MW. A new quantitative scale for clinical scar assessment. Plast Reconstr Surg. 1998;102(6):1954–61.
11. Crowe JM, Simpson K, Johnson W, Allen J. Reliability of photographic analysis in determining change in scar appearance. J Burn Care Rehabil. 1998;19(2):183–6.
12. Draaijers LJ, Tempelman FR, Botman YA, Tuinebreijer WE, Middelkoop E, Kreis RW, van Zuijlen PP. The patient and observer scar assessment scale: a reliable and feasible tool for scar evaluation. Plast Reconstr Surg. 2004;113(7):1960–5.
13. Masters M, McMahon M, Svens B. Reliability testing of a new scar assessment tool, Matching Assessment of Scars and Photographs (MAPS). J Burn Care Rehabil. 2005;26(3):273–84.
14. Singer AJ, Arora B, Dagum A, Valentine S, Hollander JE. Development and validation of a novel scar evaluation scale. Plast Reconstr Surg. 2007;120(7):1892–7.
15. Hultman CS, Friedstat JS, Edkins RE, Cairns BA, Meyer AA. Laser resurfacing and remodeling of hypertrophic burn scars: the results of a large, prospective, before-after cohort study, with long-term follow-up. Ann Surg. 2014;260(3):519–29.
16. Hultman CS, Edkins RE, Lee CN, Calvert CT, Cairns BA. Shine on: review of laser- and light-based therapies for the treatment of burn scars. Dermatol Res Pract. 2012;2012:243651.
17. Nguyen TA, Feldstein SI, Shumaker PR, Krakowski AC. A review of scar assessment scales. Semin Cutan Med Surg. 2015;34(1):28–36.
18. Idriss N, Maibach HI. Scar assessment scales: a dermatologic overview. Skin Res Technol. 2009;15(1):1–5.
19. Ogawa R, Akaishi S, Akita S, Okabe K, Shimizu T, Sunaga A, Tosa Y, Nagao M, Yamawaki S. JSW Scar Scale Working Group. Japan Scar Workshop (JSW) Scar Scale 2015. Available online at. http://www.scarkeloid.com/en/index.html.
20. Ogawa R. Keloid and hypertrophic scars are the result of chronic inflammation in the reticular dermis. Int J Mol Sci. 2017;18(3):606.
21. Zhu X, Zhuo S, Zheng L, Lu K, Jiang X, Chen J, Lin B. Quantified characterization of human cutaneous normal scar using multiphoton microscopy. J Biophotonics. 2010;3(1-2):108–16.
22. Amadeu TP, Braune AS, Porto LC, Desmoulière A, Costa AM. Fibrillin-1 and elastin are differentially expressed in hypertrophic scars and keloids. Wound Repair Regen. 2004;12(2):169–74.
23. Goodman GJ. Postacne scarring: a review of its pathophysiology and treatment. Dermatol Surg. 2000;26(9):857–71.
24. Zhu X, Zhuo S, Zheng L, Jiang X, Chen J, Lin B. Quantification of scar margin in keloid different from atrophic scar by multiphoton microscopic imaging. Scanning. 2011;33(4):195–200.
25. Tanriverdi-Akhisaroglu S, Menderes A, Oktay G. Matrix metalloproteinase-2 and -9 activities in human keloids, hypertrophic and atrophic scars: a pilot study. Cell Biochem Funct. 2009;27(2):81–7.
26. Gillard JA, Reed MW, Buttle D, Cross SS, Brown NJ. Matrix metalloproteinase activity and immunohistochemical profile of matrix metalloproteinase-2 and -9 and tissue inhibitor of metalloproteinase-1 during human dermal wound healing. Wound Repair Regen. 2004;12(3):295–304.
27. Ehrlich HP, Desmoulière A, Diegelmann RF, Cohen IK, Compton CC, Garner WL, Kapanci Y, Gabbiani G. Morphological and immunochemical differences between keloid and hypertrophic scar. Am J Pathol. 1994;145(1):105–13.
28. Clark JA, Turner ML, Howard L, Stanescu H, Kleta R, Kopp JB. Description of familial keloids in five pedigrees: evidence for autosomal dominant inheritance and phenotypic heterogeneity. BMC Dermatol. 2009;9:8.
29. Machesney M, Tidman N, Waseem A, Kirby L, Leigh I. Activated keratinocytes in the epidermis of hypertrophic scars. Am J Pathol. 1998;152(5):1133–41.
30. Niessen FB, Schalkwijk J, Vos H, Timens W. Hypertrophic scar formation is associated with an increased number of epidermal Langerhans cells. J Pathol. 2004;202(1):121–9.
31. Niessen FB, Andriessen MP, Schalkwijk J, Visser L, Timens W. Keratinocyte-derived growth factors play a role in the formation of hypertrophic scars. J Pathol. 2001;194(2):207–16.
32. Rossiello L, D'Andrea F, Grella R, Signoriello G, Abbondanza C, De Rosa C, Prudente M, Morlando M, Rossiello R. Differential expression of cyclooxygenases in hypertrophic scar and keloid tissues. Wound Repair Regen. 2009;17(5):750–7.
33. Mustoe TA, Gurjala A. The role of the epidermis and the mechanism of action of occlusive dressings in scarring. Wound Repair Regen. 2011;19(Suppl 1):s16–21.
34. Rockwell WB, Cohen IK, Ehrlich HP. Keloids and hypertrophic scars: a comprehensive review. Plast Reconstr Surg. 1989;84(5):827–37.
35. Friedman DW, Boyd CD, Mackenzie JW, Norton P, Olson RM, Deak SB. Regulation of collagen gene expression in keloids and hypertrophic scars. J Surg Res. 1993;55(2):214–22.
36. Bertheim U, Hellström S. The distribution of hyaluronan in human skin and mature, hypertrophic and keloid scars. Br J Plast Surg. 1994;47:483–9.
37. Nagata H, Ueki H, Fibronectin MT. Localization in normal human skin, granulation tissue, hypertrophic scar, mature scar, progressive systemic sclerotic skin, and other fibrosing dermatoses. Arch Dermatol. 1985;121:995–9.
38. Louw L. Keloids in rural black South Africans. Part 1: general overview and essential fatty acid hypotheses for keloid formation and prevention. Prostaglandins Leukot Essent Fatty Acids. 2000;63(5):237–45.
39. Sun LM, Wang KH, Lee YC. Keloid incidence in Asian people and its comorbidity with other fibrosis-related diseases: a nationwide population-based study. Arch Dermatol Res. 2014;306(9):803–8.
40. Ogawa R, Okai K, Tokumura F, Mori K, Ohmori Y, Huang C, Hyakusoku H, Akaishi S. The relationship between skin stretching/contraction and pathologic scarring: the important role of mechanical forces in keloid generation. Wound Repair Regen. 2012;20(2):149–57.
41. Ogawa R, Akaishi S, Huang C, Dohi T, Aoki M, Omori Y, Koike S, Kobe K, Akimoto M, Hyakusoku H. Clinical applications of basic research that shows reducing skin tension could prevent and treat abnormal scarring: the importance of facial/subcutaneous tensile reduction sutures and flap surgery for keloid and hypertrophic scar reconstruction. J Nippon Med Sch. 2011;78:68–76.

42. Huang C, Miyazaki K, Akaishi S, Watanabe A, Hyakusoku H, Ogawa R. Biological effects of cellular stretch on human dermal fibroblasts. J Plast Reconstr Aesthet Surg. 2013;66(12):e351–61.
43. Bagabir R, Byers RJ, Chaudhry IH, et al. Site-specific immunophenotyping of keloid disease demonstrates immune upregulation and the presence of lymphoid aggregates. Br J Dermatol. 2012;167:1053–66.
44. Ong CT, Khoo YT, Mukhopadhyay A, et al. Comparative proteomic analysis between normal skin and keloid scar. Br J Dermatol. 2010;162:1302–15.
45. Khoo YT, Ong CT, Mukhopadhyay A, et al. Upregulation of secretory connective tissue growth factor (CTGF) in keratinocyte-fibroblast coculture contributes to keloid pathogenesis. J Cell Physiol. 2006;208:336–43.
46. Nakaoka H, Miyauchi S, Miki Y. Proliferating activity of dermal fibroblasts in keloids and hypertrophic scars. Acta Derm Venereol. 1995;75:102–4.
47. Uitto J, Perejda AJ, Abergel RP, et al. Altered steady-state ratio of type I/III procollagen mRNAs correlates with selectively increased type I procollagen biosynthesis in cultured keloid fibroblasts. Proc Natl Acad Sci U S A. 1985;82:5935–9.
48. Kischer CW, Hendrix MJ. Fibronectin (FN) in hypertrophic scars and keloids. Cell Tissue Res. 1983;231:29–37.
49. Ogawa R, Akaishi S, Hyakusoku H. Differential and exclusive diagnosis of diseases that resemble keloids and hypertrophic scars. Ann Plast Surg. 2009;62(6):660–4.
50. James WD, Berger TG, Butler DF, Tuffanelli DL. Nodular (keloidal) scleroderma. J Am Acad Dermatol. 1984;11(6):1111–4.
51. Sabater-Marco V, Pérez-Vallés A, Berzal-Cantalejo F, Rodriguez-Serna M, Martinez-Diaz F, Martorell-Cebollada M. Sclerosing dermatofibrosarcoma protuberans (DFSP): an unusual variant with focus on the histopathologic differential diagnosis. Int J Dermatol. 2006;45(1):59–62.
52. Martin L, Combemale P, Dupin M, Chouvet B, Kanitakis J, Bouyssou-Gauthier ML, Dubreuil G, Claudy A, Grimand PS. The atrophic variant of dermatofibrosarcoma protuberans in childhood: a report of six cases. Br J Dermatol. 1998;139(4):719–25.
53. Kamath NV, Ormsby A, Bergfeld WF, House NS. A light microscopic and immunohistochemical evaluation of scars. J Cutan Pathol. 2002;29(1):27–32.
54. Aiba S, Tabata N, Ishii H, Ootani H, Tagami H. Dermatofibrosarcoma protuberans is a unique fibrohistiocytic tumour expressing CD34. Br J Dermatol. 1992;127(2):79–84.
55. Altman DA, Nickoloff BJ, Fivenson DP. Differential expression of factor XIIIa and CD34 in cutaneous mesenchymal tumors. J Cutan Pathol. 1993;20(2):154–8.
56. Burns RA, Roy JS, Woods C, Padhye AA, Warnock DW. Report of the first human case of lobomycosis in the United States. J Clin Microbiol. 2000;38(3):1283–5.
57. Paniz-Mondolfi AE, Reyes Jaimes O, Dávila Jones L. Lobomycosis in Venezuela. Int J Dermatol. 2007;46(2):180–5.
58. Okada E, Maruyama Y. Are keloids and hypertrophic scars caused by fungal infection? Plast Reconstr Surg. 2007;120(3):814–5.
59. Francesconi VA, Klein AP, Santos AP, Ramasawmy R, Francesconi F. Lobomycosis: epidemiology, clinical presentation, and management options. Ther Clin Risk Manag. 2014;10:851–60.
60. Moshref SS, Mufti ST. Keloid and hypertrophic scars: comparative histopathological and immunohistochemical study. JKAU: Med Sci. 2010;17(3):3–22.
61. Lee JY, Yang CC, Chao SC, Wong TW. Histopathological differential diagnosis of keloid and hypertrophic scar. Am J Dermatopathol. 2004;26(5):379–84.
62. Huang C, Akaishi S, Hyakusoku H, Ogawa R. Are keloid and hypertrophic scar different forms of the same disorder? A fibroproliferative skin disorder hypothesis based on keloid findings. Int Wound J. 2014;11(5):517–22.
63. Boyce DE, Ciampolini J, Ruge F, Murison MS, Harding KG. Inflammatory-cell subpopulations in keloid scars. Br J Plast Surg. 2001;54:511–6.
64. Mohammadi AA, Seyed Jafari SM, Hosseinzadeh M. Early Marjolin's ulcer after minimal superficial burn. Iran J Med Sci. 2013;38:69–70.
65. Aydoğdu E, Yildirim S, Aköz T. Is surgery an effective and adequate treatment in advanced Marjolin's ulcer? Burns. 2005;31:421–31.
66. Copcu E. Marjolin's ulcer: a preventable complication of burns? Plast Reconstr Surg. 2009;124:156e–64e.
67. Gul U, Kilic A. Squamous cell carcinoma developing on burn scar. Ann Plast Surg. 2006;56(4):406–8.
68. Pekarek B, Buck S, Osher LA. Comprehensive review on Marjolin's ulcers: diagnosis and treatment. J Am Col Certif Wound Spec. 2011;3(3):60–4.
69. Ogawa B, Chen M, Margolis J, Schiller FJ, Schnall SB. Marjolin's ulcer arising at the elbow: a case report and literature review. Hand (N Y). 2006;1(2):89–93.
70. Smith J, Mello LF, Nogueira Neto NC, Meohas W, Pinto LW, Campos VA, Barcellos MG, Fiod NJ, Rezende JF, Cabral CE. Malignancy in chronic ulcers and scars of the leg (Marjolin's ulcer): a study of 21 patients. Skeletal Radiol. 2001;30(6):331–7.
71. Kowal-Vern A, Criswell BK. Burn scar neoplasms: a literature review and statistical analysis. Burns. 2005;31:403–13.
72. Huang C, Ogawa R. Fibroproliferative disorders and their mechanobiology. Connect Tissue Res. 2012;53(3):187–96.
73. Huang C, Holfeld J, Schaden W, Orgill D, Ogawa R. Mechanotherapy: revisiting physical therapy and recruiting mechanobiology for a new era in medicine. Trends Mol Med. 2013;19(9):555–64.

Acne Scars: How They Form and How to Undo Them

8

Acne Scars

Mi Ryung Roh and Kee Yang Chung

8.1 Introduction

Acne is a very common skin disease, with an estimated prevalence of >80% in adolescence [1]. Acne is one of the main but temporary concerns of juveniles but the consequence can be a life-long problem if it results in scar formation due to uncontrolled inflammation. Scarring often results in a substantial negative impact on patients' overall function and social well-being [2]. Acne scars are associated with decreased self-confidence, including perception of decreased employability and embarrassment, and are negatively perceived by society [3, 4], thereby justifying the need for early and effective treatments. Although scarring can occur with any type of acne [5], early treatment of inflammatory and nodulocytic acne is the most important way to prevent acne scars. Scars that develop during the early years of adolescent acne may persist through lifetime and in some cases worsen with normal aging or photodamage [6]. Once scar develops, treating them can be very difficult, time consuming, financially burdensome, and often incomplete. The degree of success in acne scar treatment greatly depends on the modality of treatment according to acne scar type. Therefore, knowledge of the different acne scar types and their relationship with skin anatomy and histology along with various treatment modalities are essential to make appropriate treatment decisions.

8.2 Pathogenesis of Acne Related to Scar Formation

Acne is a chronic inflammatory disease of the pilosebaceous unit. The pathogenesis of acne is currently attributed to multiple factors such as increased sebum production, alteration in the quality of sebum lipids, regulation of cutaneous steroidogenesis, androgen activity, interactions with neuropeptides, exhibition of pro- and anti-inflammatory properties, follicular hyperkeratinization, and the proliferation of *Propionibacterium acnes* within the follicle [7, 8]. The increased sebum excretion is a major concurrent event associated with the development of acne. Sebaceous gland lipids exhibit direct pro- and anti-inflammatory properties, whereas the induction of 5-lipoxygenase and cyclooxygenase-2 pathways in sebocytes leads to the production of pro-inflammatory lipids [9]. Furthermore, hormones like androgens control the sebaceous gland size and sebum secretion. Keratinocytes and sebocytes may be activated by *P. acnes* via Toll-like receptor (TLR), CD14, and CD1 molecules [10], which may stimulate the secretion of cytokines such as interleukin (IL)-6 and IL-8 by follicular keratinocytes and IL-8 and IL-12 in macrophages, giving rise to inflammation [11]. Certain *P. acnes* species may induce an immunological reaction by stimulating the production of sebocyte and keratinocyte antimicrobial peptides, which play an important role in the innate immunity of the follicle [12]. Inflammatory lesions have a propensity to form scars as they heal. In some circumstances, excessive production of collagenase and elastase in the course of the inflammatory process results in unwanted breakdowns of collagen and elastic fibers, which cause the skin surface to sink down, leading to atrophic scars [13, 14]. Alternatively, there may be an overproduction of collagen itself, leading to hypertrophic scars or keloids [13, 14]. Type and severity of the scar varies according to the degree of inflammation, extent of tissue damage, and duration of tissue damage [15, 16]. Therefore, treatment of each type of scar requires understanding of the pathophysiology of the inflammatory process.

8.3 Classification of Acne Scars

Acne scars are classified into atrophic, hypertrophic, or keloidal, with atrophic being the most common accounting for 75% of all scars [13]. Atrophic scars are further classified

M. R. Roh (✉) · K. Y. Chung
Department of Dermatology and Cutaneous Biology Research Institute, Yonsei University College of Medicine, Seoul, Korea
e-mail: karenroh@yuhs.ac; kychung@yuhs.ac

© Springer Nature Singapore Pte Ltd. 2020

R. Ogawa (ed.), *Total Scar Management*, https://doi.org/10.1007/978-981-32-9791-3_8

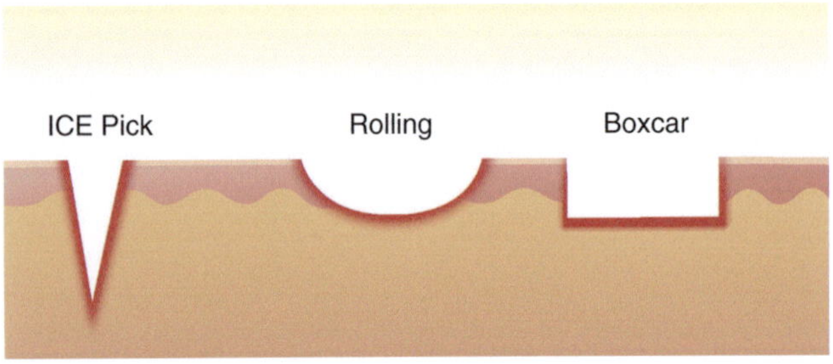

Fig. 8.1 Classification of atrophic acne scars

into ice pick, rolling, and boxcar scars based on their appearance (Fig. 8.1) [14, 17]. Ice pick scars are narrow (<2 mm), deep, sharply marginated epithelial tracts that extend vertically to the deep dermis or subcutaneous tissue. The surface opening is usually, but not always, wider than the deeper infundibulum as the scar tapers from the surface to its deepest apex. Rolling scars are formed by dermal tethering of otherwise relatively normal-appearing skin and are usually wider than 4–5 mm. Abnormal fibrous anchoring of the dermis to the subcutis leads to a rolling or undulating appearance of the overlying skin that casts superficial shadow. Although they tend to be shallow, correction of the subdermal component is essential for treatment success. Boxcar scars are round to oval depressions with sharply demarcated vertical edges, similar to varicella scars. They are clinically wider at the surface than ice pick scars and do not taper to a point at the base. They may be shallow (0.1–0.5 mm) or deep (≥5 mm) and are most often 1.5–4.0 mm in diameter. Other less common types of scars, such as hypertrophic or keloidal scars, and sinus tracts may occur with more severe and deeper inflammation.

8.4 Treatment of Acne Scars

There are numerous procedures for improving and correcting acne scars. However, treatment of acne scars must be individually prescribed for each patient depending on the types of scars they present with. Often, combination of procedures is required to obtain the best result as individual patients commonly display more than one scar type and even have a combination of atrophic, hypertrophic, and keloid scars, plus active inflammatory lesions [13, 18]. Traditionally, obtaining patient history is essential with evaluation of recent isotretinoin use and history of keloid or hypertrophic scar formation. Recently, a systematic review of the safety of procedural interventions performed either concurrently with the systemic isotretinoin therapy or immediately following the cessation was conducted. Based on the available literature, mechanical dermabrasion and fully ablative lasers are not recommended in the setting of systemic isotretinoin treatment; however, there was insufficient evidence to support delaying most acne treatment modalities, including fractional ablative and nonablative laser procedures, superficial chemical peels, and manual dermabrasion [19]. Therefore, on the basis of this information, for some patients and some conditions, an informed decision may lead to earlier and potentially more effective interventions for acne scar treatment.

8.5 Laser Therapy

Laser therapy has been a continuously evolving treatment option for acne scars. Although laser has great therapeutic potential, achieving the optimal balance between efficacy and side effects has been challenging. Traditional ablative lasers emit light at wavelengths targeting absorption by water molecules in the skin. This results in the generation of heat and elimination of the epithelium, papillary dermis, and, in some cases, the reticular dermis [20], and ultimately re-epithelialization, collagen synthesis, and remodeling occur (Fig. 8.2). The ablative 10,600 nm CO_2 laser and 2940 nm Er:YAG have shown significant and sustained clinical improvement with a single treatment session in acne scars (Fig. 8.3) [21, 22]. However, while these lasers are effective, due to the complete removal of the superficial cutaneous layers, there is significant recovery time which limits its use these days when patients ask for minimal downtime. It is also common for patients to experience persistent erythema, edema, oozing, crusting after treatment, and post-inflammatory hyperpigmentation in patients with darker skin type [23].

Therefore, the most widely used treatment for atrophic acne scars is fractional laser resurfacing. Fractional lasers create numerous, discrete columns of thermal damage with intervening untreated areas. Each treated area, known as the microscopic treatment zone (MTZ), spans an area of 100–300 μm and penetrates deeply into the tissue, up to 1500 μm (Fig. 8.2) [24, 25]. Through the creation of these MTZs, fractional lasers induce dermal remodeling and, in the case of ablative fractional lasers, re-epithelialization. Healing is

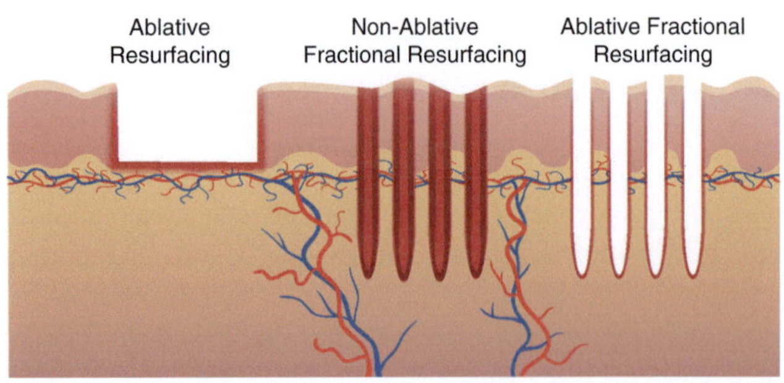

Fig. 8.2 Schematic figure for the zone of damage in ablative and fractional lasers

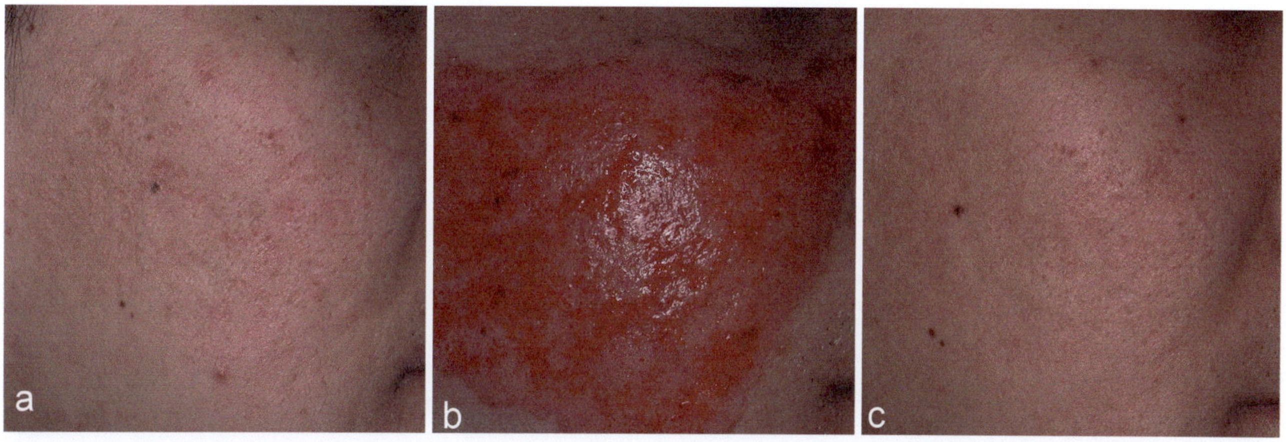

Fig. 8.3 Clinical photo of an acne scar patient before (**a**), post-laser (**b**), and after (**c**) ablative 2940 nm Er:YAG laser treatment

augmented by migration of unaffected keratinocytes from untreated areas [25]. Among these technologies, fractional nonablative lasers, fractional ablative CO_2 and Er:YAG lasers, and fractional radiofrequency (RF) devises have been most successful in improving acne scars. However, in most cases, patients need to undergo a series of treatment sessions, and the best results are often obtained when laser therapy is combined with other treatment modalities [18]. The 1550 nm fractional erbium-doped laser was the first available fractional laser system and it has been demonstrated to be beneficial in the treatment of acne scars [26]. Since it is a nonablative laser, the 1550 nm fractional laser leaves the epidermis intact. As a result, post-procedure erythema, edema, bleeding, crusting, infection, and scarring are less of a concern than with ablative fractional lasers. However, like other nonablative lasers, multiple treatment sessions are necessary. The fractional 1550 nm erbium laser is also safe to use in patients with all skin types but the clinical results may be more modest in patients with darker skin types [27]. Ablative fractional lasers include fractional 10,600 nm CO_2 laser, fractional 2940 nm Er:YAG laser, and fractional 2790 nm yttrium-scandium-gallium-garnet (YSGG) laser. Among these, ablative fractional 10600 nm CO_2 laser has been most widely used for acne scar treatment with successful results (Fig. 8.4) [24]. A comparative review found that success rates for atrophic scar treatment could be higher with ablative lasers (using CO_2 or Er:YAG lasers), but there was a trade-off in terms of prolonged erythema and higher incidences of post-inflammatory hyperpigmentation (92% vs. 13% with nonablative laser therapy) [28]. Acne scars often show erythema which can be treated with either 585 or 595 nm pulsed dye lasers in skin type I to V or intense pulsed light (IPL) in skin type I to IV [29]. Dyschromia or post-inflammatory hyperpigmentation (PIH) associated with acne can be treated with Q-switched (QS) alexandrite or Nd:YAG lasers in all skin types.

8.6 Fractional Radiofrequency Therapy

Fractional radiofrequency (RF) therapy [30] is a noninvasive method of tissue tightening that can be used for all types of atrophic scars. High-frequency energy is delivered into the skin causing water in the skin to heat up, stimulating the wound healing response. The resulting collagen remodeling, neocollagenesis, and neoelastogenesis improve the appearance of the skin. RF uses an array of small bipolar electrodes further decreasing the propensity for discomfort during the procedure. RF treatment alone for acne scars showed an improvement of 25–75% in 3–4 treatment sessions [31]. Although these results are not as dramatic as fractional ablative CO_2 lasers when used alone, side effects such as post-inflammatory pigmentation are uncommon which allows the rationale for combining treatment with other lasers to obtain better results. Combination of RF and nonablative laser treatments for acne scars can offer significant results in a wide array of skin types without the risk of major side effects while offering quicker recovery times and the ability to treat deeper scars than using RF treatments alone.

8.7 Chemical Reconstruction of Skin Scars (CROSS) Technique

CROSS method is a technique for the treatment of atrophic acne scars using an applicator to deeply deliver trichloroacetic acid (TCA) in high concentration. The technique was developed to induce neosynthesis of dermal components such as collagen, elastin, and ground substances [32]. The technique basically consists of firmly pressing down an applicator soaked in TCA on atrophic acne scars to produce a confluent frost. After 5–6 courses of treatment, 80–85% of the patients showed good clinical response using 65% TCA, whereas 90–95% of the patients presented with good clinical response

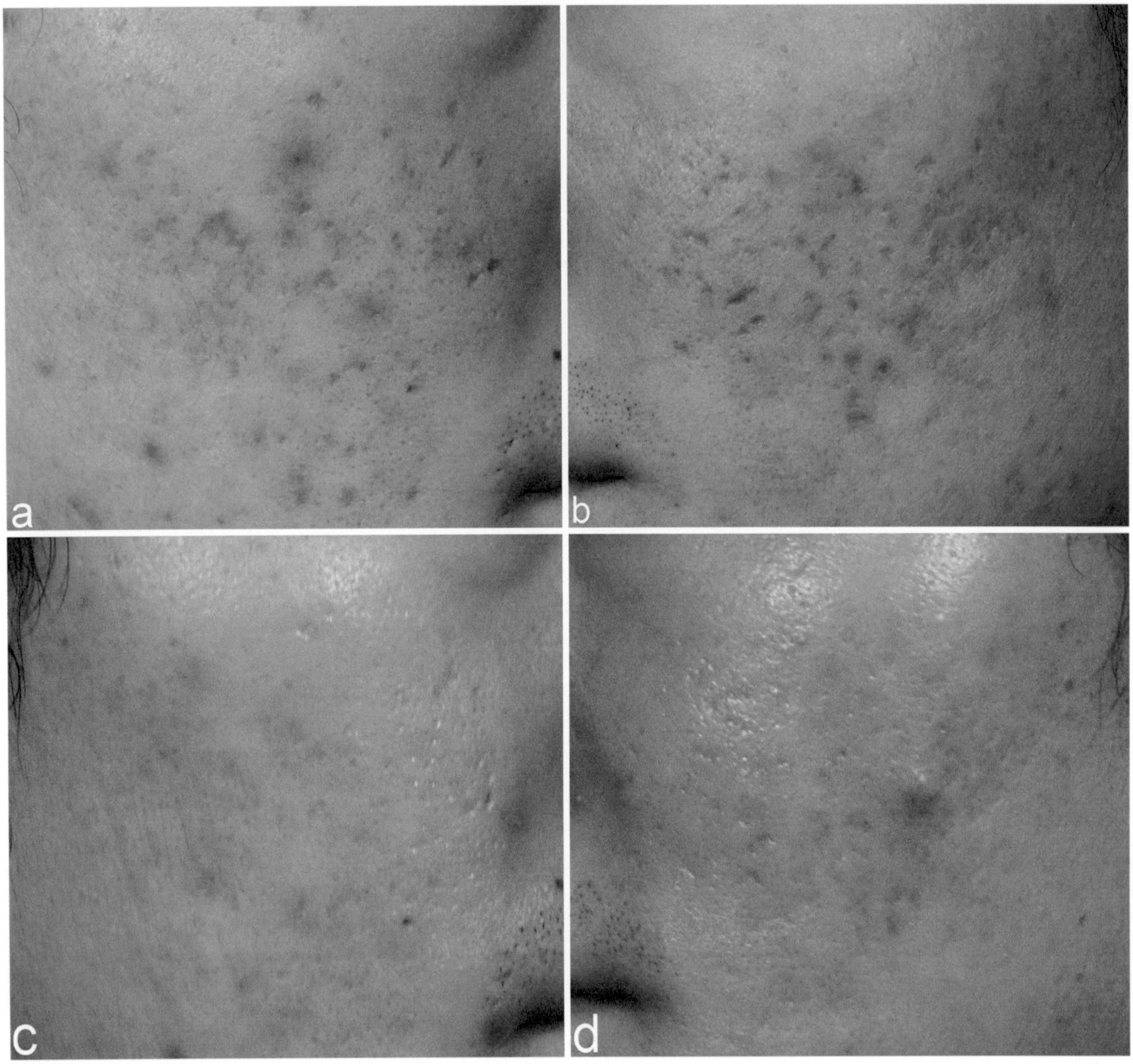

Fig. 8.4 Clinical photo of an acne scar patient before (**a**, **b**) and after (**c**, **d**) ablative fractional 10,600 nm CO_2 laser treatment

using 100% TCA (Fig. 8.5) [33]. Multiple sessions of treatment are required for better outcome. Side effects include posttreatment erythema which resolves over 2–8 weeks, and post-inflammatory hyperpigmentation which spontaneously disappears in about 6 weeks. This technique can be used for deep sharply demarcated scars such as ice pick and boxcar scars in combination with other treatment modalities.

8.8 Dermabrasion

Since the early 1900s, dermabrasion has been employed to physically remove the superficial skin layers, allowing healing to occur with a more cosmetically acceptable results. Through use of either a rotating motorized hand piece with a wire brush or a diamond-tipped hand piece, the procedure removes the epidermis and part of the dermis. The procedure requires local and sometimes general anesthesia because of significant pain [23]. Dermabrasion is effective in treating superficial atrophic scars, such as rolling or boxcar scars. However, the procedures have many potential complications, which are often operator and technique dependent. Erythema, photosensitivity, post-inflammatory pigmentation alterations, especially hypopigmentation, and post-procedural hypertrophic scarring are complications which can be permanent [34]. Although this procedure has fallen out of favor with the advent of resurfacing lasers, it is still useful in certain circumstances where other treatment options are unavailable.

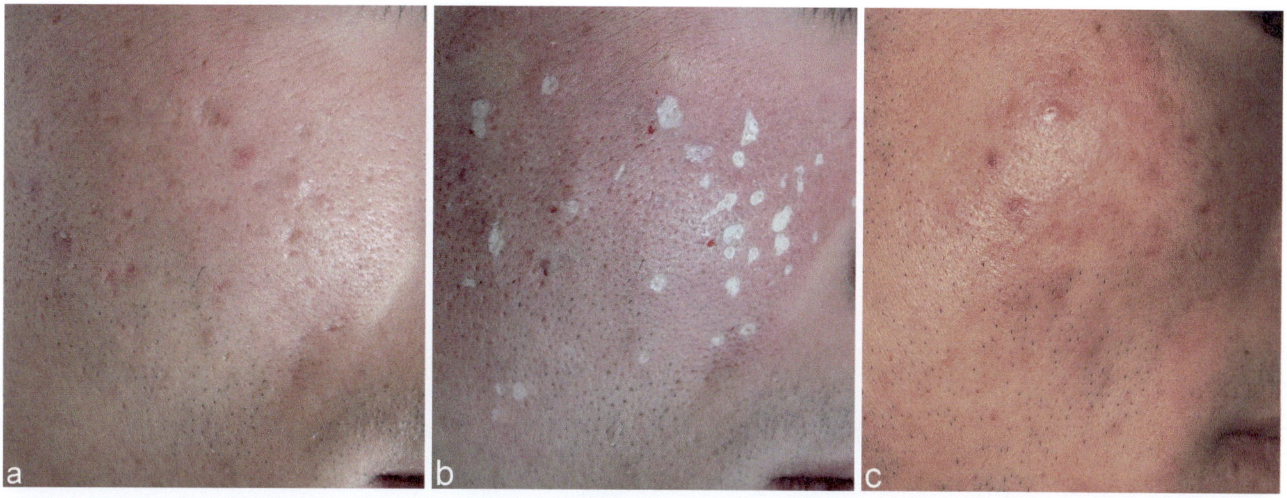

Fig. 8.5 Clinical photo of an acne scar patient before (**a**), post-CROSS (**b**), and after (**c**) CROSS treatment

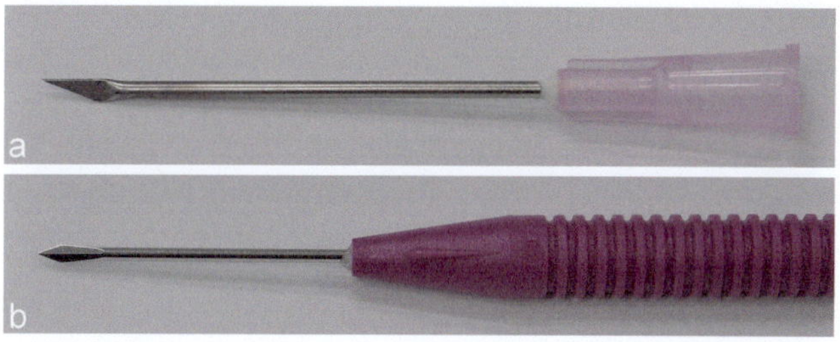

Fig. 8.6 Hypodermic needles used for subcision: (**a**) Nokor needle, (**b**) cataract blade

8.9 Subcutaneous Incision (Subcision)

Subcutaneous incision (subcision) is a simple surgical technique which uses various kinds of hypodermic needles (Fig. 8.6) inserted through a small puncture in the skin surface to undermine fibrous bands that cause depression of the scar. The releasing effect of the incisions and new connective tissue formed during the course of normal wound healing may add volume helping to achieve a flatter, more regular surface (Fig. 8.7). Subcision can be applied to rolling scars in combination with dermal fillers, fractional lasers, or CROSS for the treatment of atrophic acne scars.

8.10 Dermal Fillers

The injection of dermal fillers to improve acne scars is based on soft tissue augmentation. Hyaluronic acid fillers (HAFs) are the most commonly used filler for correction of atrophic acne scars. HAFs have shown to induce a characteristic extracellular matrix (ECM) response which stimulates collagen production [35]. Dermal fillers can be used either alone or in combinations with other procedures such as subcision, microneedling, fractional lasers, and chemical peels. The outcome and longevity of the tissue augmentation depend not only on the filler type and injection technique but also on scar type. Best results have been obtained with fillers for rolling and boxcar scars [36].

8.11 Punch Techniques

Punch excisions have been shown to be effective for nondistensible deep ice pick and boxcar scars [13, 18]. Punch excision removes a pitted scar with a straight-walled disposable punch or hair transplant punch that is slightly larger than the scar being treated. The goal is to trade a larger, deeper scar for a smaller, linear closure that would be less noticeable and possibly fade with time [5]. Punch elevation combines the techniques of punch excision and grafting without the risk of skin color or texture mismatch. This technique is usually used for boxcar scars and after the scar has been isolated from the surrounding skin, it is elevated to be slightly raised against the bordering tissue. Retraction of the grafted tissue occurs during the healing phase, resulting in a leveled surface [16]. In punch replacement grafting, the scar is discarded and is replaced with a slightly larger full-thickness skin graft, usually from the postauricular area. This technique is suitable for sharp-walled or deep ice pick scars [37].

8.12 Microneedling

Microneedling, also known as percutaneous collagen induction (PCI), is a minimally invasive procedure that uses fine needles to puncture the epidermis. Modern microneedling devices contain multiple fine needles, typically 0.5–1.5 mm in length, located on a barrel and rolled on the skin to create

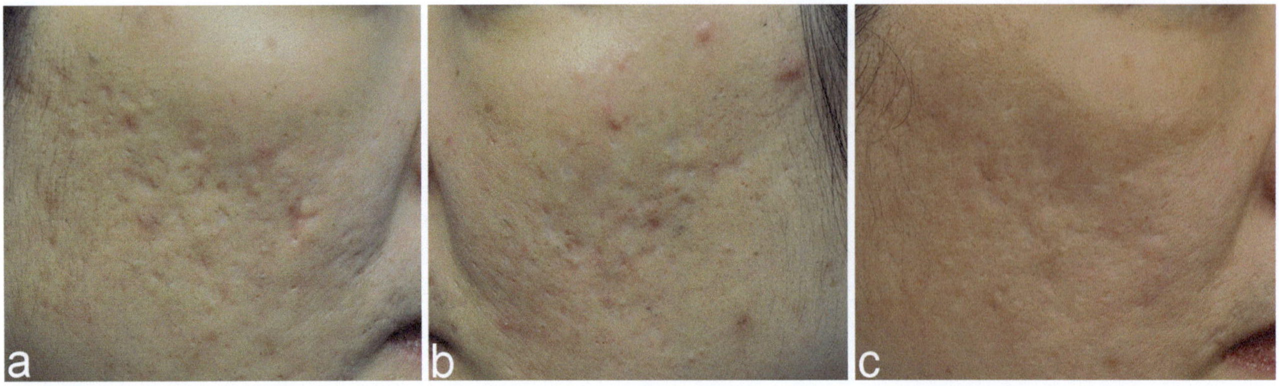

Fig. 8.7 Clinical photo showing improvement of rolling scars before (**a**, **b**) and after (**c**, **d**) subcision treatment

numerous punctures into the stratum corneum and the papillary dermis [38]. The procedure creates an even distribution of pinpoint bleeding, causing multiple microbruises in the dermis, which initiates a complex of cascade of growth factors ultimately resulting in collagen production. Microneedling has been most extensively studied for acne scar treatment. A recent review concluded that although studies analyzed were heterogenous in design, there is moderate evidence to support the use of microneedling as monotherapy for acne scars, especially rolling scars [39, 40]. Microneedling is associated with a low rate of side effects. Side effects are rare and temporary, with transient post-procedure erythema being the most common.

8.13 Combination Treatment

A number of treatment modalities are available and the choice for the individual patient is determined mainly by the type of scars present. Also most patient present with multiple types of acne scars. Therefore, single treatment modality for acne scars have less than ideal results requiring combination treatment. Ablative fractional lasers may offer the best compromise between efficacy and adverse effects. Nonablative lasers may be considered in patients with milder scars or who prefer to avoid ablative treatment. PDLs and intense pulse light systems can be utilized for erythematous acne scars or hypertrophic acne scars, and can be combined with other modalities to more completely address the atrophic defect. For all types of acne scars on the face, fractional ablative laser, fractional RF therapy, or microneedling can be used as an initial treatment modality. For erythematous acne scars, PDL or IPL can be applied. Dyschromia or post-inflammatory pigmentation associated with acne can be reduced with pigment laser such as laser toning. Following procedures may be applied for specific types of acne when improvement is limited with the above treatment modalities. For ice pick scars, CROSS and punch technique can be used. For rolling scars, subcision with or without dermal fillers can be used. In boxcar scars, CROSS or punch technique can be additionally used. Since acne scars are very complex and variable even in an individual patient, the appropriate choice of treatment modality for a given patient should take into account the extent of scarring, type and morphology of scars, as well as the patient's skin type. Additional patient goals and expectations regarding treatment timeline, number of treatment sessions, length of recovery time, and projected outcomes should be clearly discussed in order to optimize treatment experience and patient satisfactions.

References

1. Goulden V, Stables GI, Cunliffe WJ. Prevalence of facial acne in adults. J Am Acad Dermatol. 1999;41:577–80.
2. Koo JY, Smith LL. Psychologic aspects of acne. Pediatr Dermatol. 1991;8:185–8.
3. Dreno B, Tan J, Kang S, Rueda MJ, Torres Lozada V, Bettoli V, et al. How people with facial acne scars are perceived in society: an online survey. Dermatol Ther (Heidelb). 2016;6:207–18.
4. Chuah SY, Goh CL. The impact of post-acne scars on the quality of life among young adults in Singapore. J Cutan Aesthet Surg. 2015;8:153–8.
5. Goodman GJ, Baron JA. The management of postacne scarring. Dermatol Surg. 2007;33:1175–88.
6. Rivera AE. Acne scarring: a review and current treatment modalities. J Am Acad Dermatol. 2008;59:659–76.
7. Zouboulis CC. Acne and sebaceous gland function. Clin Dermatol. 2004;22:360–6.
8. Zouboulis CC, Bohm M. Neuroendocrine regulation of sebocytes—a pathogenetic link between stress and acne. Exp Dermatol. 2004;13(Suppl 4):31–5.
9. Alestas T, Ganceviciene R, Fimmel S, Muller-Decker K, Zouboulis CC. Enzymes involved in the biosynthesis of leukotriene B4 and prostaglandin E2 are active in sebaceous glands. J Mol Med (Berl). 2006;84:75–87.
10. Nagy I, Pivarcsi A, Kis K, Koreck A, Bodai L, McDowell A, et al. *Propionibacterium acnes* and lipopolysaccharide induce the expression of antimicrobial peptides and proinflammatory cytokines/chemokines in human sebocytes. Microbes Infect. 2006;8:2195–205.
11. Kurokawa I, Danby FW, Ju Q, Wang X, Xiang LF, Xia L, et al. New developments in our understanding of acne pathogenesis and treatment. Exp Dermatol. 2009;18:821–32.

12. Koreck A, Pivarcsi A, Dobozy A, Kemeny L. The role of innate immunity in the pathogenesis of acne. Dermatology. 2003;206:96–105.
13. Fabbrocini G, Annunziata MC, D'Arco V, De Vita V, Lodi G, Mauriello MC, et al. Acne scars: pathogenesis, classification and treatment. Dermatol Res Pract. 2010;2010:893080.
14. Jacob CI, Dover JS, Kaminer MS. Acne scarring: a classification system and review of treatment options. J Am Acad Dermatol. 2001;45:109–17.
15. Rao J. Treatment of acne scarring. Facial Plast Surg Clin North Am. 2011;19:275–91.
16. Thiboutot D, Gollnick H, Bettoli V, Dreno B, Kang S, Leyden JJ, et al. New insights into the management of acne: an update from the Global Alliance to Improve Outcomes in Acne group. J Am Acad Dermatol. 2009;60:S1–50.
17. Lacarrubba F, Verzi AE, Tedeschi A, Catalfo P, Nasca MR, Micali G. Clinical and ultrasonographic correlation of acne scars. Dermatol Surg. 2013;39:1683–8.
18. Fife D. Practical evaluation and management of atrophic acne scars: tips for the general dermatologist. J Clin Aesthet Dermatol. 2011;4:50–7.
19. Spring LK, Krakowski AC, Alam M, Bhatia A, Brauer J, Cohen J, et al. Isotretinoin and timing of procedural interventions: a systematic review with consensus recommendations. JAMA Dermatol. 2017;153:802–9.
20. Fitzpatrick RE, Rostan EF, Marchell N. Collagen tightening induced by carbon dioxide laser versus erbium: YAG laser. Lasers Surg Med. 2000;27:395–403.
21. Walia S, Alster TS. Prolonged clinical and histologic effects from CO2 laser resurfacing of atrophic acne scars. Dermatol Surg. 1999;25:926–30.
22. Woo SH, Park JH, Kye YC. Resurfacing of different types of facial acne scar with short-pulsed, variable-pulsed, and dual-mode Er:YAG laser. Dermatol Surg. 2004;30:488–93.
23. Alster TS, Lupton JR. Prevention and treatment of side effects and complications of cutaneous laser resurfacing. Plast Reconstr Surg. 2002;109:308–16. discussion 17–8.
24. Cho SB, Lee SJ, Kang JM, Kim YK, Chung WS, Oh SH. The efficacy and safety of 10,600-nm carbon dioxide fractional laser for acne scars in Asian patients. Dermatol Surg. 2009;35:1955–61.
25. Geronemus RG. Fractional photothermolysis: current and future applications. Lasers Surg Med. 2006;38:169–76.
26. Alster TS, Tanzi EL, Lazarus M. The use of fractional laser photothermolysis for the treatment of atrophic scars. Dermatol Surg. 2007;33:295–9.
27. Mahmoud BH, Srivastava D, Janiga JJ, Yang JJ, Lim HW, Ozog DM. Safety and efficacy of erbium-doped yttrium aluminum garnet fractionated laser for treatment of acne scars in type IV to VI skin. Dermatol Surg. 2010;36:602–9.
28. Ong MW, Bashir SJ. Fractional laser resurfacing for acne scars: a review. Br J Dermatol. 2012;166:1160–9.
29. Zaleski-Larsen LA, Fabi SG, McGraw T, Taylor M. Acne scar treatment: a multimodality approach tailored to scar type. Dermatol Surg. 2016;42(Suppl 2):S139–49.
30. Cameli N, Mariano M, Serio M, Ardigo M. Preliminary comparison of fractional laser with fractional laser plus radiofrequency for the treatment of acne scars and photoaging. Dermatol Surg. 2014;40:553–61.
31. Simmons BJ, Griffith RD, Falto-Aizpurua LA, Nouri K. Use of radiofrequency in cosmetic dermatology: focus on nonablative treatment of acne scars. Clin Cosmet Investig Dermatol. 2014;7:335–9.
32. Cho SB, Park CO, Chung WG, Lee KH, Lee JB, Chung KY. Histometric and histochemical analysis of the effect of trichloroacetic acid concentration in the chemical reconstruction of skin scars method. Dermatol Surg. 2006;32:1231–6. discussion 6.
33. Lee JB, Chung WG, Kwahck H, Lee KH. Focal treatment of acne scars with trichloroacetic acid: chemical reconstruction of skin scars method. Dermatol Surg. 2002;28:1017–21. discussion 21.
34. Hirsch RJ, Lewis AB. Treatment of acne scarring. Semin Cutan Med Surg. 2001;20:190–8.
35. Wang F, Garza LA, Kang S, Varani J, Orringer JS, Fisher GJ, et al. In vivo stimulation of de novo collagen production caused by cross-linked hyaluronic acid dermal filler injections in photodamaged human skin. Arch Dermatol. 2007;143:155–63.
36. Wollina U, Goldman A. Fillers for the improvement in acne scars. Clin Cosmet Investig Dermatol. 2015;8:493–9.
37. Goodman G. Post acne scarring: a review. J Cosmet Laser Ther. 2003;5:77–95.
38. Aust MC, Reimers K, Repenning C, Stahl F, Jahn S, Guggenheim M, et al. Percutaneous collagen induction: minimally invasive skin rejuvenation without risk of hyperpigmentation-fact or fiction? Plast Reconstr Surg. 2008;122:1553–63.
39. Alam M, Han S, Pongprutthipan M, Disphanurat W, Kakar R, Nodzenski M, et al. Efficacy of a needling device for the treatment of acne scars: a randomized clinical trial. JAMA Dermatol. 2014;150:844–9.
40. Hou A, Cohen B, Haimovic A, Elbuluk N. Microneedling: a comprehensive review. Dermatol Surg. 2017;43:321–39.

9 Pediatric Burns and Scars

Mark Fisher

9.1 Introduction

Wound healing through childhood is a poignant story reflecting the underlying biology, potential, and limitations of the developing child who has been wounded. Familiarity with the interweaving factors at play is important to guide physicians and surgeons in the care of the scarred child. In broad strokes this includes:

1. The scar itself
2. Physical growth and development
3. Cognitive, social, and emotional development

The scar itself is generally the same in children and adults in biology and natural history. The crux of the pediatric scar is the way the scar interacts with the developing body. Numerous classic developmental milestones affect the natural history of a scar as well as therapeutic planning. Figure 9.1a, b provides a general overview of this timeline with some surgical considerations.

9.2 Developmental Overview

In the first year of life, growth is rapid and begins to decelerate to an extent after the second year. Proportions are also distinctive with the head comprising 19% TBSA (total body surface area) in the first year of life but with relatively small thighs. These proportions make extensive scarring of the face and scalp more difficult as a greater proportion of total body surface area is involved. Throughout life the trunk including the buttocks and perineum comprises the largest surface area of the body staying about 1/3 of body. By puberty, body proportions have changed primarily due relative changes in the thigh and head size. From a reconstructive standpoint, starting at age 9–10 the thigh has become a larger donor site, and reconstructive needs for the head are less demanding as it has become a smaller fraction of total body surface area (Fig. 9.2) [1]. Indeed, at this point BSA of the head has halved from 19% to 10%.

Brain growth is rapid with the cranial vault reaching 85% of adult growth by age 3. Ear growth is similarly rapid with 85% of growth achieved by age 4. From a reconstructive standpoint however, total ear construction necessitating a full rib construct is reserved until age 10 when cartilage is adequate and contralateral ear growth is complete. Puberty begins around age 10 in girls and age 11 in boys with growth velocity peaking at about 12 and 14, respectively. During this period of rapid growth and development, children can experience profound tension and exacerbation of scarring with loss of range of motion. Thelarche occurs with the onset of puberty and is largely complete within 2–4 years reaching final maturity by age 18. Skeletal maturity occurs at around 14 years of age for girls, and around 17 years for boys. This is also the timing at which facial growth is largely complete, making orthognathic and nasal surgery practical.

9.3 Cognitive, Social, Emotional Considerations

In addition to the physical dimension, it is important to understand the impact of scarring and surgery on the developing child from a social, emotional, and cognitive perspective. Scars and the burden of care entailed in their treatment can be substantial. The period of life between 6 months and 4 years of life has been suggested as a time where medical interventions can be particularly stressful due to immature coping ability [2].

Recently, considerable attention has been directed to the risk of anesthetic neurotoxicity in the developing brain. Neuronal apoptosis and reduced synaptic sprouting have been demonstrated in a developing rat brain model exposed to general anesthesia [3]. Teenagers with a history of a general

M. Fisher (✉)
The University of Iowa Hospitals and Clinics, Iowa City, IA, USA
e-mail: mark-d-fisher@uiowa.edu

© Springer Nature Singapore Pte Ltd. 2020
R. Ogawa (ed.), *Total Scar Management*, https://doi.org/10.1007/978-981-32-9791-3_9

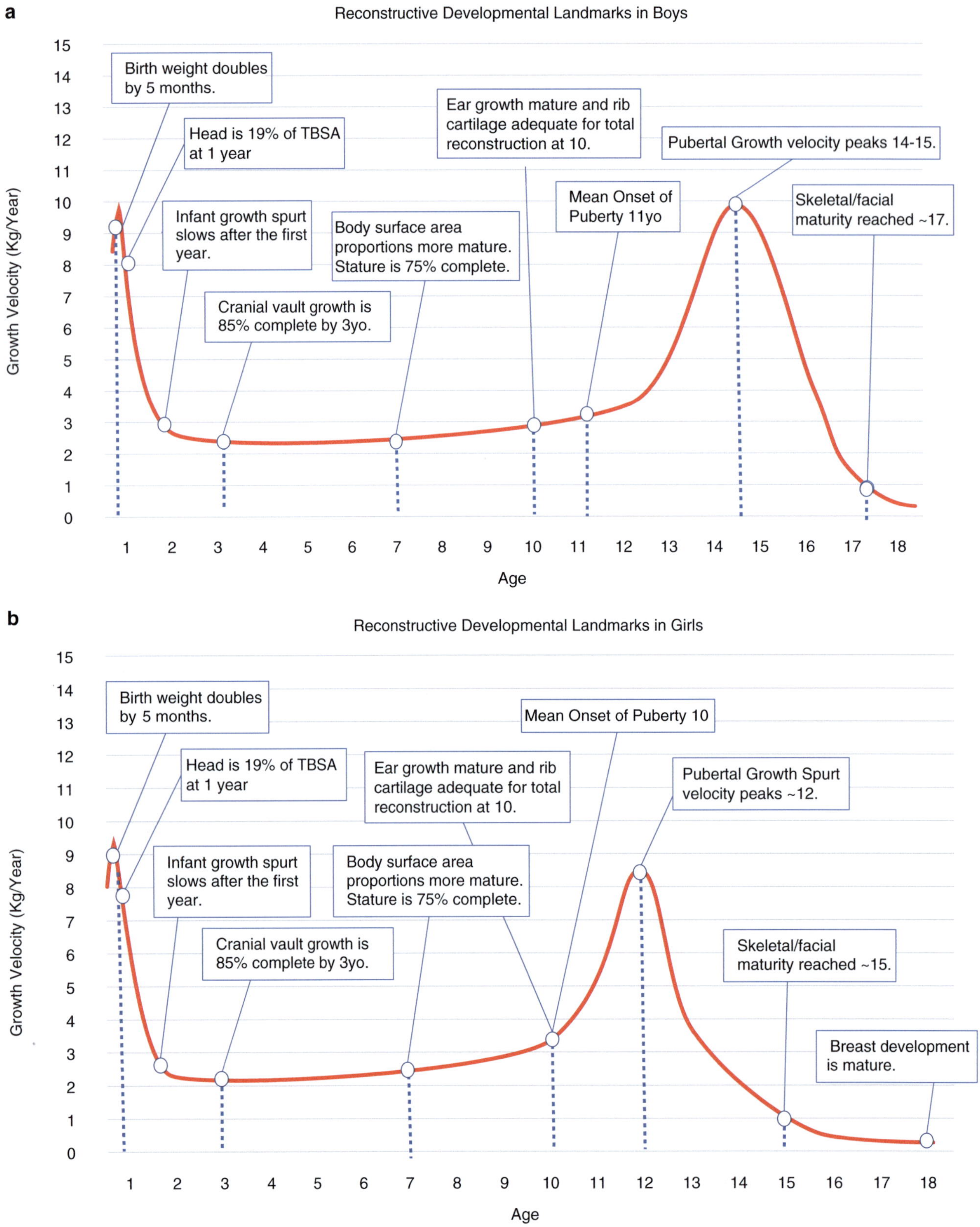

Fig. 9.1 Growth and development milestones are key considerations in long-term planning of reconstruction

Fig. 9.2 Changes in body surface area are key to keep in mind and anticipate: note two points illustrated here as a representation of the Lund Browder Chart. The trunk and arms stay relatively stable over time. The small child has a large head and small thighs. The adult has a relatively smaller head, and larger thighs

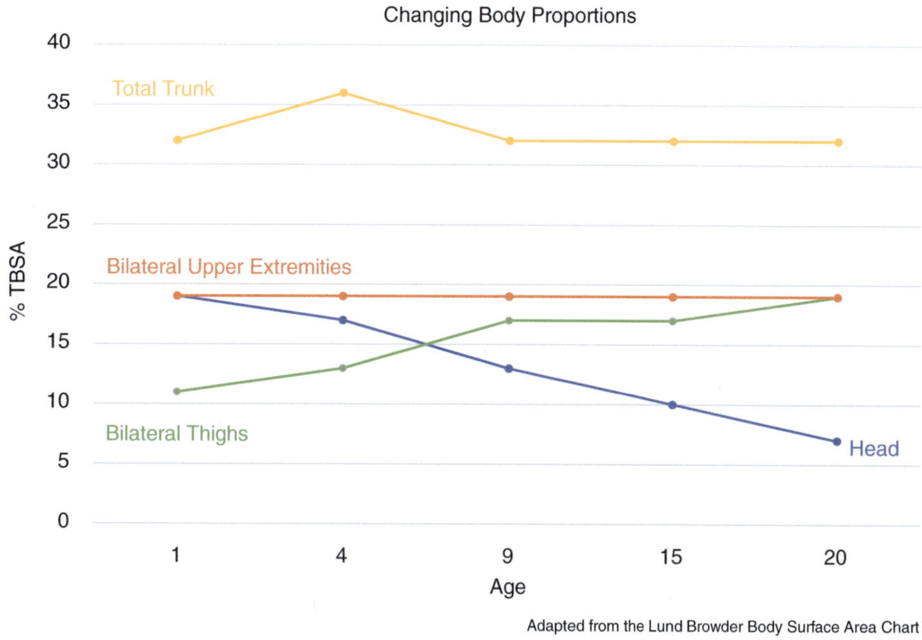

anesthetic prior to age 4 were shown to have a nearly 1% decrement in mean IQ over controls in one Swedish population-based study. But the best data presently available on the subject to date came out in 2015. The General Anesthesia compared to Spinal Anesthesia (GAS) trial reported initial data on a randomized controlled trial in neonates undergoing herniorrhaphy. No difference was demonstrated at 2 years in Bayley Scales of Infant and Toddler Development [4]. Best evidence to date thus supports offering elective surgery including general anesthesia to even the smallest child if a strong indication is present.

The psychological impact of scarring on children has been well attested in the literature. Pediatric burn survivors report higher emotional and behavioral problems with lower health-related quality of life scores, particularly related to appearance [5]. Facial scarring, in particular, is associated with impaired social interactions and development [6, 7]. That disfiguring scars can cause suffering is self-evident, but predicting the impact of a scar on a given patient is difficult. A systematic review of studies aimed at measuring the impact of scarring in 2011 demonstrated mixed results relating to body image, with some children with burns reporting higher body image than unburned controls [8]. Similar findings raise questions about the validity of our measurements and have stimulated the development of new measures though these are still in development [9–11]. Ultimately, the social and emotional impact of scars in children must not be ignored. In addition to the above considerations, the anatomic and physiologic distinctives of children are also important.

9.4 Pediatric Skin

The developing fetus has the well-known ability to create new skin without scar following an excisional injury. Unfortunately, at 24 weeks of gestation, this ability begins to disappear [12]. Hence, scarring occurs even in the youngest injured child. Figure 9.3 demonstrates a neonate with cutis aplasia congenita who healed ultimately with considerable scar.

At birth, neonatal skin contains all five strata of mature skin although there are multiple distinctions relative to adults. The skin in early infancy is delicate, lacking tensile strength. It is also sensitive to mechanical stimulation as evidenced by vasospasm which has been noted in flaps for the very young [13]. The risk of desiccation is also increased due to a high ratio of surface area to mass and the relatively ineffective barrier function of neonatal skin. After 6 months of age, children begin to heal wounds with exuberant scarring. Multiple factors likely contribute to this phenomenon. Injury and inflammation in the deep reticular dermis per se correlates with the development of hypertrophic scar and keloid [14, 15]. Since pediatric skin is thin, the reticular dermis is more easily injured, leading to an increased risk for untoward scarring. Repetitive tension also leads to wound fibrosis via multiple pro-inflammatory mechanisms including mechano-transduction pathways [16]. Growing children are active and have relatively tight skin that can be rendered pathologically tight with small wounds. Hence, tension is a major contributor to pathologic scarring in children. Keloids also occur in children but are less common in earlier childhood [17]. On

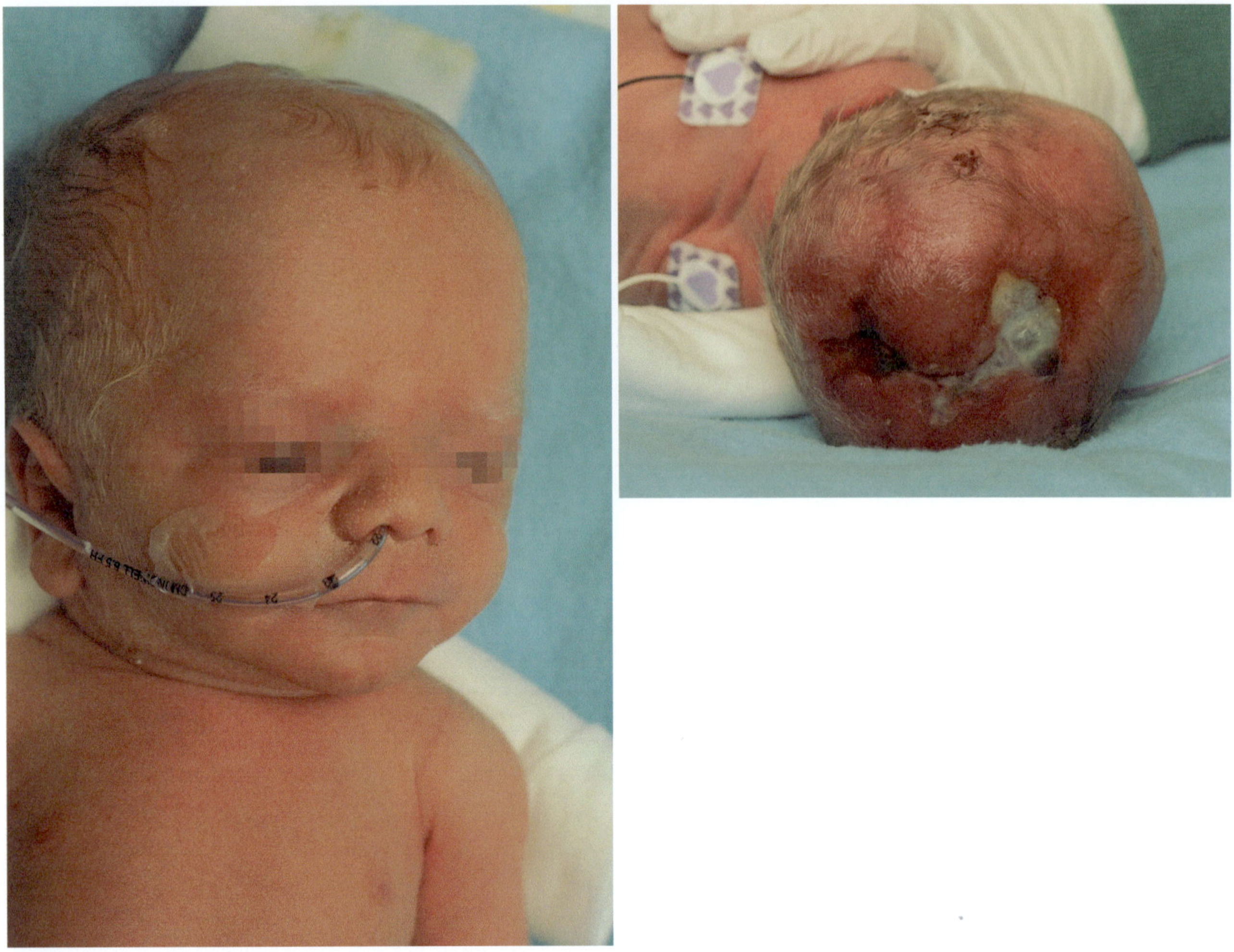

Fig. 9.3 Scarless wound healing unfortunately, is already gone in the neonatal period. This child with cutis aplasia congenita healed with considerable scar

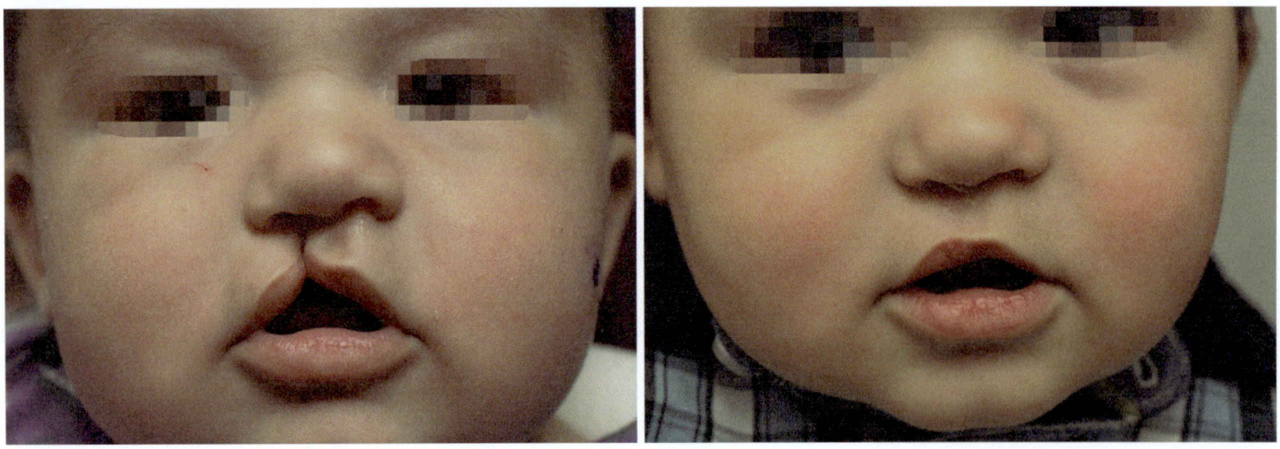

Fig. 9.4 Although growing children have great physiologic potential to create hypertrophic scars when tissues are under tension, ideal conditions can result in minimal scars as we often see in our cleft lip patients

the other hand, when tension is relieved, excellent healing and minimal scarring can be anticipated with regularity as we know from routine surgery such as cleft repairs. Figure 9.4 demonstrates a unilateral incomplete cleft repair performed at 4 months of age with very little discernible scar subsequently.

In sum, multiple factors make pathologic scarring the natural consequence of an injury in children. Their skin is thin, making injuries to the deep dermis relatively easy, tension arises easily, and children have the physiologic reserve necessary to create a powerful contracting scar. It is also important to recognize the interaction between these factors with growth as well.

9.5 Fundamentals of Pediatric Scar Evaluation

Evaluation of scar by anatomic area will be discussed in further detail below, but overall principles are treated here. As previously stated, there is currently no widely accepted child-specific measure for scar. But the most commonly used is the Vancouver scar scale, which includes vascularity, pigmentation, pliability, and height. Additional detail should include the anatomic structures involved. In children, any effect on growth and development should be noted. The overall examination is then used to quantify the amount of tissue deficit. Finally, the patient's and family's perception of the scar should also be documented, including symptoms of pain or pruritus. Figure 9.5 provides a sample scar evaluation including these areas.

Subjective scar tightness is a valuable piece of information but it can be variable. Bilmire noted that children with burns who complain of feelings of tightness during rapid growth often report spontaneous amelioration with time, suggesting a capacity to stretch and grow in response to tension [18].

The key question for any scar is, "How much tissue is missing?" Untoward scars *without* a paucity of tissue are amenable to simpler measures such as compression, splinting, massage, steroids, silicone sheeting, and, in the case of keloids, radiation. Selective cases may be excised and closed if technique or postoperative relief of tension were inadequate. To determine the need for additional tissue, a combination of palpation and passive manipulation of the affected part through the range of motion provides a vivid sense of the missing tissue, often to the square centimeter. It is helpful to imagine the size of the defect that would result if the scarred tissue were incised and released with restoration of full range of motion and relief of tension. It can be difficult to manipulate a child in this fashion in clinic due to anxiety and pain. But efforts should be made to obtain thorough preoperative examinations for improved planning. Child life specialists can be invaluable in this regard during clinic visits.

For children with major scarring, such as in burns, multidisciplinary teams with excellent communication provide best care. When great breadth and depth of expertise is coupled with streamlined, rapid, efficient care, a critical mass is achieved that makes true centers of excellence.

Sample Basic Scar Evaluation

Anatomy:

- **Location:** Anterior thorax extending through anterior axillary fold, biceps, and dorsal forearm in a continuous band.
- **Structures Involved:** Skin, subcutaneous fat, with tethering extending to deep fascia in thorax and axilla.
- **Tissue Deficit:** ~10cm^2 in the axilla

Vancouver Scar Scale:

- Vascularity: Pink
- Pigmentation: Hyperpigmentation
- Pliability: Yielding
- Height: <5mm

Growth and Development

- Nipple areola complex lost but no growth restriction.

Patient & Family Report: "The scar on his armpit seems tight, but it doesn't seem to bother him. He's a little embarrassed to take his shirt off at the pool. He has no pain, but does scratch at times."

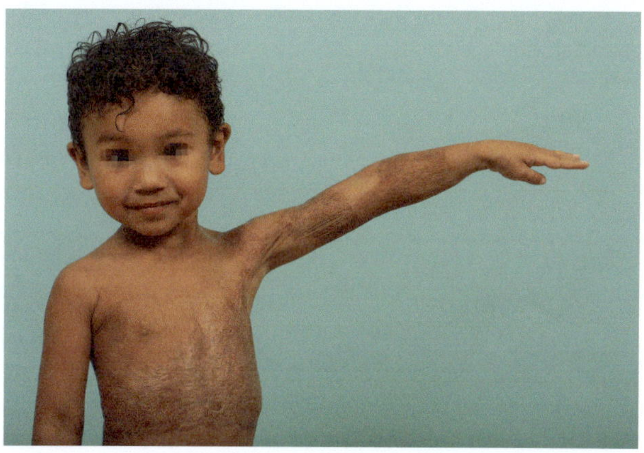

Fig. 9.5 Scar assessment in children should systematically take into consideration the unique variable of psychosocial and physical growth and development

With respect to developing a plan, the reconstructive ladder continues to be a relevant concept for pediatric scars. This is the dictum that for a given problem, options of lower complexity should be considered before options of higher complexity. But scars are often complex problems best treated by multiple modalities of varying levels of complexity. Hence, multiple rungs on the ladder may be employed in parallel or in series. We may also find ourselves climbing up and down the ladder depending on the evolving needs of the patient over time. For instance, a given patient may undergo laser and local tissue rearrangement in the same operation.

9.6 Face and Scalp

9.6.1 Growth and Development

The developing craniofacial skeleton grows by a combination of intramembranous and endochondral ossification with most of vault growth complete in early childhood whereas much of facial growth proceeds into the teen years. Cicatricial impairment of craniofacial growth occurs in the face, particularly the nose and jaws, resulting in cross bites, open bites, constricted arch forms, and impaired jaw movement and speech [19, 20]. Principles of facial scar management in children are therefore:

1. Prevent growth impairment and deformity through timely intervention while developing.
2. Aim for definitive correction when growth is stable, e.g., at skeletal maturity.

9.6.2 Analysis of the Scarred Face

Once scarring has produced a significant deformity in a child, analysis of the problem is key. Severe facial scarring can be a complex, daunting web of interconnected problems. Breaking things down systematically can help to identify actionable reconstructive aims amenable to prioritization. A systematic approach to the scarred face should include analysis of the impact scarring has had on:

1. Cover
2. Defining landmarks
3. Facial expression
4. Volumes
5. Breathing
6. Feeding
7. Speech

One must address each of these areas effectively and with appropriate prioritization. The classic mistake is to prioritize surface scar while inadvertently distorting facial landmarks resulting in a net deformity for the patient.

9.6.2.1 Cover

Cover in the face and head includes the skin and the complex system of fascial layers including the galea aponeurotica, superficial mesoaponeurotic system (SMAS), and platysma. These of course relate intrinsically to the deeper fascial structures and planes of the head, face, and neck. A thorough discussion of these layers is beyond the scope of this chapter but must be thoroughly understood when deeper and more extensive scars are present.

9.6.2.2 Defining Facial Landmarks

Defining landmarks of the face include points and contours of high contrast to which the viewer's eye is naturally drawn, defining the face. Every portraitist understands the importance of getting these right. If the facial landmarks are correct, many other imperfections are overlooked. Conversely, if facial landmarks are distorted, severe deformity is obvious. Key points of high contrast in the face include:

1. Palpebral fissures particularly as they intersect with the iris.
2. Eyebrows.
3. Nostrils and alar base with their shadows.
4. Oral commissures and the shadow below the upper lip.

The importance of these landmarks becomes apparent, for example, when tension results in cicatricial ectropion, medial canthal webbing, asymmetrical alar bases, or loss of the upper lip contours due to dentoskeletal deformity, microstomia, or direct deformity of the mouth. Figure 9.6 demonstrates that simplification of a face to only the key high contrast landmarks preserves the likeness. The corollary to this observation is that even small deformities of these landmarks can disfigure the face.

9.6.2.3 Facial Volumes

Volumes of the face refer to the three-dimensional shape of the face. These are dependent on dentoskeletal support and soft tissue bulk and provide the foundation of the face. Severe scarring in the developing face can warp and restrain facial growth. When this occurs, the scar must be taken into consideration when correction of facial volumes is planned. For example, a child with an Angle class III dentoskeletal relationship due to scar who requires a Le Fort I advancement will require correction of enveloping cicatrix to facilitate orthognathic surgery and minimize the risk of relapse. The patient in Fig. 9.7 demonstrates such a case: dense scarring has restricted upper and lower jaw growth resulting in malocclusion and an Angle class III relationship which will require orthognathic surgery to name a single point. But the scar must be addressed potentiate this process.

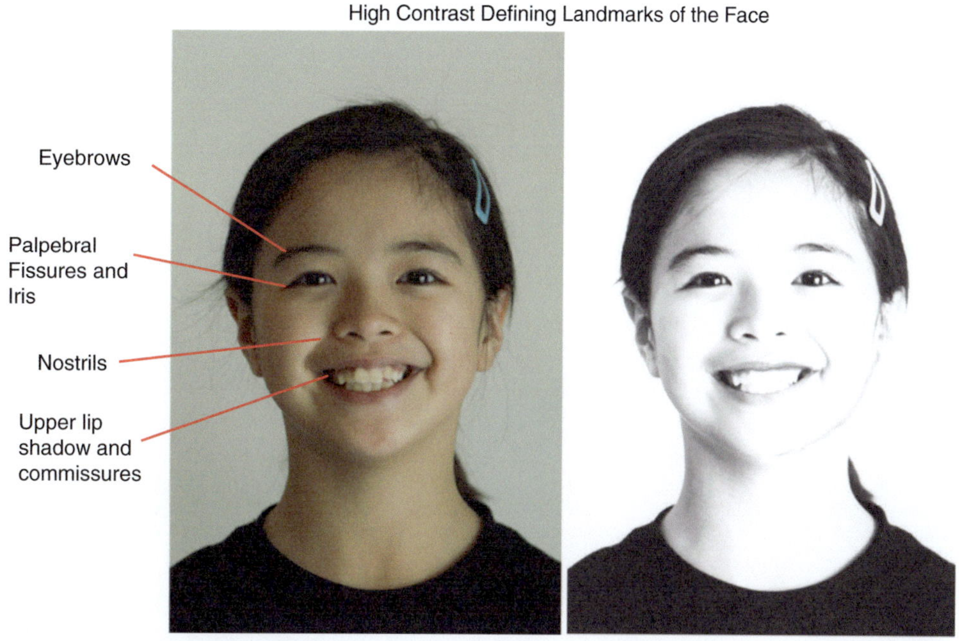

Fig. 9.6 The high-contrast simplification on the right demonstrates key defining landmarks. Small perturbations in the eyelids, nostrils, oral commissures can have a profound impact on appearance

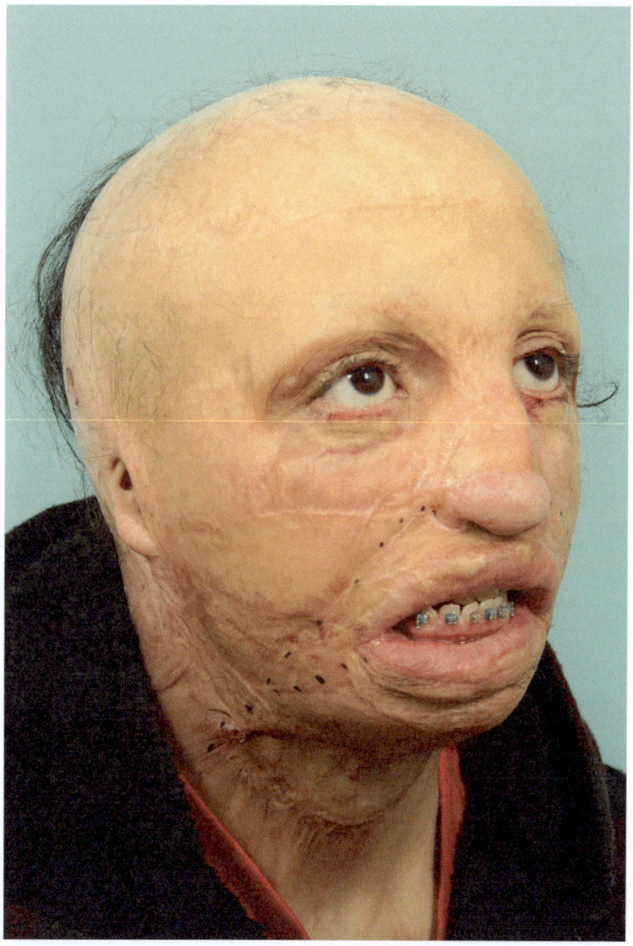

Fig. 9.7 Severe scar present from early childhood has created volumetric deformities through the restraint of dentoskeletal growth. A full and natural reconstruction will require normalization of volume relationships through orthognathic surgery

Figure 9.8, a girl with Treacher Collins syndrome, was treated with emphasis on correcting stigmatizing volume relationships including orthognathic surgery, custom malar implants of PEEK, periorbital fat grafting, and a rhinoplasty.

9.6.2.4 Facial Expression

Scarring can also impair facial expression due to sclerosis of either deep or superficial components of the mechanism of facial expression. This includes the facial nerve, muscles of facial expression, the superficial musculoaponeurotic system (SMAS), and the overlying skin. Derangement of facial expression can manifest as tethering with animation or, in the worst cases, profound loss of expression due to a mask of scar as in Fig. 9.9.

9.6.2.5 Breathing, Feeding, Speech, Hearing

On occasion, extensive scar such as in massive burn can impair breathing, feeding, speech, and hearing through contractures and obliteration involving the mouth, neck, and ears. These functional concerns should be treated with the highest priority.

9.6.3 Treatment of Facial Scar

Facial reconstructive techniques in children are principally the same as in adults. Scars with no tissue deficit benefit from laser and adjunctive medications. Donelan's series of PDL with local tissue rearrangement for the face demonstrates the power of combining these techniques [21].

With more severe scarring, additional tissue must be provided. When this is the case, the full gamut of surgical

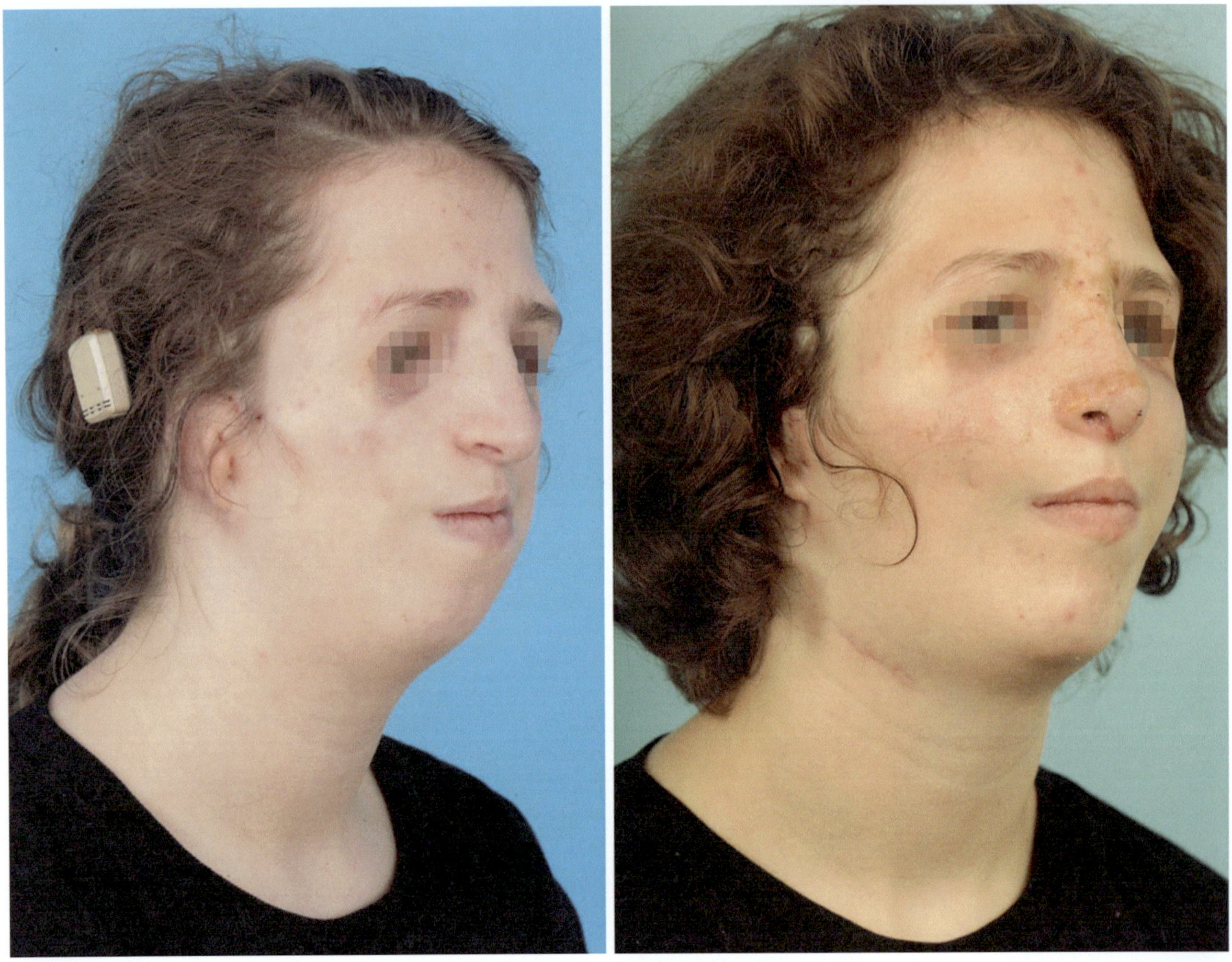

Fig. 9.8 A girl with Treacher Collins syndrome, was treated with emphasis on correcting stigmatizing volume relationships including orthognathic surgery, custom malar implants of PEEK, periorbital fat grafting, and a rhinoplasty

techniques must be considered employing the reconstructive elevator concept, described by Gottlieb [22]. This is a modification of the ladder concept emphasizing that the best reconstructive choice may not necessarily be the lowest feasible rung on the ladder.

Importantly, laser and less invasive techniques can ameliorate the deficit, making subsequent reconstruction less demanding. When a substantial skin deficit is present in the face, options include full-thickness skin grafting ideally from above the clavicles as for cicatricial ectropion. When larger grafts are needed, tissue expansion may provide needed tissue. When very large grafts are needed for the face, the issue of color match may become less important as these tend to be massive injuries where color will not be normal regardless. Regional and free flaps are also important in this area.

Tissue expansion for pediatric facial scarring and reconstruction is a key tool, but a significant rate of extrusion, infection, and iatrogenic deformities have cooled the ardor of many surgeons. Neale et al. published a series of 37 cases of pediatric tissue expansion for the face and neck in 1992 representing the Cincinnati Shrine experience at the time [23]. The article is an excellent and thoughtful summary of design principles for facial tissue expansion. A few key points include:

1. Advancing expanded skin above the mandibular border should be done with caution because of the risk of distortion.
2. Flaps with vertical closures may have to be revised because of subsequent contraction.
3. Rotating down is preferable to rotating up when possible.

Bauer on the other hand has demonstrated a 20-year experience 995 tissue expander-based reconstructions throughout the body with an exceedingly low complication rate as reviewed in his 2004 report [24]. Expanded flaps are used for the cheek, neck, and forehead with expanded full-

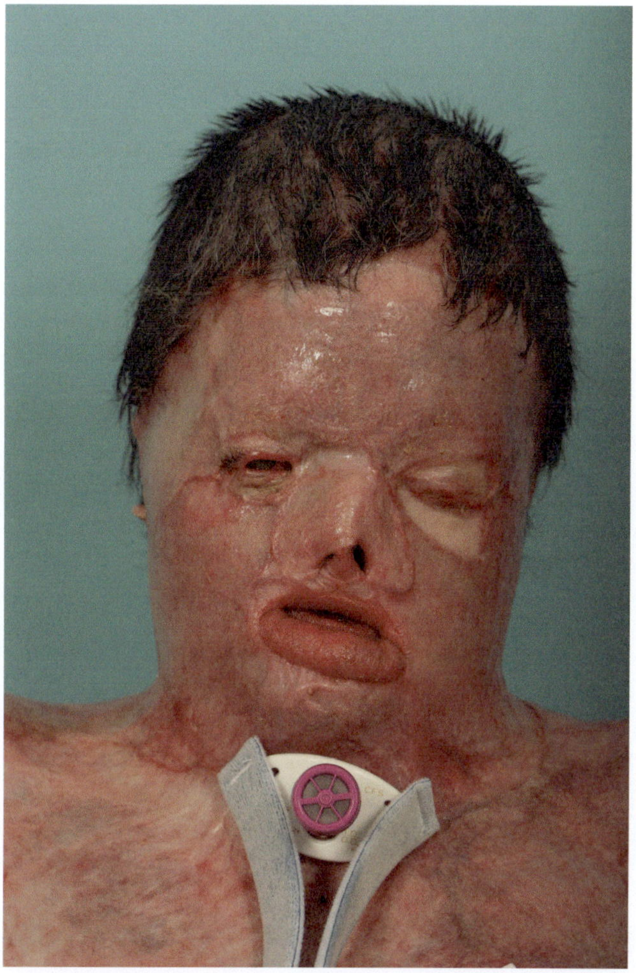

Fig. 9.9 In the most severe facial scarring cases, facial animation is lost leading to a mask-like appearance lacking expression

thickness grafts for the periorbital and nasal areas. Tension deformities of facial landmarks with expanded flaps are avoided by using transpositional designs as opposed to advancement flaps in a way that resembles medially based cervicofacial flaps.

A critical point underlying both of these reports is that normal location of face-defining landmarks is a *sine qua non* of a normal appearing face. If our efforts to reduce scar result in distortion of face-defining landmarks, then a net deformity will be perceived.

Inspiring series of superthin flaps have been described around the world for the neck and face particularly in the work of Hyakusoku and Ogawa [25, 26]. Children may be prime candidates for these techniques in North America as they are less likely to be obese. Conventional fasciocutaneous flaps are also good options but they may require multiple debulking operations. Reconstruction of a supple soft tissue envelope makes dentoskeletal and nasal reconstruction possible in severe cases. Once this has been achieved, standard techniques of orthognathic surgery and rhinoplasty are employed.

9.7 Neck

The neck is a relatively small body part in children and adults and there is little to mention from a developmental standpoint. Yet, it is an important reconstructive problem as severe scarring of the neck can have profound aesthetic and functional results when tension and fibrosis distort the face or limit range of motion. Indeed, prolonged impairment of range of motion can result in strabismus and other ocular problems [27].

In children, even the most trivial injury to neck skin can hypertrophy and become pruritic due to neck motion and tension. Standard basic therapies such as laser and steroids can be successful. But local tissue rearrangement is quite effective and should be added early if improvement is not observed.

Scarring of greater severity in the neck are those with a tissue deficit and with involvement of deep structures. Tissue deficit in the neck is defined when the skin envelope is too tight to permit functional range of motion. When this is the case, deep structures involvement is common. Just under the skin is the superficial cervical fascia investing the platysma which can be quite scarred and fibrotic. In exceptionally contracted necks, the confluence of fascial layers in and above the carotid sheath are key components of the contracture that must be addressed. Adequate release requires thorough understanding of neck anatomy. Also important is the understanding of how the neck extends. Fifty percent of neck extension is accomplished between the occiput and C1 and 50% of rotation occurs between C1 and C2. This emphasizes the importance of the upper anterior neck in providing range of motion. An interesting corollary is that tracheostomies do not need to be moved to accomplish release.

If a tissue deficit has been identified, the source of replacement tissue must be considered. Skin grafting with or without dermal replacement template is a consideration. In the 1980s, Waymack et al. reported a series of 143 children treated with incision and skin grafting. A 63% recurrence rate was reduced to 17% if splinting for over a year could be done. Dermal templates have been suggested as a means of reducing recurrence but data is limited. Frame et al. described a recurrence rate in the 25% range with an infection rate of about 20% with the use of Integra® for releases throughout the body [28]. Figus et al. reported a case series demonstrating excision of scar followed by Integra® and skin grafting with compelling early results [29]. The real efficacy, durability, and infection rates related to dermal substitutes are not known. But this approach is certainly on the reconstructive ladder and is an important option when there is a paucity of available donor.

When regional tissue is available, one recalls classic series presented over the years by surgeons such as Spence [30], Feldman [31], and Bauer [24], who have demonstrated the power of tissue expansion in the chest and shoulders for neck release. Griskevich has demonstrated the efficacy of multiple large local flaps in the neck and other areas [32, 33]. Figure 9.10 demonstrates how expanded transpositional flaps (outlined in red) from the upper back and shoulder can reduce the tension experienced by the face from the chest resulting in de-escalation of facial scar. This case also demonstrates how demanding and recalcitrant facial and cervical scar can be as additional attention is clearly needed.

At the top of the reconstructive ladder, Hyakusoku and Ogawa have demonstrated the power of huge thin flaps for neck and face reconstruction [34, 35]. These remarkable flaps are made possible by a dermal bridge for augmented venous outflow, a distal venous supercharge to permit efficient linear flow, and thinning which may reduce the physiologic requirements on the flap. One challenge that has yet to be clearly worked out in the literature is how to apply these techniques in the obese. A more traditional approach employing free tissue transfer was reported by Angrigiani in 1994 documenting powerful total anterior neck resurfacing in 86 patients using extended scapular-parascapular flaps with an average of 3 debulking operations [36]. Considering the quality of the final outcome, its durability and resistance to recurrence, flap-based neck reconstruction has much to commend it.

9.8 Axilla

From a developmental standpoint, there is not much to mention regarding the pediatric axilla. The chest and upper extremity compose a constant fraction of total body surface area through life. The main developmental consideration relates to breast development.

When considering extremities in general, a key principle is that the more proximal the contracture, the greater the impact on limb function. Hence, loss of shoulder range of motion profoundly impacts upper extremity function. Also important is the proximity of the breast with consequent effacement of breast development in larger axillary scars. Multiple authors have offered classification schemes for axillary scarring and contracture. But the common theme is that axillary scar and contracture may involve any of the following:

1. Anterior axillary fold
2. Posterior axillary fold
3. Dome
4. Surrounding tissues of the back or chest

The extent of involvement will drive decision-making. As Bilmire has advised, a feeling of tightness per se does not

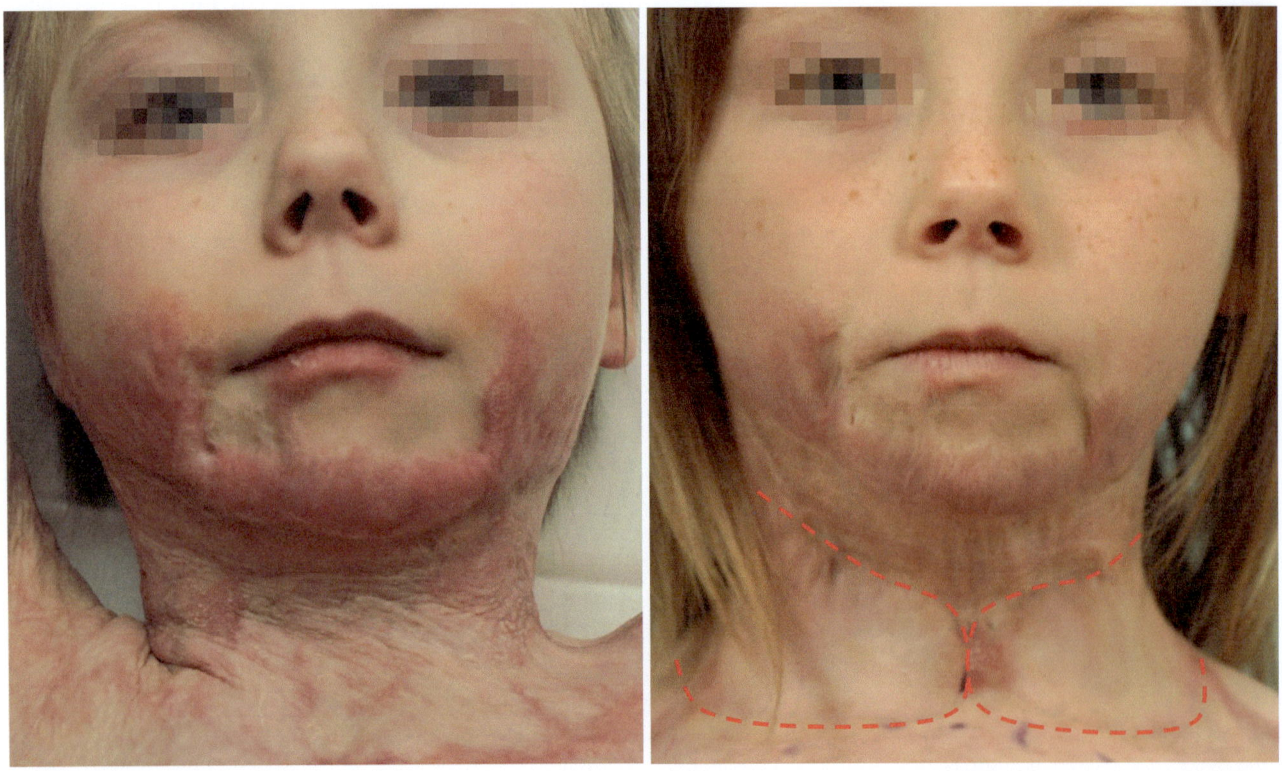

Fig. 9.10 When regional flaps are introduced into a tense scarred area, tension is diminished resulting in improvement in scar in the surrounding tissues. Note the improvement in the facial scars after introduction of bilateral supraclavicular flaps

require operative intervention in the growing child [18]. But important goals of surgery are as follows:

- To maintain full range of motion
- To preserve anatomical landmarks such as the nipple areola complex
- To prevent and treat complications of scar such as itching, pain, and ulceration

Along these lines, Greenhalgh showed that release of axillary contractures "as soon as they appear" had similar long-term outcomes in comparison to a more conservative approach waiting for scar maturation prior to intervention [37].

Incision, release of scar, and split-thickness skin grafting is one option reported by Palmieri et al. demonstrating durable results in children with TBSA averaging 40% [38]. Similarly, Greenhalgh's series noted above also featured incision and grafting with durable results. But there are downsides to skin grafting to provide axillary releases. The reconstructive principle of replacing like with like would suggest that full-thickness skin and subcutaneous tissue would provide a superior axillary release if possible. Many authors feel that skin grafting has a tendency to experience relapse, and the results may not be aesthetically ideal.

Scarring and contracture involving a single axillary fold is frequently treated with local tissue rearrangement. Multiple powerful flap designs are available, including one or more z-plasties, the ¾ z-plasty of Huang, the trapezoidal flaps of Grishkevich, and the square-flap of Ogawa [39–42] depicted in Fig. 9.11. Isolated bands in the axilla are particularly apt to correction through local flaps since thin, pliable adjacent tissue tends to be available within the dome of the axilla close by in the arm. When scarring is more widespread across much of the axilla, surface area requirements may exceed the ability of local tissue rearrangement. In this case, regional or more distant options should be considered. A wide variety of flaps based on the subscapular system have been used for this indication, including the parascapular, scapular, a bilobed combination of both of these flaps, and the thoracodorsal artery perforator flap [41, 43–51]. Tissue expansion has also been used in combination with these techniques to aid in donor site closure. Based on excellent results demonstrated in the series noted above, there are clearly multiple ways to skin this cat.

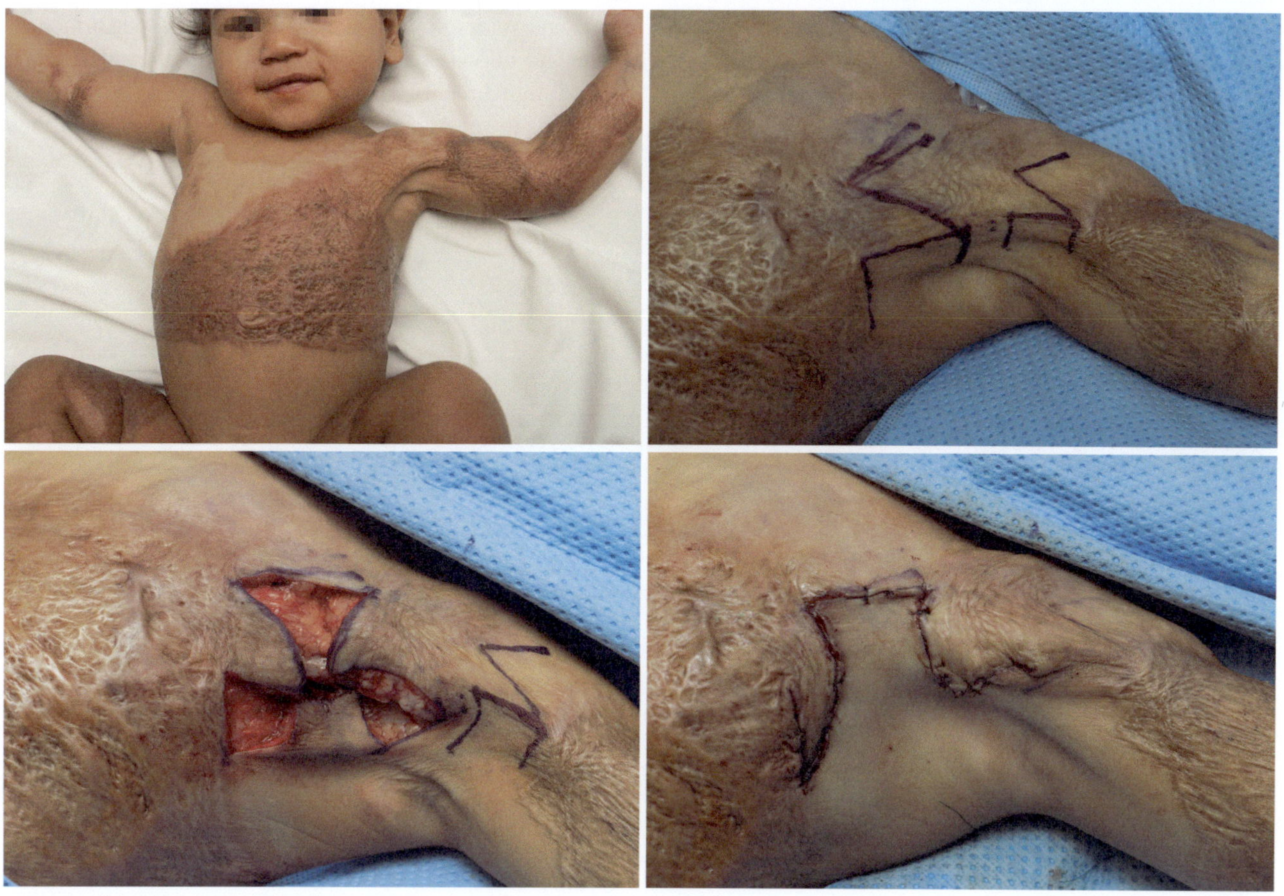

Fig. 9.11 The dome of the axilla is usually spared and provides a good source of skin for local tissue rearrangement. The square-flap as described by Ogawa is a good choice

The downside of flap reconstruction in the axilla that is most often cited is excessive bulk that may require subsequent debulking. In the most severe cases where there is a global paucity of donor options, thoughts turn to incisional release and skin grafting with or without dermal matrix. Just such a case was described by Figus et al. [29].

9.9 Hand

The hand early in life is flexible and tolerant of scar demonstrating an ability to bounce back without stiffness after prolonged deformity. Ossification of epiphyses begins in the first year of life and is not complete until the late teens. The risks of stiffness as a sequel of trauma or immobilization increases in older children but remains less than that of adults. The compliance of the pediatric hand, however, can also manifest by the extreme deformity that can result from uncontrolled scar. Very little difference is noted between treatment algorithms for pediatric versus adult hand scarring. But the ability of the pediatric hand to recover from severe scarring does open some options that would be less likely to succeed in adults. For instance, McCauley et al. reported the radical release of the hands of six children with a history of electrical injury with subsequent sural nerve grafting up to 2 years after injury with good results [52]. Laser has been somewhat disappointing in palmar scar in adults. This may be less so in children.

9.10 Thorax and Breast

Pediatric considerations in scars of the thorax come into play when the size and depth of the scar are large enough to impact breast development, ventilation, and range of motion. The breast bud lies just below the areola and measures around 5 mm in diameter. Scars or wounds near this must be judiciously treated in a way that does not endanger the breast bud. A concerted effort must also be made to protect the breast from deforming tension. This is particularly the case as thelarche approaches between 9 and 12 years of age with the onset of puberty and ovarian stimulation. Interestingly, the breast bud may be present even in the absence of a discernible areola [53].

Smaller and more superficial scars are addressed with laser, local tissue rearrangement, and steroids or other adjuncts. As previously noted, laser also has a role in the comprehensive treatment of extensive scars. The patient in Fig. 9.12 has an extensive immature scar involving the axilla, anterior, and lateral thorax. In this case, a combination of pulsed dye laser and fractional CO_2 laser ameliorated much of the scar leaving a tissue deficit in the axilla proper which was treated with regional flaps in another stage.

When scar is extensive, the developing breast parenchyma can become trapped, resulting in considerable discomfort. Incisional release of the scarred envelope is performed as needed to allow expansion. This is most often performed at the inframammary fold, but incisions should be added as necessary to release the breast. Resultant wounds are then

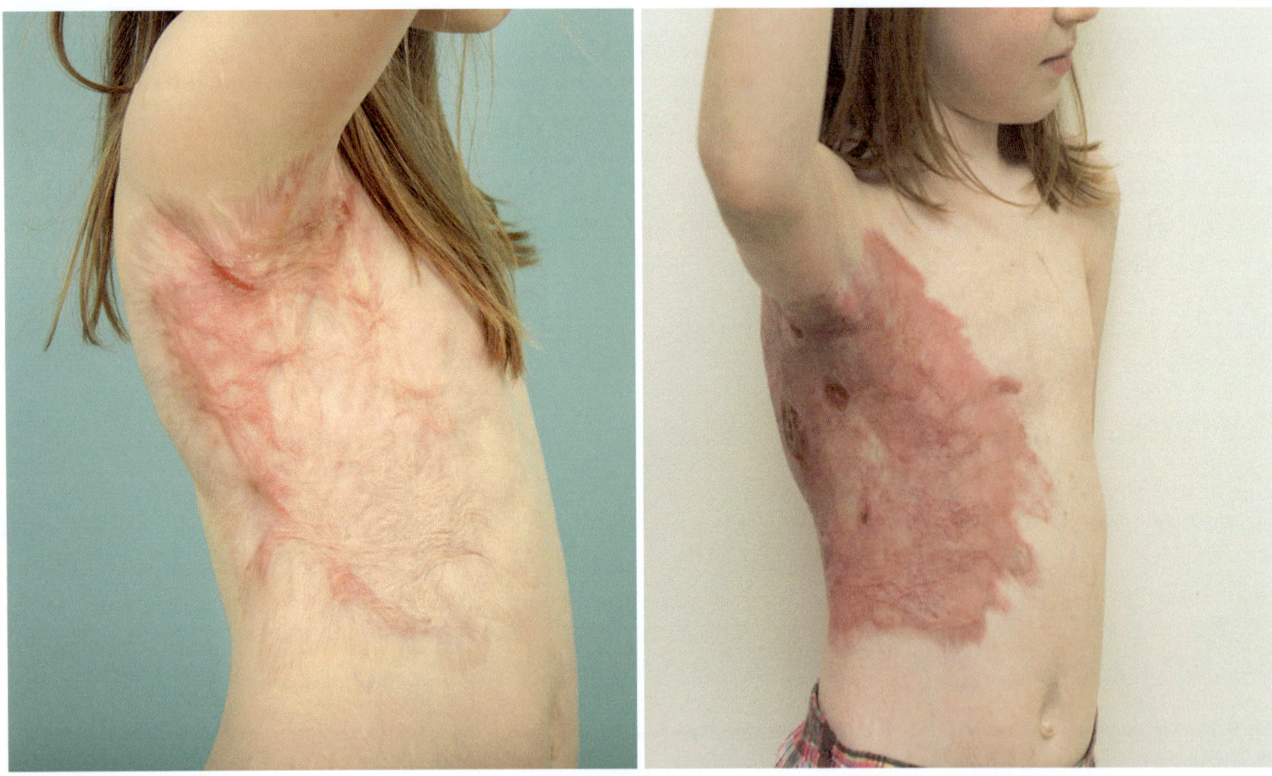

Fig. 9.12 Axillary and flank scars in girls can create tension effects on the breast bud. Local flaps and laser are good options early on to protect the breast bud from derangement. Yet many of these children will require formal breast reconstruction in a subsequent stage

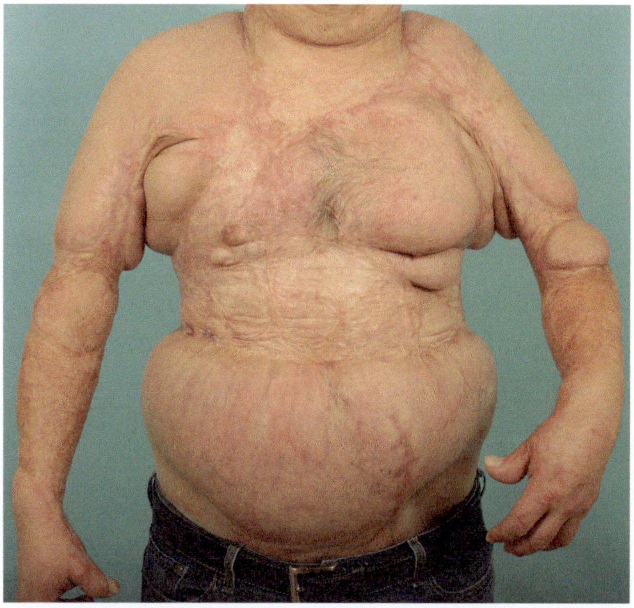

Fig. 9.13 When left untreated, pediatric scars of the chest can prevent normal thoracic expansion

grafted with split-thickness skin grafts. Of course the entire gamut of breast reconstructive techniques are available with the goal of concluding definitive reconstruction once parenchymal development is complete in the late teens.

With respect to range of motion and ventilation, it remains only to emphasize that a constricting envelope of scar can impair both. Figure 9.13 demonstrates burn scars from childhood not treated into adulthood that restrict thoracic expansion.

When thoracic scar is large enough to embarrass either ventilation or range of motion, it is also difficult to eliminate. In these cases, laser and incisional release much like an escharotomy followed by skin grafting is the mainstay of therapy. Tissue expanded free fasciocutaneous flaps for breast reconstruction are also considerations. Fat grafting has been conjectured as a tool to provide a subcutaneous release and reconstruction of a gliding plane. But significant data is not yet available to evaluate this hypothesis.

9.11 Lower Extremity

From a developmental standpoint, the lower extremities are relatively small early on but comprise an increasing proportion of total body surface area over time. This is particularly true of the thighs as previously shown. Extensive scarring such as from burns can produce limb length discrepancies [54]. As in other areas, limitation in range of motion is an important indicator for intervention. Paucity of tissue also manifests in chronic ulcerations particularly over the knees, pretibial areas, and Achilles.

Lower extremity scarring is followed regularly through childhood and is treated as in adults with laser, local tissue rearrangement, and flaps if needed. Interestingly, we have observed spontaneous closure of ulcerations with laser alone. This may be owing to improved perfusion from diminished tension.

9.11.1 Laser

Laser therapy for scar has become standard therapy for children with symptomatic scars [21, 55–59]. But to date, there is very little data to indicate concrete differences between their use in children versus adults. One potential exception may be scars of the palm of the hand. Flexion contractures of the palm of the hand have been found to be recalcitrant to laser therapy in many adults. This is likely multifactorial, but one factor is likely the thickness of the scar. This is less an issue in children due to the thinness of their skin. And indeed, anecdotal experience comports with this finding: children with palmar scars do respond to an extent to laser. Additionally, children with scar may benefit from repeat rounds of laser treatment later in life should growth and tension stimulate recurrence of scar pathobiology.

Pulsed dye laser improves inflammatory qualities of scar including redness, friability, and pruritus, hastening the maturation process. Depending on the child, PDL can be performed without sedation. Donelan's 2010 review is oft-cited and provides some reasonable starting settings [60]:

- Spot size: 7 or 10 mm spot size.
- Pulse duration 1.5 ms.
- Fluence:
  - 5–8 J/cm^2 with the 7 mm handpiece.
  - 4–5 J/cm^2 with the 10 mm handpiece.
- Cryogenic cooling settings of 30-ms spray and 20 ms delay.

Similarly, fractionated CO_2 laser has become standard therapy to treat thickened scars in children. Settings depend on the thickness of the scar and a given scar may benefit from a combination of settings and densities. Figure 9.14 provides

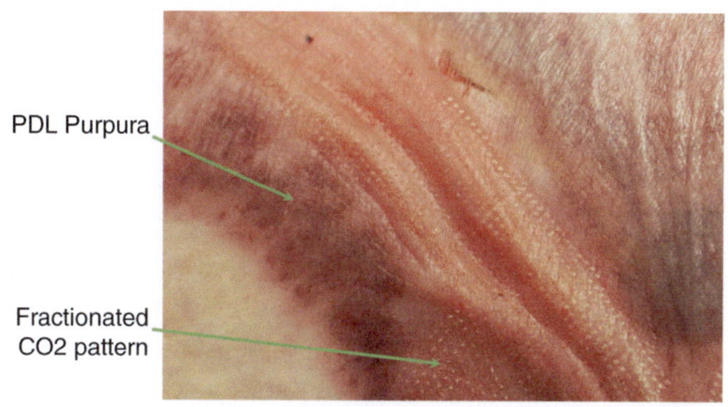

Fig. 9.14 PDL and fractionated CO_2 laser are commonly used in children. This close-up view demonstrated the purpura of PDL and the laser pattern of CO_2 laser

a close-up view of CO_2 and pulsed dye laser patterns used on the same occasion.

Adjuncts to laser including topical, injected corticosteroids or antimetabolites are also valuable tools still being examined for efficacy.

9.12 Conclusion

In summary, children have the capacity to cope with considerable scarring due to their inherent resilience. But optimal care can be very challenging due to the dynamic nature of the pediatric frame and their special needs from a social, emotional, and cognitive standpoint. May we all exert the diligence and care our pediatric patients deserve.

References

1. Lund CCBN. The estimation of areas of burns. Surg Gynecol Obstet. 1944;79:352–8.
2. Perrin E. In: Carey W, editor. Developmental-behavioral pediatrics.4th ed. Philadelphia, PA: Saunders/Elsevier; 2009. p. 329–36.
3. Sanchez V, Feinstein SD, Lunardi N, Joksovic PM, Boscolo A, Todorovic SM, et al. General anesthesia causes long-term impairment of mitochondrial morphogenesis and synaptic transmission in developing rat brain. Anesthesiology. 2011;115(5):992–1002.
4. Davidson AJ, Disma N, de Graaff JC. Neurodevelopmental outcome at 2 years of age after general anaesthesia and awake-regional anaesthesia in infancy (GAS): an international multicentre, randomised controlled trial (vol 387, pg 239, 2015). Lancet. 2016;387(10015):228.
5. Maskell J, Newcombe P, Martin G, Kimble R. Psychosocial functioning differences in pediatric burn survivors compared with healthy norms. J Burn Care Res. 2013;34(4):465–76.
6. Van Loey NEE, Van Song MJM. Psychopathology and psychological problems in patients with burn scars—epidemiology and management. Am J Clin Dermatol. 2003;4(4):245–72.
7. Ye EM. Psychological morbidity in patients with facial and neck burns. Burns. 1998;24(7):646–8.
8. Lawrence JW, Mason ST, Schomer K, Klein MB. Epidemiology and impact of scarring after burn injury: a systematic review of the literature. J Burn Care Res. 2012;33(1):136–46.
9. Tyack Z, Ziviani J, Kimble R, Plaza A, Jones A, Cuttle L, et al. Measuring the impact of burn scarring on health-related quality of life: development and preliminary content validation of the Brisbane Burn Scar Impact Profile (BBSIP) for children and adults. Burns. 2015;41(7):1405–19.
10. Finlay V, Burrows S, Kendell R, Berghuber A, Chong V, Tan J, et al. Modified Vancouver Scar Scale score is linked with quality of life after burn. Burns. 2017;43(4):741–6.
11. DeJong HM, Phillips M, Edgar DW, Wood FM. Patient opinion of scarring is multidimensional: an investigation of the POSAS with confirmatory factor analysis. Burns. 2017;43(1):58–68.
12. Lorenz HP, Longaker MT, Perkocha LA, Jennings RW, Harrison MR, Adzick NS. Scarless wound repair: a human fetal skin model. Development. 1992;114(1):253–9.
13. Clarke HM, Upton J, Zuker RM, Manktelow RT. Pediatric free tissue transfer—an evaluation of 99 cases. Can J Surg. 1993;36(6):525–8.
14. Huang C, Akaishi S, Hyakusoku H, Ogawa R. Are keloid and hypertrophic scar different forms of the same disorder? A fibroproliferative skin disorder hypothesis based on keloid findings. Int Wound J. 2014;11(5):517–22.
15. Huang C, Murphy GF, Akaishi S, Ogawa R, et al. Plast Reconstr Surg Glob Open. 2013;1(4):e25-e.
16. Leavitt T, Hu MS, Marshall CD, Barnes LA, Lorenz HP, Longaker MT. Scarless wound healing: finding the right cells and signals. Cell Tissue Res. 2016;365(3):483–93.
17. Marco Romanelli VD, Miteva M, Romanelli P. Dermal hypertrophies. In: Bolognia J, Jorizzo JL, Schaffer JV, editors. Dermatology. 3rd ed. Philadelphia ; London: Elsevier Saunders; 2012. p. 1621.
18. Bilmire D. Pediatric plastic surgery. In: Bentz ML, editor. Stamford, Conn.: QMP; 2008. p. 267–307.
19. Hashem FK, Al Khayal Z. Oral burn contractures in children. Ann Plast Surg. 2003;51(5):468–71.
20. Nahlieli O, Kelly JP, Baruchin AM, Benmeir P, Shapira Y. Oromaxillofacial skeletal deformities resulting from burn scar contractures of the face and neck. Burns. 1995;21(1):65–9.
21. Donelan MB, Parrett BM, Sheridan RL. Pulsed dye laser therapy and z-plasty for facial burn scars—the alternative to excision. Ann Plast Surg. 2008;60(5):480–6.
22. Gottlieb LJ, Krieger LM. From the reconstructive ladder to the reconstructive elevator. Plast Reconstr Surg. 1994;93(7):1503–4.
23. Neale HW, Kurtzman LC, Goh KBC, Billmire DA, Yakuboff KP, Warden G. Tissue expanders in the lower face and anterior neck in pediatric burn patients—limitations and pitfalls. Plast Reconstr Surg. 1993;91(4):624–31.
24. Bauer BS, Margulis A. The expanded transposition flap: shifting paradigms based on experience gained from two decades of pediatric tissue expansion. Plast Reconstr Surg. 2004;114(1):98–106.
25. Hyakusoku H, Takizawa Y, Murakami M, Gao JH, Takekoshi A, Fumiiri M. Versatility of the free or pedicled superficial cervical artery skin flaps in head and neck burns. Burns. 1993;19(2):168–73.
26. Vinh VQ, Van Anh T, Tien NG, Hyakusoku H, Ogawa R. Bipedicled "superthin" free perforator flaps for facial burn scar reconstruction: expanded scope of superthin flaps: a case series. Plast Reconstr Surg Glob Open. 2015;3(8):e493-e.
27. Kraft SP. In: Lambert SR, Lyons CJ, editors. Taylor & Hoyt's pediatric ophthalmology and strabismus. 5th ed. Edinburgh; New York: Elsevier; 2017. p. 992–5.
28. Frame JD, Still J, Lakhel-LeCoadou A, Carstens MH, Lorenz C, Orlet H, et al. Use of dermal regeneration template in contracture release procedures: a multicenter evaluation. Plast Reconstr Surg. 2004;113(5):1330–8.
29. Figus A, Leon-Villapalos J, Philp B, Dziewulski P. Severe multiple extensive postburn contractures: a simultaneous approach with total scar tissue excision and resurfacing with dermal regeneration template. J Burn Care Res. 2007;28(6):913–7.
30. Spence RJ. Experience with novel uses of tissue expanders in burn reconstruction of the face and neck. Ann Plast Surg. 1992;28(5):453–64.
31. Feldman J. Reconstruction of the burned face in children. In: Serafin D, Georgia NG, editors. St. Louis: Mosby; 1984.
32. Grishkevich VM. Trapeze-flap plasty: effective method for postburn neck contracture elimination. Burns. 2010;36(3):383–8.
33. Grishkevich VM, Grishkevich M, Menzul V. Postburn neck anterior contracture treatment in children with scar-fascial local trapezoid flaps: a new approach. J Burn Care Res. 2015;36(3):E112–E9.
34. Hyakusoku H, Orgill DP, Téot L, Pribaz JJ, Ogawa R. Color atlas of burn reconstructive surgery. Berlin, Heidelberg: Springer; 2010. https://doi.org/10.1007/978-3-642-05070-1. SpringerLink (Online service).
35. Vinh VQ, Van Anh T, Gia Tien N, Hyakusoku H, Ogawa R. Reconstruction of neck and face scar contractures using occipito-cervico-dorsal supercharged "super-thin flaps": a retrospective analysis of 82 cases in Vietnam. Burns. 2018;44:462–7.
36. Angrigiani C. Aesthetic microsurgical reconstruction of anterior neck burn deformities. Plast Reconstr Surg. 1994;93(3):507–18.

37. Greenhalgh DG, Gaboury T, Warden GD. The early release of axillary contractures in pediatric patients with burns. J Burn Care Rehabil. 1993;14(1):39–42.
38. Sison-Williamson M, Bagley A, Petuskey K, Takashiba S, Palmieri T. Analysis of upper extremity motion in children after axillary burn scar contracture release. J Burn Care Res. 2009;30(6):1002–6.
39. Lars Peter Kamholz TH. Reconstruction of burn deformities an overview. Edinburgh; New York: Saunders Elsevier; 2012. Available from: https://www.clinicalkey.com/dura/browse/bookChapter/3-s2.0-C20090425133.
40. Grishkevich VM. Postburn shoulder medial-adduction contracture: anatomy and treatment with trapeze-flap plasty. Burns. 2013;39(2):341–8.
41. Ogawa R, Hyakusoku H, Murakami M, Koike S. Reconstruction of axillary scar contractures—retrospective study of 124 cases over 25 years. Br J Plast Surg. 2003;56(2):100–5.
42. Huang C, Ogawa R. Three-dimensional reconstruction of scar contracture-bearing axilla and digital webs using the square flap method. Plast Reconstr Surg Glob Open. 2014;2(5):e149-e.
43. Agarwal R, Chandra R. Latissimus dorsi myocutaneous flap reconstruction of neck and axillary burn contractures. Plast Reconstr Surg. 2000;106(5):1216.
44. Asuku ME, Ibrahim A, Ijekeye FO. Post-burn axillary contractures in pediatric patients: a retrospective survey of management and outcome. Burns. 2008;34(8):1190–5.
45. Chen BG, Xu MH, Chai JK, Song HF, Gao QW. Surgical treatment of severe or moderate axillary burn scar contracture with transverse island scapular flap and expanded transverse island scapular flap in adult and pediatric patients—a clinical experience of 15 cases. Burns. 2015;41(4):872–80.
46. Er E, Ucar C. Reconstruction of axillary contractures with thoracodorsal perforator island flap. Burns. 2005;31(6):726–30.
47. Hallock GG, Okunski WJ. The parascapular fasciocutaneous flap for release of the axillary burn contracture. J Burn Care Rehabil. 1987;8(5):387–90.
48. Hallock GG. A systematic approach to flap selection for the axillary burn contracture. J Burn Care Rehabil. 1993;14(3):343–7.
49. Kim DY, Cho SY, Kim KS, Lee SY, Cho BH. Correction of axillary burn scar contracture with the thoracodorsal perforator-based cutaneous island flap. Ann Plast Surg. 2000;44(2):181–7.
50. Kulahci Y, Sever C, Uygur F, Oksuz S, Sahin C, Duman H. Pre-expanded pedicled thoracodorsal artery perforator flap for postburn axillary contracture reconstruction. Microsurgery. 2011;31(1):26–31.
51. Turkaslan T, Turan A, Dayicioglu D, Ozsoy Z. Uses of scapular island flap in pediatric axillary burn conractures. Burns. 2006;32(7):885–90.
52. McCauley RL. Reconstruction of the pediatric burned hand. Hand Clin. 2009;25(4):543.
53. McCauley RL, Beraja V, Rutan RL, Huang TT, Abston S, Rutan TC, et al. Longitudinal assessment of breast development in adolescent female patients with burns involving the nipple-areolar complex. Plast Reconstr Surg. 1989;83(4):676–80.
54. Frantz CH, Delgado S. Limb-length discrepancy after third-degree burns about foot and ankle—report of 4 cases. J Bone Joint Surg. 1966;A 48(3):443.
55. Bailey JK, Burkes SA, Visscher MO, Whitestone J, Kagan RJ, Yakuboff KP, et al. Multimodal quantitative analysis of early pulsed-dye laser treatment of scars at a pediatric burn hospital. Dermatol Surg. 2012;38(9):1490–6.
56. Blome-Eberwein S, Gogal C, Weiss MJ, Boorse D, Pagella P. Prospective evaluation of fractional CO2 laser treatment of mature burn scars. J Burn Care Res. 2016;37(6):379–87.
57. Hultman CS, Friedstat JS, Edkins RE, Cairns BA, Laser Resurfacing MAA. Remodeling of hypertrophic burn scars the results of a large, prospective, before-after cohort study, with long-term follow-up. Ann Surg. 2014;260(3):519–32.
58. Krakowski AC, Totri CR, Donelan MB, Shumaker PR. Scar management in the pediatric and adolescent populations. Pediatrics. 2016;137(2):e20142065.
59. Liuzzi F, Chadwick S, Shah M. Paediatric post-burn scar management in the UK: a national survey. Burns. 2015;41(2):252–6.
60. Parrett BM, Donelan MB. Pulsed dye laser in burn scars: current concepts and future directions. Burns. 2010;36(4):443–9.

Dermal Substitutes and Negative-Pressure Wound Therapy for Burns and Scars

10

J. Genevieve Park and Joseph A. Molnar

10.1 Historical Overview

Burn care has undergone a significant evolution in the last several decades that has led to both improved patient survival and greater challenges for the reconstructive surgeon. Much of the improved survival was due to advances in critical care medicine, but coincident changes in management of the burn wound also played an important role. Historically, burn wounds were allowed to sit and demarcate over weeks, leading to sepsis. Wide acceptance of the technique of early excision and grafting minimized this problem and improved survival [1–5]. With this advancement, a new problem emerged: how to cover the large burn with minimal donor sites [6, 7]. The standard treatment evolved to become meshed, split-thickness skin graft over the wound, which led to scarring and contracture due to the replacement of full-thickness skin loss with minimal dermis [8]. In an effort to increase survival of larger percent body surface area burns, meshing ratios became larger and grafts became thinner in order to allow rapid re-harvesting of the donor site. All of this led to greater and greater problems of scarring, contracture, and poor functionality. More patients survived larger burns but the concern was also how to make the patient functional and cosmetically acceptable to make life worth living [9].

Advancements in the 1970s included the development of cultured epithelium and progressive use of allograft and xenograft to deal with this problem of coverage [10, 11]. Xenograft and allograft only allowed temporary coverage until donor sites could be repeatedly re-harvested for definitive coverage. The observation that sometimes the dermis would become incorporated into the wound led to the discovery that the epidermis contained the most antigenic portion of the allograft, and if this was removed, the allogenic dermis could be left in the wound with the hope of improving functional and cosmetic outcomes [11, 12]. The result was progressive attempts to develop decellularized dermis that could be placed in the burn wound to replace the lost dermis of a full-thickness burn and later cover with the patient's own epidermis or keratinocytes grown in culture [10, 11, 13, 14].

The dream of cultured epithelium was to replace the limitation of donor site availability. Unfortunately, it was found that the result often was an unstable, friable epidermis that led to considerable scarring and contracture [15–17]. Furthermore, cultured keratinocytes had a high cost in terms of time, expense, and complexity of cell expansion [16]. There was some success in culturing keratinocytes directly on top of synthetic dermis or allograft (to be used as a composite graft), but this was time consuming as well as costly [18]. There was some success in healing full-thickness wounds with allograft, followed by sheets of CEA, with reportedly 87–100% take, with 4 years of follow-up [14]. Wainwright performed a pilot study comparing split-thickness skin graft alone to AlloDerm and split-thickness skin graft, side-by-side, in three patients, and they showed that the functional and cosmetic results of the AlloDerm group were superior at 3 months. This was attributed to the acellular dermal allograft allowing a more mature and continuous dermis to form. In the meshed split-thickness skin graft sites, in comparison, immature collagen matrix was seen in open areas of mesh, which later made scarring worse [12].

An entirely different approach to coverage of the burn wound was to completely bioengineer a skin substitute. Burke and Yannas wished to develop a skin substitute for burn patients that would resemble skin, rather than scar, when fully healed [19, 20]. The bioengineered skin substitute was designed to have two layers, just as normal skin has two layers: dermis and epidermis. The dermal layer was made of cross-linked bovine collagen and shark chondroitin 6-sulfate (glycosaminoglycan) with control of such proper-

J. G. Park · J. A. Molnar (✉)
Department of Plastic and Reconstructive Surgery, Wake Forest School of Medicine, Winston-Salem, NC, USA
e-mail: jmolnar@wakehealth.edu

© Springer Nature Singapore Pte Ltd. 2020
R. Ogawa (ed.), *Total Scar Management*, https://doi.org/10.1007/978-981-32-9791-3_10

ties as cross-linking and porosity to control cellular ingrowth and degradation [21]. The temporary "epidermis" was made of silicone to prevent desiccation and provide mechanical protection to the underlying dermal substitute. This product had the advantage of rapid coverage of the excised burn wound while providing a dermis that would allow thinner split-thickness skin grafts for rapid re-harvest of donor sites.

The first reported use of Burke and Yannas's bi-layered artificial skin (later called Integra) came in 1981, when it was used to treat patients with 50–90% total body surface area (TBSA) burns [22]. Tompkins et al. performed a retrospective study of adults with massive burn injuries and showed that improved survival was associated with the use of artificial skin, likely due to the ability to cover excised wounds earlier when autograft donor sites are limited [7].

While originally designed to be a lifesaving product, the hope was that dermal substitutes would also provide a functionally and cosmetically superior outcome compared to the standard of split-thickness skin graft alone. The initial published study showed that collagen arrangement in healed Integra skin resembled normal dermis rather than scar [22]. Patients and physicians also subjectively thought it was more normal than split-thickness skin graft, with 72% patients preferring the skin reconstructed with artificial dermis 1 year after reconstruction [23]. Investigators noted that the use of artificial dermis decreased the likelihood of unfavorable scars, and that when used with a meshed autograft, the resulting skin did not have the characteristic "crocodile skin" showing the meshed pattern [22, 23].

In the 1980s, clinicians reported that it was difficult to work with Integra, with reported take rate as low as 43%, often attributed to fluid collection below the silastic layer [22–24]. In a prospective, multicenter study of 106 patients, immediate coverage with standard of care (split-thickness skin graft or allograft) resulted in take rate of 79%, whereas immediate coverage with Integra resulted in only 62% take rate [23]. A retrospective review of 89 consecutive patients treated with Integra for hypertrophic scars found that fluid collected under the silastic layer in 14% of cases and there was microbial colonization or infection in 20% of cases [25]. Daily vigilance and wound care to prevent rampant infection was required. A variety of investigations concentrated on developing the ideal dressing to optimize success [26].

A new device became available in the 1990s that helped solve this problem. The use of a dressing that enabled subatmospheric pressure application to the wound became known as negative-pressure wound therapy (NPWT) or topical negative pressure (TNP) [27, 28]. It accelerated the ingrowth of granulation tissue, decreased edema, and decreased bacterial colonization in a variety of circumstances by an uncertain mechanism [29]. Schneider et al. demonstrated this as a convenient and effective way to secure skin grafts as it conformed to the wound, eliminated dead space, removed excess fluid, and could be used as a splint (Fig. 10.1) [28, 30].

It was logical to think that a device that worked so well on skin grafts might also work well with an artificial skin substitute. Early efforts showed excellent results in complicated reconstructive wounds showing take rates approaching

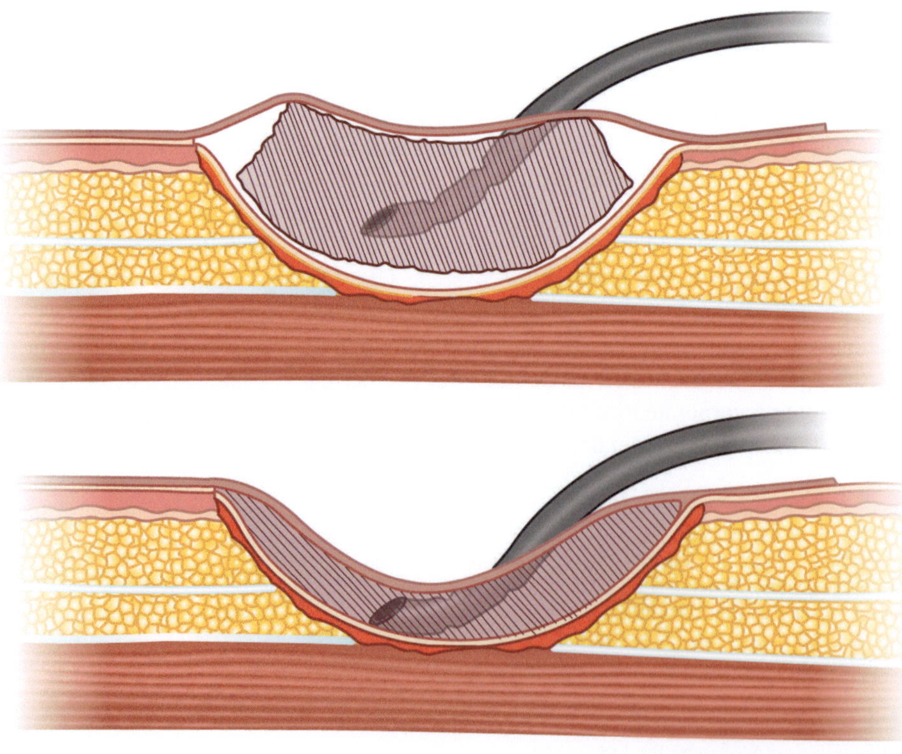

Fig. 10.1 The properties of NPWT that improved the take of skin graft made it a logical dressing for a skin substitute. A dermal substitute or skin graft is placed between the wound bed and the NPWT dressing (top). Application of subatmospheric pressure eliminates dead space and prevents shearing (bottom). Reproduced from [28]. Images used with permission of the Wake Forest Department of Plastic and Reconstructive Surgery

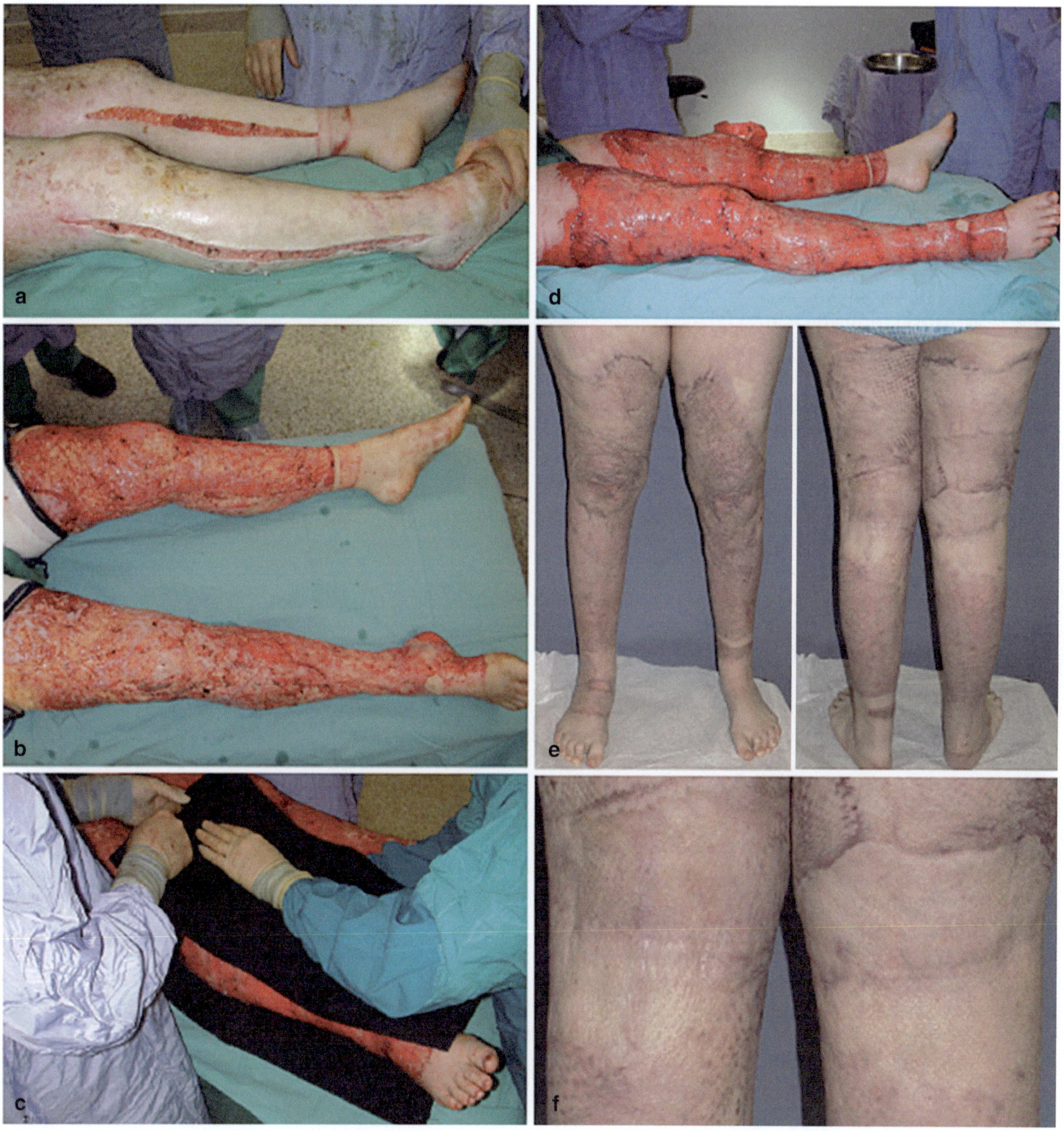

Fig. 10.2 A 15-year-old female with (**a**) bilateral circumferential full-thickness burns of lower extremities. (**b**) Operative excision to fat. (**c**) Integra placed and wrapped with NPWT device. (**d**) Integra incorporated at 1 week in preparation for skin grafting. (**e**) Result at 6 months. (**f**) Close-up of popliteal fossae showing lack of contractures. 1:1 meshed skin was used in this area and 1:3 or greater in other areas. Images used with permission of the Wake Forest Department of Plastic and Reconstructive Surgery.

100% [29, 31, 32]. Jeschke et al., in a prospective randomized trial, demonstrated that large wounds could be covered by Integra, with an engraftment rate of 98% when used in conjunction with NPWT and fibrin glue [32]. The use of NPWT and fibrin glue also decreased the time interval between Integra placement and skin grafting by over 50% [32]. Molnar et al. (2004) found similar results without fibrin glue [29]. These improvements also resulted in decreased length of stay of patients treated with Integra instead of conventional split-thickness skin graft in large burns [33]. It also allowed for ease of use in reconstructive patients as outpatients [34]. A multicenter, randomized, controlled trial of 86 patients showed that the use of NPWT did not significantly affect the take of the dermal substitute (Matriderm) or the subsequent skin graft, but it did improve the quality of scar [35]. Figure 10.2 shows a 15-year-old girl who sustained bilateral, circumferential, full-thickness leg burns. Her burns were excised to fat and covered with Integra. She underwent NPWT and delayed split-thickness skin grafting. She had an excellent functional result at 6 months.

After initial success in covering acute burn wounds, dermal substitutes were quickly adapted to solve other clinical situations, including hypertrophic scars and keloids, traumatic wounds, soft tissue defects after oncologic resection, and chronic wounds.

10.2 Wound Healing Using Dermal Substitutes

This section is a simplified review of concepts that may help the clinician better understand reconstruction of skin using a dermal substitute. Our hope is that this insight will aid the clinician in identifying the right applications of this method, and enable the clinician to troubleshoot some issues that may come up.

Reconstruction of normal skin is a lofty goal. Normal skin consists of two layers, the epidermis and the dermis, separated by a basement membrane. The major cell type in the epidermis is the keratinocyte, and this cell is critical to the barrier function of skin. The epidermis also contains melanocytes, which provide pigmentation to the skin. The epidermis and dermis are separated by a thin basement membrane, an interdigitating connection consisting of epidermal rete and dermal papillae. The main cell type in the dermis is the fibroblast, which is responsible for maintaining and remodeling the extracellular matrix, primarily made up of collagen and proteoglycans. In normal dermis, the collagen fibrils are randomly oriented. The dermis also contains adnexal structures, including hair follicles and sweat glands. Dermal substitutes do not recreate normal skin, but they can allow a wound to heal with some of the properties of normal skin: protection from infection, evaporative losses, and adequate pliability and elasticity that does not restrict movement or growth.

Normal wound healing proceeds through three overlapping phases: inflammation (days 2–5), proliferation (days 4–14), and remodeling (8 days to 1 year). During the inflammation phase, growth factors and cytokines attract neutrophils and monocytes to the area of injury. Monocytes differentiate into macrophages, which remove debris, engulf bacteria, and secrete cytokines and growth factors critical to the proliferation phase of wound healing. During the proliferation phase, fibroblasts and keratinocytes migrate into the wound. Keratinocytes begin to re-epithelialize the skin, while fibroblasts begin to secrete collagen and other proteins, including proteoglycans and glycosaminoglycans, creating an immature extracellular matrix. Some fibroblasts differentiate into myofibroblasts, which promote wound contraction. Fibroblasts also secrete enzymes that function to modify and increase turnover of the extracellular matrix in the remodeling phase. Collagen becomes aligned in mature scar.

Healing full-thickness wounds by secondary intention relies on wound contraction for wound closure, which leads to thick, fibrous, non-pliable skin. Histological studies demonstrate a normal-appearing epithelium and scant, abnormal dermis. Deep partial-thickness wounds, which retain some dermis, exhibit robust contraction and can result in unfavorable scars, including hypertrophic scars, contractures, and keloids. An abnormal dermis characterizes hypertrophic scars and keloids: hypertrophic scar contains nodular areas with myofibroblasts and randomly oriented collagen, and keloids have thick collagen fibers packed closely together [36].

The presence of adequate and "normal" dermis can prevent unfavorable scar formation, retain pliability, and reduce contraction. Skin grafts provide a wound with normal dermis and epidermis, and thicker grafts (with more dermis) have decreased wound contraction. A dermal substitute is designed as a scaffold to promote the formation of a thicker dermis, and thus prevent the formation of an unfavorable, abnormal scar [19, 22, 37]. Studies in the 1980s demonstrated that this did indeed work: placing the right scaffold in a wound bed resulted in the host's fibroblasts populating the scaffold and slowly replacing the scaffold with an extracellular matrix similar to that of normal dermis, often called a "neodermis" [22, 38, 39]. Living allogenic cells, integrated into some dermal substitutes, are replaced by the host's own cells after several weeks; their main function may be to secrete growth factors [40, 41]. An epidermis integrated with the neodermis forms after the placement of a thin, epithelial skin graft [42].

NPWT appears to accelerate the "take" of dermal substitute, but the mechanism is not fully understood [29, 43]. In open wounds, NPWT immediately increases blood flow, increases the rate of granulation tissue formation, and decreases bacterial load [27]. Further studies have shown that it promotes wound healing by macrodeformation, microdeformation, fluid removal, and altering cell signaling factors in the wound [44–47]. It is postulated, but not proven, that NPWT increases the growth and proliferation of cells in a dermal substitute by the same mechanisms. After 3 days of NPWT, there is increased vascularity and better adherence of Integra (unpublished data). A histological study of hypertrophic scar resurfacing with Integra seemed to show otherwise: neovascularization was not significantly different with or without NPWT [31]. NPWT may simply improve the adherence of the dermal substitute to the wound bed by removing dead space. Regardless of mechanism, NPWT has become a reliable tool to be used with dermal substitutes.

10.3 Clinical Applications of Dermal Substitutes

The initial application of dermal substitutes was in patients with massive burn injury. This technology was rapidly adopted for coverage of full-thickness wounds in other clinical scenarios as early as 2001 [39]. The use of dermal substitutes, with and without NPWT, in the reconstruction of wounds unrelated to burn injury has been extensively reviewed [41, 48, 49]. This section serves as a brief overview of some of the most common applications of dermal substitutes and NPWT in the prevention and treatment of abnormal scar.

10.3.1 Acute Burn Injury

Early excision and wound coverage has been shown to decrease mortality and accelerate recovery after burn injury [4, 50], and wound closure within 2–3 weeks has been shown to decrease the rate of hypertrophic burn scar formation [51, 52]. The most common strategy for early wound coverage is immediate placement of a meshed split-thickness skin graft, when available. However, if the patient has limited donor sites or cannot tolerate harvesting of skin grafts, a dermal substitute can be placed for immediate, temporary coverage of the excised wounds. In 1981, Burke et al. reported the successful use of Integra as a temporizing dermal matrix in patients with 50–90% TBSA burns, until skin grafting occurred weeks later [53]. Numerous studies followed, demonstrating the successful use of a variety of dermal substitutes in initial coverage of large, acute burns [11, 13, 54–56]. An example of an acute burn treated with Integra and NPWT is shown in Fig. 10.2.

Cuono et al. showed that decellularized human cadaver dermis (AlloDerm) could be used to cover excised burn wounds while autologous keratinocytes were cultured and expanded. The autologous keratinocytes were then seeded over the neodermis with successful engraftment [11, 13, 56]. A retrospective case series of massive burn patients found that the placement of AlloDerm with a split-thickness skin graft over major joints resulted in no limitation of movement in 43% of patients [55].

One of the most challenging areas to treat is the burned hand, due to its propensity to form contractures that limit functional movement. There has been success with treating acute hand burns with Integra and delayed split-thickness skin graft [57, 58]. A case series of 11 acute, full-thickness hand burns demonstrated the effectiveness of this method, with only two hands having hypertrophic scarring requiring further operation [58].

The sequelae of facial burn injury can be devastating. Hypertrophic scarring can lead to ectropion, microstomia, hypertrophic scar, in addition to poor cosmesis and social exclusion. Thus, prevention of hypertrophic scarring has been an area of clinical interest for quite some time [59]. Many clinicians have reported good results using a dermal substitute to cover acute facial burns. In a case series, 16 patients with deep facial burns underwent early excision of their burns (within 3 days of injury), followed by immediate coverage with an acellular dermal matrix and an epidermal skin graft overlay (approximately 8/1000 of an inch thickness). After this one-stage operation, the authors reported 97% take at postoperative day 14, and low rates of complications related to hypertrophic scar (one patient with microstomia, two patients with ectropion) [60]. A one-stage operation using Matriderm and a thin skin graft in both pediatric and adult facial burns has been used with encouraging results [61, 62].

NPWT over facial burns is not typically recommended due to difficulty in maintaining a seal and airway issues. However, it can be safely placed over ears. The pressure differential of 1/6 atmosphere is not harmful for tympanic membranes. It may also be safely used over eyes with a temporary tarsorrhaphy [63].

10.3.2 Sequelae of Burn Injury: Hypertrophic Scars and Contracture

Hypertrophic scars, common after deep partial-thickness and full-thickness burn injury, are pruritic, disfiguring, erythematous, and inelastic, often leading to disfigurement and the formation of contractures [64]. Hypertrophic scars form through a complex interplay of pro-fibrotic cytokines, abnormal fibroblasts and keratinocytes, and an abnormal extracellular matrix (ECM) [65]. In comparison to mature scar, the ECM of hypertrophic scar contains increased amounts of proteoglycans, glycoproteins, and type III collagen (found in immature scar), and collagen forms disorganized nodules [36]. Nonoperative treatments, such as silicone gel sheeting, pressure (compression) therapy, corticosteroid injection, cryotherapy, and laser therapy, have proven to be effective in over 50% of patients [52]. Hypertrophic scars that are refractory to conservative treatments can undergo operative intervention by excision or contracture release followed by wound coverage. Tissue expansion, local flaps (Z-plasty), regional flaps, free flaps, skin grafts, or a dermal substitute can provide wound coverage [52, 66, 67].

There are several reports of successful treatment of hypertrophic scars by resurfacing them with a dermal substitute. One of the first of reports of success with this method was using Matriderm and a skin graft (in a two-stage procedure), showing that this led to significant improvements in pliability, elasticity, and retraction of nearly all 44 scars [68]. Moiemen et al. demonstrated that Integra could be used to

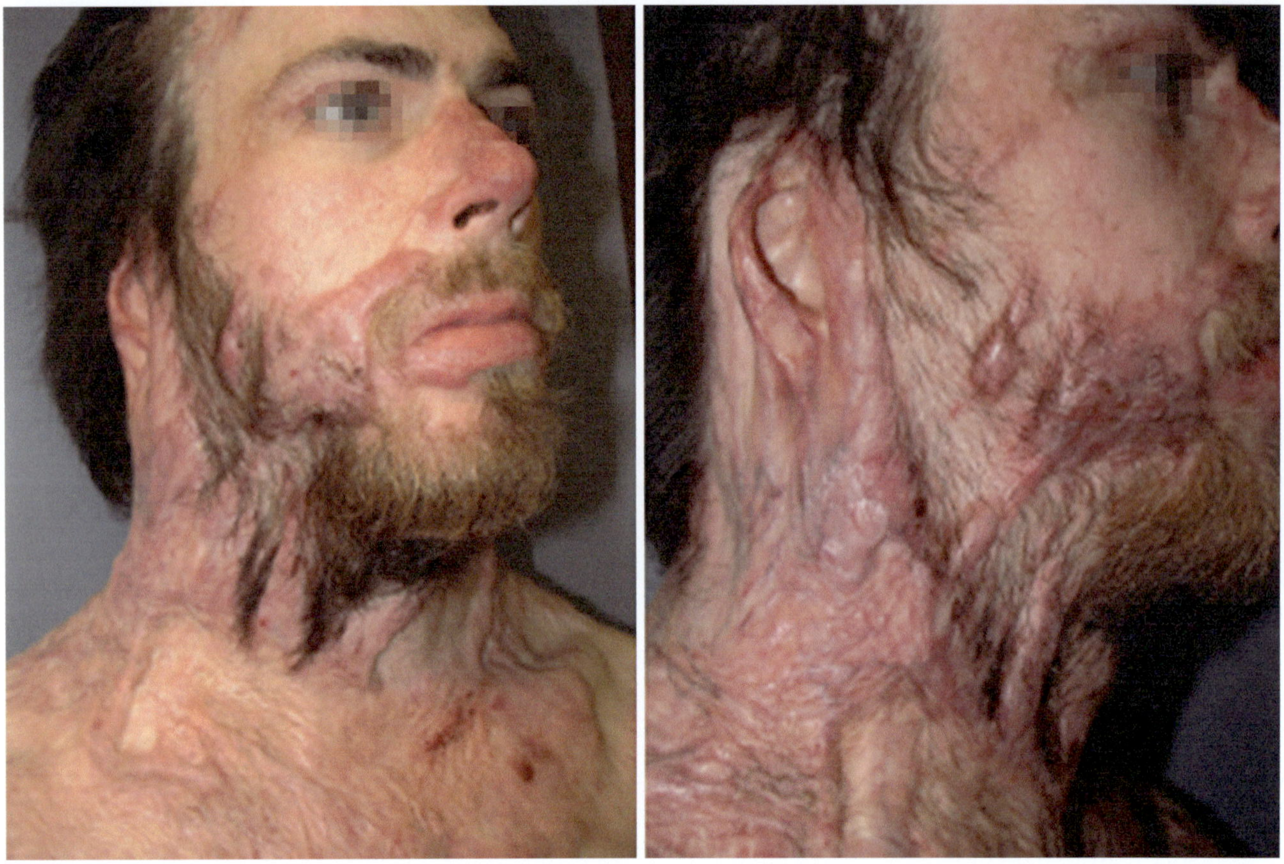

Fig. 10.3 A 23-year-old male, 1 year after burn injury with hypertrophic scar and contracture. Images used with permission of the Wake Forest Department of Plastic and Reconstructive Surgery

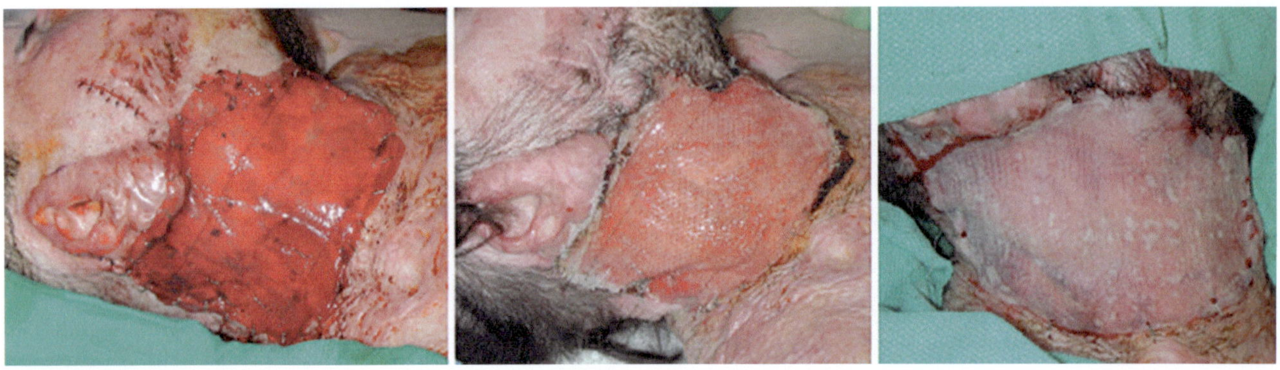

Fig. 10.4 The patient in Fig. 10.3 underwent excision of cervical scar and placement of 1:1 mesh dermal regeneration template prior to placing NPWT (left). Engraftment of Integra at 2 weeks prior to placing skin graft (middle). A 0.010-inch sheet graft was placed (right). Gauze dressing now used due to difficulty in obtaining seal in hair bearing area. Custom-made thermoplastic splint used to decrease motion for 1 week. Images used with permission of the Wake Forest Department of Plastic and Reconstructive Surgery

improve the quality of hypertrophic scars in a case study of 35 scars, and later reported over 95% take when used in conjunction with NPWT [31, 39]. Another early study of contracture releases covered by Integra reported a 25% recurrence rate over a mean of 11.4 months of follow-up. This was excellent in comparison to other studies at the time reporting 38–80% recurrence rate using full-thickness and split-thickness skin grafts [25]. Hypertrophic scars resurfaced with Integra appeared to retain their pliability and softness over more than 2 years of follow-up [42]. Figure 10.3 shows

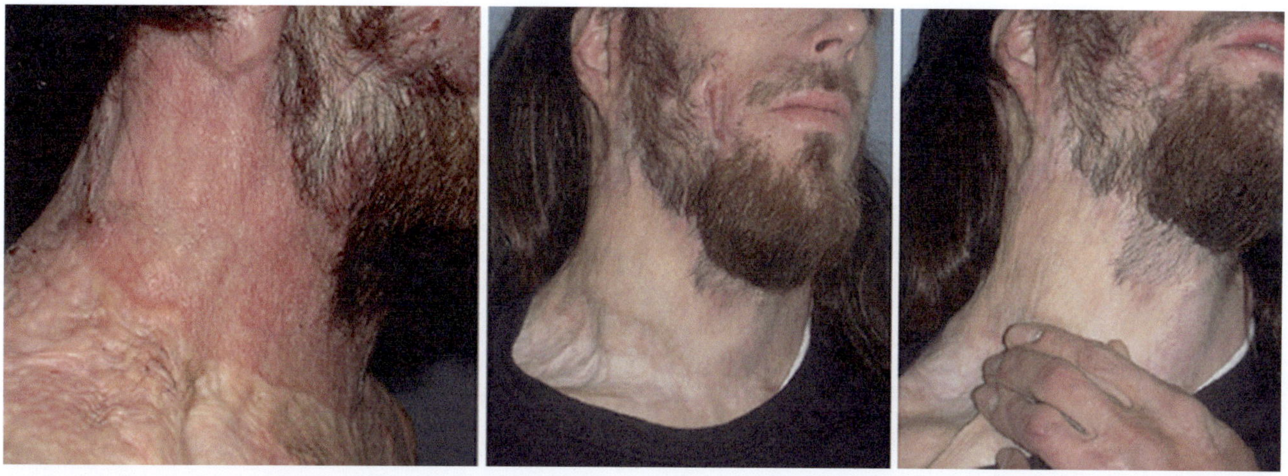

Fig. 10.5 Reconstruction of cervical hypertrophic scar with Integra. Patient in Figs. 10.3 and 10.4 at 3 months postoperatively (left). Graft remains hyperemic and skin is tight. Therapy should be continued during this period of healing. Final result at 1 year (middle, right). Improved distensibility of tissue and no recurrent scarring. Images used with permission of the Wake Forest Department of Plastic and Reconstructive Surgery

a 23-year-old man who developed a hypertrophic neck scar 1 year after his injury. The scar was excised and covered with Integra. A 0.010-inch-thick skin graft was placed 2 weeks later (Fig. 10.4). There has been no recurrence of hypertrophic scar in 2 years of follow-up (Fig. 10.5).

One of the most challenging areas to treat hypertrophic burn scars is on the hand. Contracture releases often result in open areas needing skin coverage with excellent pliability. While a full-thickness skin graft remains the standard of care, dermal substitutes have also been used to improve range of motion of the hand. The two-stage procedure of initial application of Integra, followed by a split-thickness skin graft, has been the subject of several retrospective case series, with success rates as high as 100% [57, 69–71]. In one study, over 75% of patients retain their improved range of motion over 6 months to 6 years [57]. Interestingly, some of the best results were described in a case series of nine patients who underwent two-stage reconstruction with AlloDerm (applied with fibrin glue and secured with NPWT) and split-thickness skin graft. Over 10 months of follow-up, the patients retained 83% of postoperative improvement in range of motion and web space depth [72]. A case series of patients treated with a one-stage reconstruction using Matriderm and a split-thickness skin graft reported 100% take of graft and a good functional result at 12 months of follow-up [73].

Interestingly, burned breast contractures have been treated with dermal substitutes. After release of these contractures, there is a large skin defect that would be difficult to cover with a full-thickness skin graft. Instead, Integra has been used to cover the wound. The healed skin allows for continued breast growth, and recurrent contracture is reported in only 1 of 13 reported cases [74, 75].

Pediatric hypertrophic burn scars have improved with resurfacing using a dermal substitute, with or without NPWT [76, 77]. Figure 10.6 shows a 4-year-old Asian female, who sustained burns to the left arm, axilla, and chest at 9 months of age. She developed a burn scar contracture of the left axilla and elbow, limiting her range of motion. She underwent contracture release of the axillary scar. Integra and NPWT were applied to the anterior axilla so as not to endanger breast tissue (Fig. 10.7). Seven days later, a 0.006-inch-thick skin graft was placed over the Integra. She had 100% take of skin graft and full range of motion (Fig. 10.8). There has been no recurrence of contracture in 14 years of follow-up.

10.3.3 Traumatic Injuries: Soft Tissue Loss with Exposed Bone and Tendon

Dermal substitutes and NPWT have become important tools in the treatment of traumatic injuries with exposed bone and tendon. Traumatic soft tissue and orthopedic injuries can be challenging to close. Many require placement of a flap to protect exposed tendon and bone from infection. NPWT alone was advocated as a good way to accelerate granulation tissue over exposed bone, tendon, and hardware, thus decreasing the size of the wound and providing a wound amenable to placement of a skin graft or flap [78, 79]. A retrospective series of 75 patients with lower extremity wounds initially treated with NPWT after debridement showed decreased wound size and formation of granulation tissue in 95% of patients. All wounds were amenable to split-thickness skin graft or flap closure [80]. This method was also shown to be effective to treat hand and foot degloving injuries [81]. NPWT is an effective method to prepare wound beds containing exposed bone in traumatic injuries, namely open tibial fractures, including those in pediatric patients [82–84]. NPWT and serial debridement can serve as

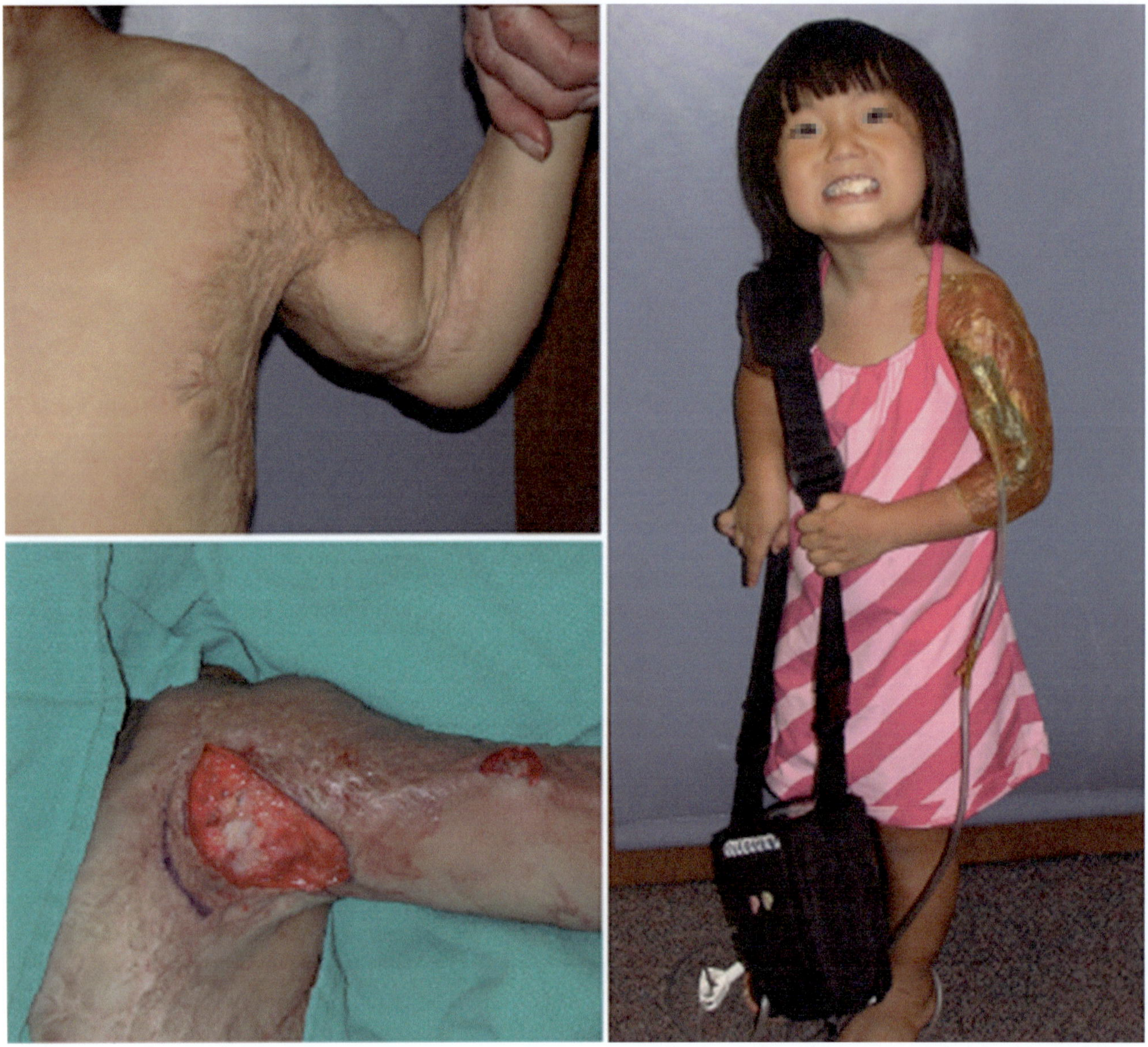

Fig. 10.6 A 4-year-old female with a fixed left axillary contracture from burn injury at 9 months of age. Shown is the maximum abduction possible (left, above). Scar released on arm and skin retracted into axilla in order to avoid damage to breast tissue (left, below). Integra was placed, dressed with NPWT, and patient was discharged home postoperatively (right). Reproduced from [34], used with permission of the Wake Forest Department of Plastic and Reconstructive Surgery

a bridge to definitive closure, and may actually decrease the time to bony union.

The combination of a dermal substitute, NPWT, and delayed split-thickness skin graft has been shown to be effective in healing traumatic wounds with exposed bone and tendon in a number of studies [29, 48, 85–87]. Figure 10.9 is an example of a deep burn injury to the ankle with exposed ligament, tendon, bone, and joint treated successfully with NPWT and dermal substitute.

This approach has also proven useful in treating complex, combat-related injuries [88, 89]. A recent retrospective review of 251 combat injuries treated at Walter Reed National Military Medical Center found that 80% of wounds healed after the first attempt at closure with Integra, NPWT, and delayed skin graft.

10.3.4 Keloids

Keloids occur when there is an aberrant wound healing response to a cutaneous injury. The pathogenesis of keloids is reviewed in this book and elsewhere [36, 90]. The end result is a benign lesion that continues to grow beyond the edges of the initial injury. Histological studies reveal a

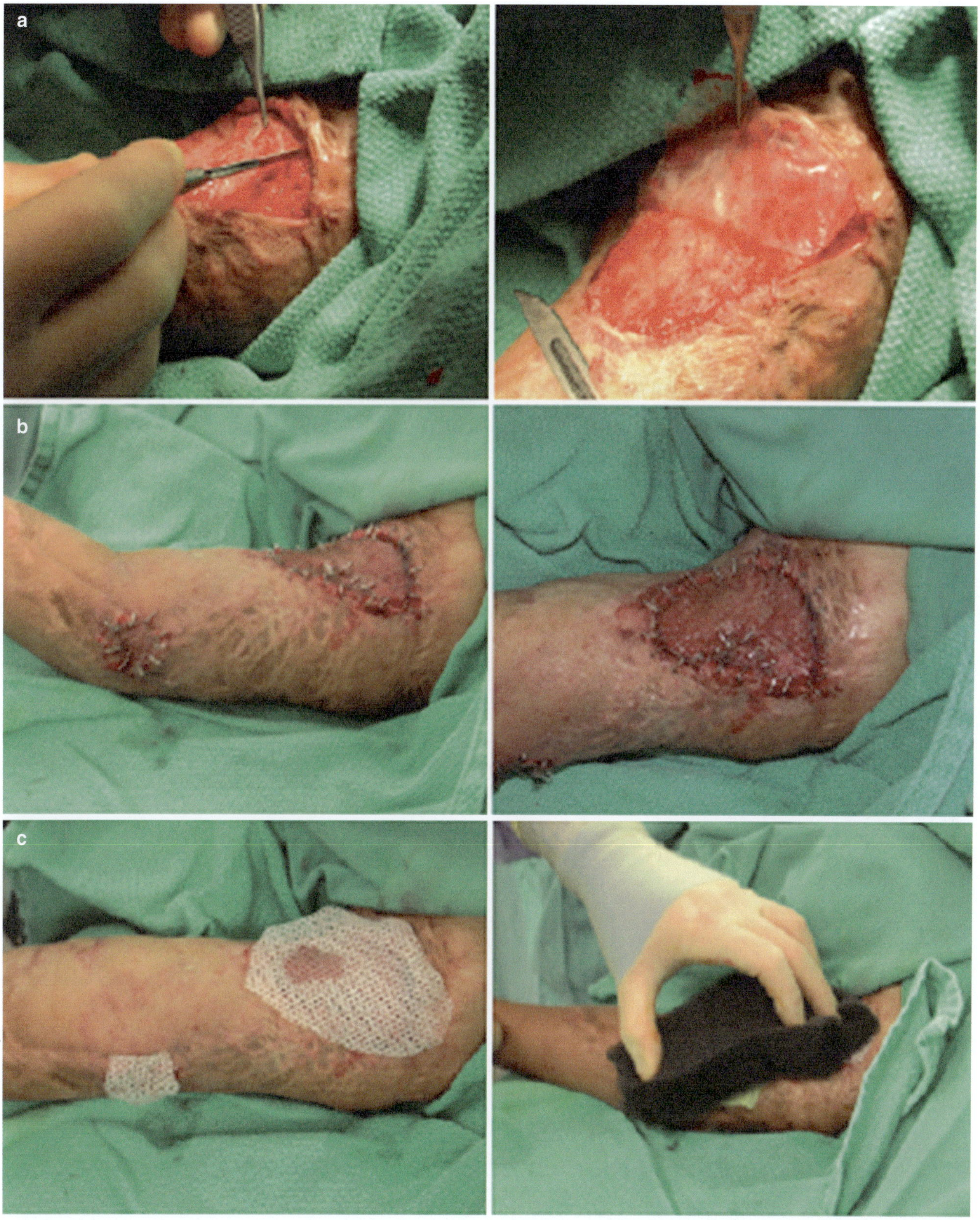

Fig. 10.7 Second-stage operation of patient in Fig. 10.6. (**a**) Integra was engrafted after 1 week of NPWT. Silicone layer removed from Integra. (**b**) Split-thickness skin graft placed on wound. (**c**) Nonadherent dressing applied. Mepitel (Molynke) was used in this case but Adaptic and Conformant may also be used. (**d**) NPWT applied and again patient treated as outpatient. Images used with permission of the Wake Forest Department of Plastic and Reconstructive Surgery

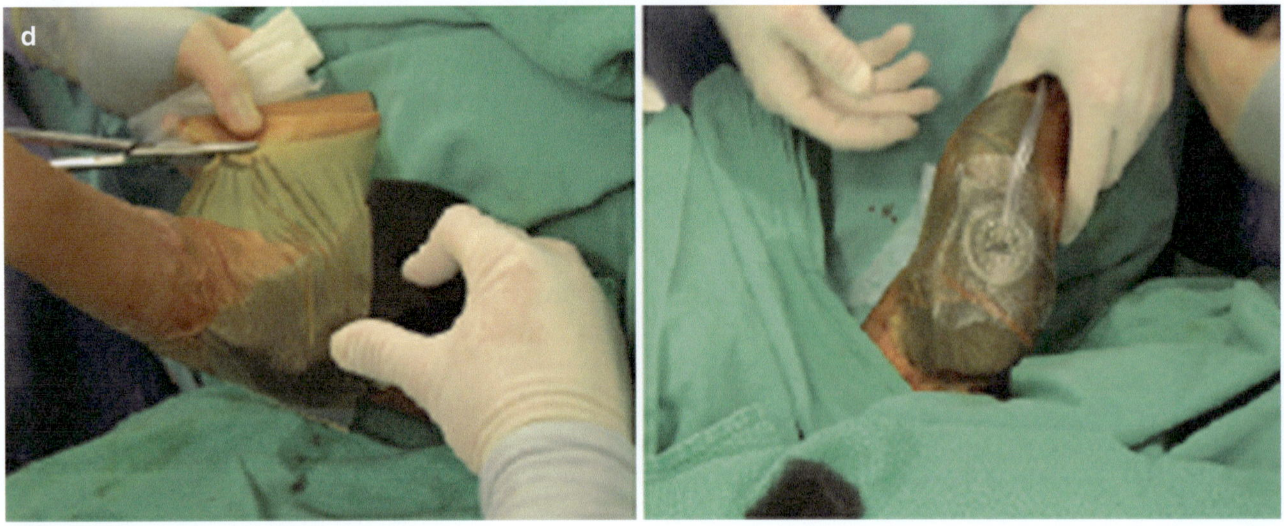

Fig. 10.7 (continued)

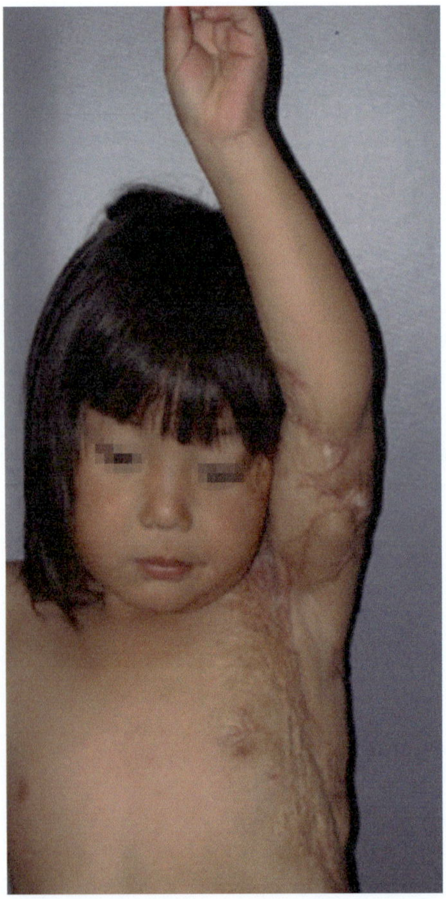

Fig. 10.8 Final result of patient seen in Figs. 10.6 and 10.7. Improved range of motion at 2 months after surgery. Images used with permission of the Wake Forest Department of Plastic and Reconstructive Surgery

normal-appearing epidermis and a markedly abnormal and thickened dermis, characterized by broad collagen bundles and fibrous bands, increased amount of proteoglycans, inflammatory infiltrate, and fibroblasts. Keloids can lead to pain, pruritis, decreased range of motion, infection, and social exclusion. Common treatments include steroid injections, fluorouracil (5-FU) injections, radiation therapy, and excision, but the rate of recurrence is notoriously high (45–100%) [91, 92].

Several case reports of successful treatment of keloids, refractory to other treatments, by excision and placement of a dermal substitute have been published. The use of Integra, followed by split-thickness or epidermal skin graft, has been reported the most often, with no recurrence in most cases over 6–24 months of follow-up [34, 70, 93–95]. An example is shown in Fig. 10.10. In some cases, recurrence is reported at the rim of the wound, which is then treated with excision and injection of 5-FU [70, 94]. Patel et al. used AlloDerm to successfully treat 8 keloids, with no recurrence in up to 48 months of follow-up [96]. There has been speculation, but no definitive evidence, that a dermal substitute provides a scaffold that promotes regeneration of a normal dermis [48]. Larger prospective studies comparing this method to the standard of care will be necessary before it gains wider acceptance.

10.3.5 Other Surgical Wounds

This method is also applicable to a variety of surgical wounds, including those that result in exposed bone or

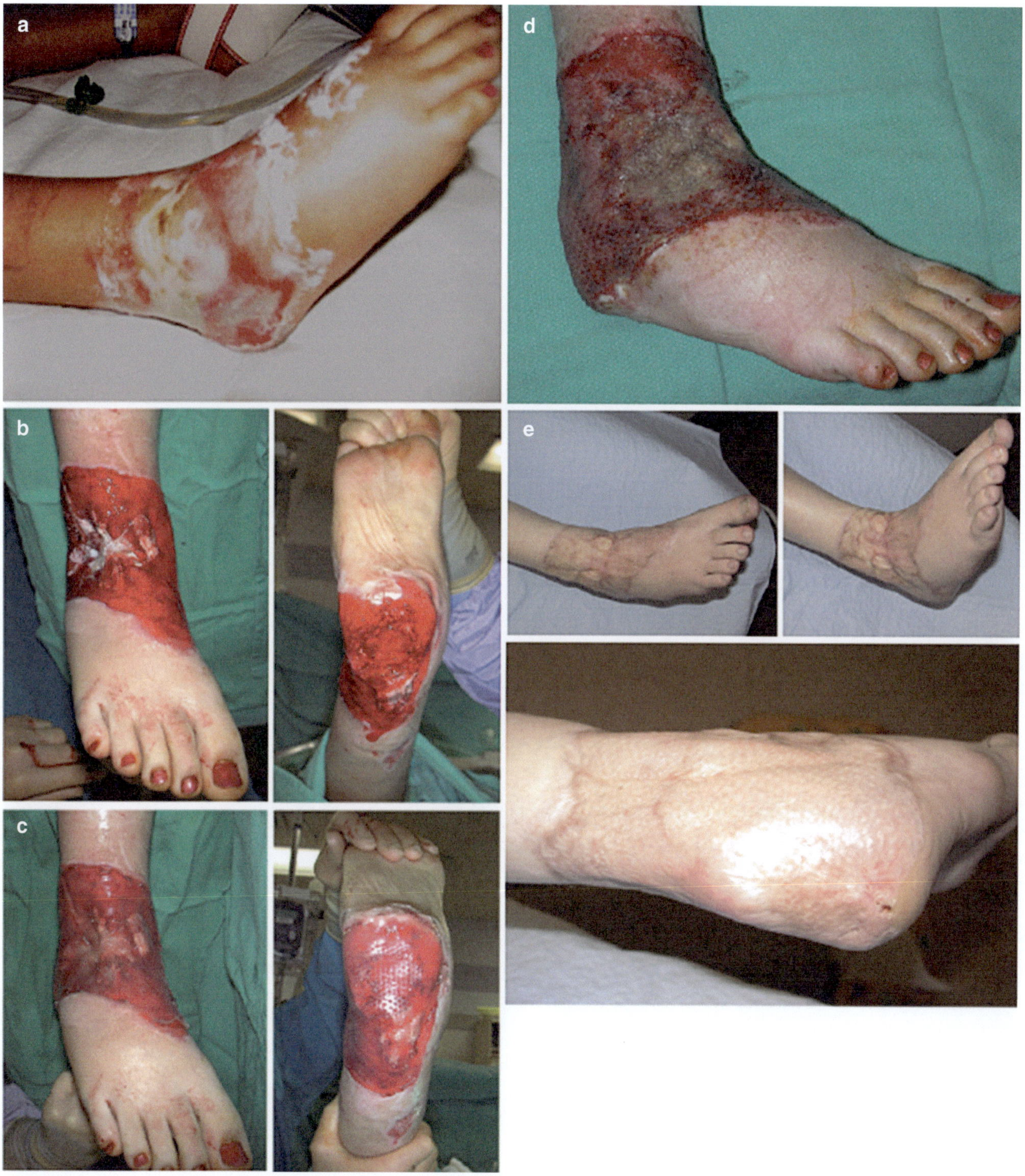

Fig. 10.9 A 16-year-old female with a deep burn from a motor vehicular accident exposing tendon, ligaments, and calcaneus (**a**, **b**). Orthopedic plan was ankle fusion due to ankle fractures. (**c**) Integra placed over wound after debridement. Treated with NPWT for 12 days. (**d**) Wound after skin grafting. NPWT was used for 5 days to aid engraftment. (**e**) Result at 6 months. No additional reconstruction was required and patient resumed all previous activities. Images used with permission of the Wake Forest Department of Plastic and Reconstructive Surgery

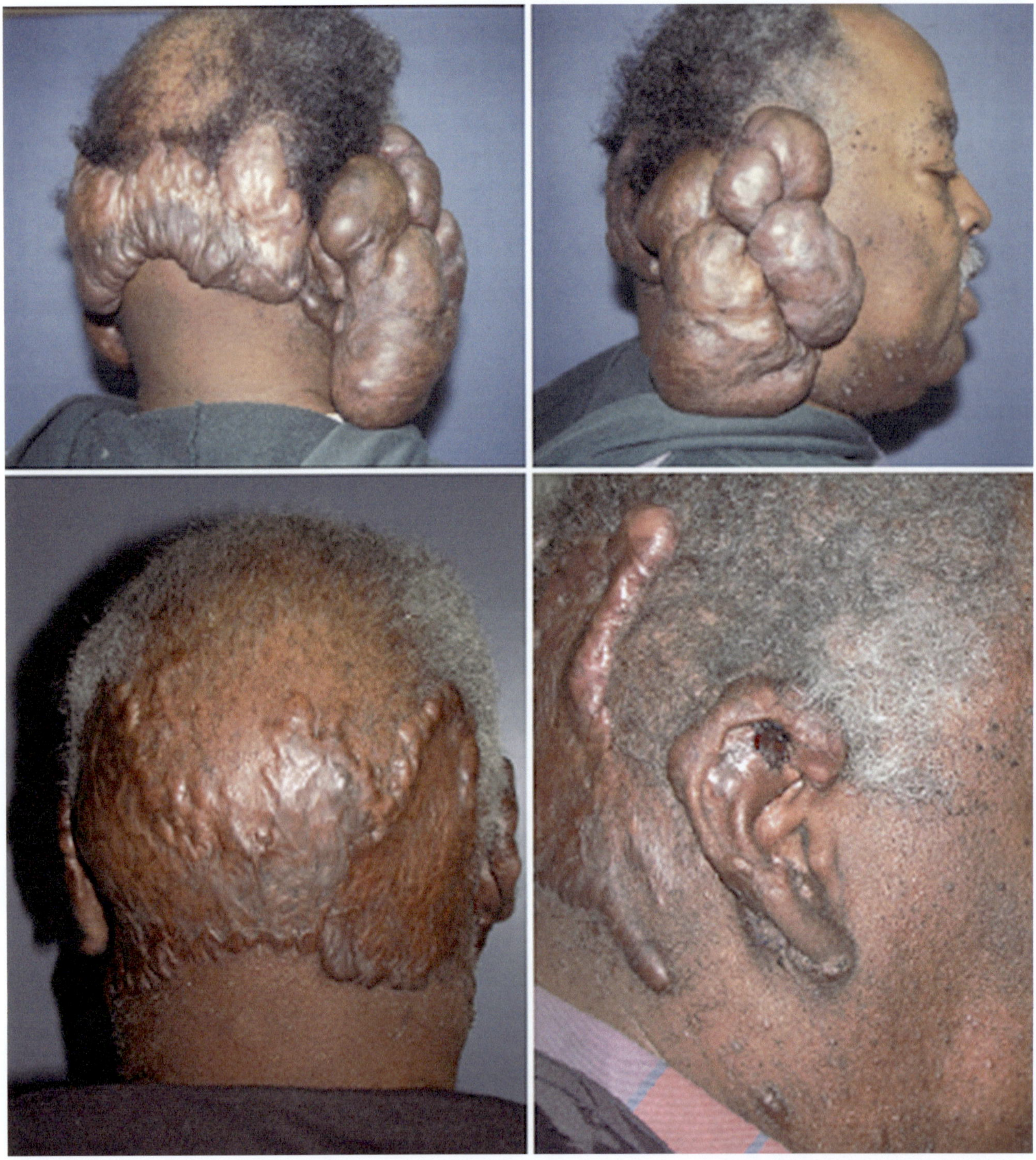

Fig. 10.10 Large keloid treated with excision, Integra, and delayed skin graft, with good result. Images used with permission of the Wake Forest Department of Plastic and Reconstructive Surgery

tendon. Not surprisingly, some the best results using dermal substitutes have been obtained in clean surgical wounds, including those with exposed bone and tendon. A common example is reconstruction of a defect after oncologic resection of skin cancer. Even wounds of the scalp, with exposed calvarium, have been successfully treated with a two-stage operation [97–99].

Dermal substitutes have also been used to improve healing of free flap donor defects, specifically the radial forearm free flap defect [87]. In a small retrospective study, Rowe et al. compared functional results of reconstruction with a skin graft alone or a composite graft consisting of a dermal substitute and a thin skin graft and found that the results using the composite graft were far superior [100]. A retrospective review of 29 patients with radial forearm free flap donor defects, who underwent two-stage reconstruction with Integra and delayed split-thickness skin graft, reported no complications and good results [101]. A pilot study of 10 patients with free flap donor site defects showed good healing using a two-stage operation and a degradable polyurethane dermal substitute [102].

10.4 Surgical Technique: Two-Stage Skin Reconstruction with a Dermal Substitute and Split-Thickness Skin Graft

The simplicity, adaptability, and reliability of this method make it attractive and accessible to many surgeons. There are many variations of this method that have been described in the literature, but we have used this particular method at our institution since the early 2000s with reliable results. This method is similar to the one provided by Integra Life Sciences [103].

10.4.1 Preparation of the Wound

The success of this method, especially in reconstructing contaminated wounds, relies heavily on a clean, healthy wound bed. Burn wounds should be excised down to healthy, viable tissue [104, 105]. Blood loss is limited by the use of tourniquets, tumescent solutions, epinephrine-soaked materials, or fascial excision, especially in large burns. The first stage of this operation is performed immediately after burn excision or other "clean" procedures, including hypertrophic scar release, keloid or oncologic resection, or flap harvest.

Contaminated wounds often benefit from serial debridement (every 24–72 h) before the first stage of this operation [106]. NPWT between debridement can help decrease bacterial colonization and promote the growth of granulation tissue [78, 84]. In a study out of Walter Reed Hospital, they found that in combat injuries treated with Integra and delayed split-thickness skin graft or flap, there were an average of three debridements to prepare wounds for the first stage of the operation [89]. Early infection can lead to poor take of the dermal substitute and prolonged wound healing, increasing the risk of an unfavorable scar.

10.4.2 Choosing a Dermal Substitute

There are a daunting number of so-called dermal substitutes commercially available today (Table 10.1). Many recent excellent reviews describe the wide variety of skin substitutes [41, 56, 107–111]. Very few guidelines for choosing the best dermal substitute exist, perhaps because there have not

Table 10.1 Examples of dermal substitutes

Product name	Manufacturer	Composition	Available size(s)	Notes	Select references
AlloDerm™ Regenerative Tissue Matrix	Allergan (Dublin, Ireland)	Lyophilized, acellular, human cadaver dermis	48–320 cm^2 0.23–3.3 mm thick		[12]
Graftjacket™	Wright Medical Technology (Middlesex, UK)	Cryopreserved, acellular, human cadaver dermis	16–32 cm^2 0.38 mm thick	Stored at room temperature	[118, 119]
PriMatrix® Dermal Repair Scaffold	Integra Life Sciences (Waltham, MA)	Decellularized fetal bovine dermis, rich in type III collagen	5–250 cm^2	5 year shelf life	[120]
Matriderm	MedSkin Solutions Dr. Suwelack AG (Billerbeck, Germany)	Non-cross-linked, bovine collagen matrix impregnated with elastin	38–624 cm^2 1 mm thick		[121–124]
Integra Dermal Regeneration Template	Integra LifeSciences, (Plainsboro, NJ)	Bovine collagen and glycosaminoglycan (shark chondroitin 6 sulfate) with semipermeable polysiloxane outer layer	25–500 cm^2 1.3 mm thick	Available with or without silastic layer	[23, 25, 29, 32]
Pelnac	Gunze Medical Materials Center (Kyoto, Japan)	Cross-linked, porcine tendon collagen	12–480 cm^2 3 mm thick	Available with or without silicone layer, store at room temperature	[43, 125, 126]
Terudermis	Olympus Terumo Biomaterials Corp. (Tokyo, Japan)	Cross-linked, bovine, dermal collagen (Type 1) with a silicone top layer	6.25–100 cm^2	Available with or without silicone layer, store at room temperature	[43, 127]
NovoSorb™ Biodegradable Temporizing Matrix	PolyNovo (Melbourne, Australia)	Biodegradable open cell polyurethane foam (0.15 mm pore size); polyurethane bonding layer; sealing polyurethane membrane	100–800 cm^2 2 mm thick	Top layer prevents overgrowth of tissue	[99, 128, 129]

been any large randomized controlled comparison studies. The production process of any particular dermal substitute is often proprietary, and clinicians must rely upon information provided by the manufacturer. On the other hand, a few dermal substitutes, including Integra and AlloDerm, have been studied extensively in the literature, from both basic science and clinical application standpoints. Integra has been used in combination with NPWT in many studies, while other dermal substitutes have not. In addition, the availability of different dermal substitutes is limited in many institutions (and countries), and the cost of the product may vary among institutions. Another consideration is the size of the wound, since most dermal substitutes are sold in a limited number of sizes. The shelf life and storage conditions may also be the limiting factors. These logistical factors may make the choice of dermal substitute very straightforward.

Dermal substitutes are often classified based on their composition. Many dermal substitutes are derived from human cadaver dermis, which is decellularized and preserved by various techniques. Most studies have been performed with AlloDerm, but theoretically, other decellularized human cadaver dermis products should function similarly. Other dermal substitutes, such as Matriderm, Integra, and Terudermis, are created from animal-derived collagen and other proteins, and are cross-linked to create sheets of gel-like material. Some dermal substitutes are derived from other animals, such as porcine tendon collagen (Pelnac) or fetal bovine collagen (PriMatrix). Lastly, there are some dermal substitutes that are completely synthetic: NovoSorb is made of biodegradable polyurethane foam.

There are also dermal substitutes that consist of multiple layers, although the majority of dermal substitutes have only one layer. Integra and Pelnac have a thin silicone layer that serves the barrier function of the epidermis, until it is removed at the second stage of the operation (Integra is also available as a single layer). NovoSorb consists of three layers: a biodegradable polyurethane foam, a bonding layer, and a sealing polyurethane membrane. When performing the two-stage operation, it is easier to use a dermal substitute with a removable, nonadherent, top layer.

10.4.3 First Stage: Application of Dermal Substitute and NPWT Dressing

Several excellent reviews of Integra placement have been published [29, 49, 77, 112, 113]. Briefly, the dermal substitute can be meshed or perforated before application to help it conform to contour irregularities in the wound. It is cut to the exact size of the wound and secured with staples, suture, fibrin glue, or a combination of these. In those patients prone to keloids, it can be sutured to the surrounding dermis to prevent formation of new keloids [94].

Negative-pressure wound therapy has become much more complex in recent years [79]. At its inception, it consisted of a porous polyurethane foam, a semipermeable adhesive film, a tube connecting the foam to the vacuum, and a vacuum pump. A variety of foams, films, and vacuum devices are now available. The purpose of the foam layer is to distribute the negative pressure evenly over the wound. There are a variety of devices that are stationary, portable, or disposable, and devices capable of applying continuous or intermittent negative pressure. When used in conjunction with a dermal substitute, the purpose of NPWT is to remove dead space or exudate between the wound bed and the dermal substitute, decrease bacterial load, and potentially accelerate vascularization and ingrowth into the dermal substitute. Thus, continuous negative pressure is recommended to maintain contact between the dermal substitute and the wound bed.

Placement of the negative-pressure dressing has been described in the literature and information provided by the manufacturer [106]. In brief, the foam is cut to the size of the wound and placed over the dermal substitute. If Integra is used, it is not necessary to place a nonadherent layer between the dermal substitute and the foam. It is not common practice to use a single-layer dermal substitute with NPWT, but not out of the realm of possibility, if there is a nonadherent layer between the dermal substitute and the foam. The foam is secured with an adhesive film. Over large or difficult areas, such as the hand or the groin, it may be necessary to use multiple pieces of foam and larger adhesive films, such as Ioban (3M, St. Paul, MN). Additional adhesive, such as Mastisol (Eloquest Healthcare, Ferndale, MI), can also help secure the dressing in moist periwound areas. Once the dressing is sealed, heavy scissors are used to cut a 1–2-cm hole in the adhesive film over the foam; the vacuum tubing is placed over this hole. Turning on the NPWT device checks the seal, and leaks are patched with another piece of adhesive film. The NPWT dressing can be left in place for 7–10 days over Integra [34].

It is often impractical to put a NPWT dressing on very small, irregular areas, such as the ear. In these cases, a bolster may be fashioned to exert even, constant pressure over the wound. Other small areas may be secured with a disposable NPWT device called the Pico (Smith and Nephew, London, UK) [114, 115]. The NPWT should continue until the second-stage operation.

10.4.4 Second Stage: Delayed Skin Graft

There is a wide range of recommended time interval between the first- and second-stage operations. Most clinicians inspect the wound periodically to assess the "take" of Integra, which should turn a salmon color and become more opaque over the course of 2–4 weeks. NPWT accelerates this process so that it occurs within 7–10 days [34].

In the second-stage operation, the silastic layer is removed, and a split-thickness skin graft is placed on top of the neodermis. The recommended thickness of the skin graft is anywhere from 0.003 to 0.016 inch. Thinner grafts are recommended when re-harvest of donor sites is anticipated. We use a skin graft thickness in the middle of that range, about 0.010–0.012 inch, for ease of handling intraoperatively and postoperatively, and have seen reliable results. The skin graft is either meshed 1:1 or minimally perforated. Then, a NPWT dressing is placed on the skin graft, as previously described [28]. The use of other skin graft techniques, including the modified Meek micrografting technique or sheets of cultured epithelium, has been described as well. After 5 days, we assess the skin graft "take" and stop NPWT. Occlusive petrolatum gauze dressing is placed over the skin graft until it is completely healed.

10.4.5 Most Common Complications with Recommended Solutions

10.4.5.1 Seroma

Occasionally, fluid collects beneath the silastic layer of Integra. Perforating or meshing Integra and applying snugly before application may prevent this problem. Once a seroma has been identified, it should be evacuated. A portion of the silastic layer can be removed for continued drainage before NPWT is restarted. The dermal substitute may be salvaged.

10.4.5.2 Hematoma

Much like seromas, a hematoma can be prevented by meticulous hemostasis prior to application of the dermal substitute. A hematoma should also be evacuated. It may be necessary to remove a portion of the dermal substitute to achieve hemostasis. This is an uncommon complication.

10.4.5.3 Infection

The best way to prevent infection is to make sure the wound bed is clean and viable (or that the burn is completely excised). Serial debridement and close monitoring of traumatic wounds is almost always necessary to ensure that the wound bed contains only viable tissue. NPWT can also decrease the risk of infection in wounds, although it has not specifically been shown to decrease infection in Integra [27, 35, 45]. The silastic layer over infected Integra can be removed, and mafenide acetate solution (Sulfamylon) dressings can help treat the infection. Of note, it is not uncommon for there to be a non-purulent exudate from a wound covered with Integra. Inexperienced clinicians with use of the product often overdiagnose infection with Integra. Areas of nonadherence of the matrix are often mistaken for infection.

10.5 Future Directions

An effective, affordable one-stage operation, with lower donor site morbidity, continues to be an enticing goal in the field of skin reconstruction. There have been several reports of complete healing after placing a split-thickness skin graft over a dermal substitute in a one-stage operation. Ingrowth of vessels from the wound bed, through Matriderm, and into the skin graft has, over the course of 15 days, been observed [116]. We have used the combination of Integra (without the silastic layer) and a split-thickness skin graft, in our practice, on particularly clean and healthy wound beds. Complete healing occurs over approximately 10–14 days (unpublished data). Cultured epithelial autograft in combination with a dermal substitute has been described. This method has minimal donor site morbidity, but it typically takes 2–3 weeks to culture enough autologous keratinocytes to cover a wound. This method is also time-intensive and requires technical skill and equipment, which is prohibitive to many clinicians. Another approach is to take a 2 cm × 2 cm skin graft, mechanically and enzymatically separate the skin cells, and resuspend them in a solution that can be sprayed on the wound bed (ReCell, Avita Medical, South Perth, Australia). This "spray skin," which contains autologous fibroblasts, keratinocytes, and melanocytes, in combination with Integra, has been used to heal full-thickness wounds in a swine model [117]. Further studies are needed to compare the long-term results of these one-stage procedures to the two-stage operation described in this chapter.

References

1. Whittaker AH. Treatment of burns by excision and immediate skin grafting. Am J Surg. 1953;85:411–7.
2. Burke JF, Bondoc CC, Quinby WC. Primary burn excision and immediate grafting: a method shortening illness. J Trauma. 1974;14:389–95.
3. Young F. Immediate skin grafting in the treatment of burns: a preliminary report. Ann Surg. 1942;116:445–51.
4. Gray DT, Pine RW, Harnar TJ, Marvin JA, Engrav LH, Heimbach DM. Early surgical excision versus conventional therapy in patients with 20 to 40 percent burns. A comparative study. Am J Surg. 1982;144:76–80.
5. Ong YS, Samuel M, Song C. Meta-analysis of early excision of burns. Burns. 2006;32:145–50.
6. Tompkins RG, Remensnyder JP, Burke JF, Tompkins DM, Hilton JF, Schoenfeld DA, Behringer GE, Bondoc CC, Briggs SE, Quinby WC. Significant reductions in mortality for children with burn injuries through the use of prompt eschar excision. Ann Surg. 1988;208:577–85.
7. Tompkins RG, Hilton JF, Burke JF, Schoenfeld DA, Hegarty MT, Bondoc CC, Quinby WC, Behringer GE, Ackroyd FW. Increased survival after massive thermal injuries in adults: preliminary report using artificial skin. Crit Care Med. 1989;17:734–40.
8. Singh M, Nuutila K, Collins KC, Huang A. Evolution of skin grafting for treatment of burns: reverdin pinch grafting to Tanner mesh grafting and beyond. Burns. 2017;43:1149–54.

9. Teich Alasia S, Castagnoli C, Calcagni M, Stella M. The influence of progress in the treatment of severe burns on the quality of life. Acta Chir Plast. 1996;38:119–21.
10. Rheinwald JG, Green H. Serial cultivation of strains of human epidermal keratinocytes: the formation of keratinizing colonies from single cells. Cell. 1975;6:331–43.
11. Cuono C, Langdon R, McGuire J. Use of cultured epidermal autografts and dermal allografts as skin replacement after burn injury. Lancet. 1986;1:1123–4.
12. Wainwright DJ. Use of an acellular allograft dermal matrix (AlloDerm) in the management of full-thickness burns. Burns. 1995;21:243–8.
13. Cuono CB, Langdon R, Birchall N, Barttelbort S, McGuire J. Composite autologous-allogeneic skin replacement: development and clinical application. Plast Reconstr Surg. 1987;80:626–37.
14. Hickerson WL, Compton C, Fletchall S, Smith LR. Cultured epidermal autografts and allodermis combination for permanent burn wound coverage. Burns. 1994;20(Suppl 1):S52–5. discussion S55–6.
15. Herzog SR, Meyer A, Woodley D, Peterson HD. Wound coverage with cultured autologous keratinocytes: use after burn wound excision, including biopsy followup. J Trauma. 1988;28:195–8.
16. Rue LW, Cioffi WG, McManus WF, Pruitt BA. Wound closure and outcome in extensively burned patients treated with cultured autologous keratinocytes. J Trauma. 1993;34:662–7. discussion 667–8.
17. Woodley DT, Peterson HD, Herzog SR, Stricklin GP, Burgeson RE, Briggaman RA, Cronce DJ, O'Keefe EJ. Burn wounds resurfaced by cultured epidermal autografts show abnormal reconstitution of anchoring fibrils. JAMA. 1988;259:2566–71.
18. Boyce ST, Hansbrough JF. Biologic attachment, growth, and differentiation of cultured human epidermal keratinocytes on a graftable collagen and chondroitin-6-sulfate substrate. Surgery. 1988;103:421–31.
19. Yannas IV, Burke JF. Design of an artificial skin. I. Basic design principles. J Biomed Mater Res. 1980;14:65–81.
20. Yannas IV, Burke JF, Gordon PL, Huang C, Rubenstein RH. Design of an artificial skin. II. Control of chemical composition. J Biomed Mater Res. 1980;14:107–32.
21. Dagalakis N, Flink J, Stasikelis P, Burke JF, Yannas IV. Design of an artificial skin. Part III. Control of pore structure. J Biomed Mater Res. 1980;14:511–28.
22. Burke JF, Yannas IV, Quinby WC, Bondoc CC, Jung WK. Successful use of a physiologically acceptable artificial skin in the treatment of extensive burn injury. Ann Surg. 1981;194:413–28.
23. Heimbach D, Luterman A, Burke J, Cram A, Herndon D, Hunt J, Jordan M, McManus W, Solem L, Warden G. Artificial dermis for major burns. A multi-center randomized clinical trial. Ann Surg. 1988;208:313–20.
24. Dantzer E, Braye FM. Reconstructive surgery using an artificial dermis (Integra): results with 39 grafts. Br J Plast Surg. 2001;54:659–64.
25. Frame JD, Still J, Lakhel-LeCoadou A, Carstens MH, Lorenz C, Orlet H, Spence R, Berger AC, Dantzer E, Burd A. Use of dermal regeneration template in contracture release procedures: a multicenter evaluation. Plast Reconstr Surg. 2004;113:1330–8.
26. Grant I, Green C, Martin R. Strategies to improve the take of commercially available collagen/glycosaminoglycan wound repair material investigated in an animal model. Burns. 2001;27:699–707.
27. Morykwas MJ, Argenta LC, Shelton-Brown EI, McGuirt W. Vacuum-assisted closure: a new method for wound control and treatment: animal studies and basic foundation. Ann Plast Surg. 1997;38:553–62.
28. Schneider AM, Morykwas MJ, Argenta LC. A new and reliable method of securing skin grafts to the difficult recipient bed. Plast Reconstr Surg. 1998;102:1195–8.
29. Molnar JA, Defranzo AJ, Hadaegh A, Morykwas MJ, Shen P, Argenta LC. Acceleration of integra incorporation in complex tissue defects with subatmospheric pressure. Plast Reconstr Surg. 2004;113:1339–46.
30. Scherer LA, Shiver S, Chang M, Meredith JW, Owings JT. The vacuum assisted closure device: a method of securing skin grafts and improving graft survival. Arch Surg. 2002;137:930–3. discussion 933–4.
31. Moiemen NS, Yarrow J, Kamel D, Kearns D, Mendonca D. Topical negative pressure therapy: does it accelerate neovascularisation within the dermal regeneration template, Integra? A prospective histological in vivo study. Burns. 2010;36:764–8.
32. Jeschke MG, Rose C, Angele P, Füchtmeier B, Nerlich MN, Bolder U. Development of new reconstructive techniques: use of Integra in combination with fibrin glue and negative-pressure therapy for reconstruction of acute and chronic wounds. Plast Reconstr Surg. 2004;113:525–30.
33. Ryan CM, Schoenfeld DA, Malloy M, Schulz JT, Sheridan RL, Tompkins RG. Use of Integra artificial skin is associated with decreased length of stay for severely injured adult burn survivors. J Burn Care Rehabil. 2002;23:311–7.
34. Park CA, Defranzo AJ, Marks MW, Molnar JA. Outpatient reconstruction using integra* and subatmospheric pressure. Ann Plast Surg. 2009;62:164–9.
35. Bloemen MCT, van der Wal MBA, Verhaegen PDHM, Nieuwenhuis MK, van Baar ME, van Zuijlen PPM, Middelkoop E. Clinical effectiveness of dermal substitution in burns by topical negative pressure: a multicenter randomized controlled trial. Wound Repair Regen. 2012;20:797–805.
36. Ehrlich HP, Desmoulière A, Diegelmann RF, Cohen IK, Compton CC, Garner WL, Kapanci Y, Gabbiani G. Morphological and immunochemical differences between keloid and hypertrophic scar. Am J Pathol. 1994;145:105–13.
37. Soller EC, Tzeranis DS, Miu K, So PTC, Yannas IV. Common features of optimal collagen scaffolds that disrupt wound contraction and enhance regeneration both in peripheral nerves and in skin. Biomaterials. 2012;33:4783–91.
38. Stern R, McPherson M, Longaker MT. Histologic study of artificial skin used in the treatment of full-thickness thermal injury. J Burn Care Rehabil. 1990;11:7–13.
39. Moiemen NS, Staiano JJ, Ojeh NO, Thway Y, Frame JD. Reconstructive surgery with a dermal regeneration template: clinical and histologic study. Plast Reconstr Surg. 2001;108: 93–103.
40. Hu S, Kirsner RS, Falanga V, Phillips T, Eaglstein WH. Evaluation of Apligraf persistence and basement membrane restoration in donor site wounds: a pilot study. Wound Repair Regen. 2006;14:427–33.
41. Lazic T, Falanga V. Bioengineered skin constructs and their use in wound healing. Plast Reconstr Surg. 2011;127(Suppl 1):75S–90S.
42. Moiemen N, Yarrow J, Hodgson E, Constantinides J, Chipp E, Oakley H, Shale E, Freeth M. Long-term clinical and histological analysis of integra dermal regeneration template. Plast Reconstr Surg. 2011;127:1149–54.
43. Eo S, Kim Y, Cho S. Vacuum-assisted closure improves the incorporation of artificial dermis in soft tissue defects: Terudermis(®) and Pelnac(®). Int Wound J. 2011;8:261–7.
44. Labler L, Rancan M, Mica L, Härter L, Mihic-Probst D, Keel M. Vacuum-assisted closure therapy increases local interleukin-8 and vascular endothelial growth factor levels in traumatic wounds. J Trauma. 2009;66:749–57.
45. Anghel EL, Kim PJ. Negative-pressure wound therapy. Plast Reconstr Surg. 2016;138:129S–37S.
46. Huang C, Leavitt T, Bayer LR, Orgill DP. Effect of negative pressure wound therapy on wound healing. Curr Probl Surg. 2014;51:301–31.

47. Lalezari S, Lee CJ, Borovikova AA, Banyard DA, Paydar KZ, Wirth GA, Widgerow AD. Deconstructing negative pressure wound therapy. Int Wound J. 2016;14:649–57.
48. Yannas IV, Orgill DP, Burke JF. Template for skin regeneration. Plast Reconstr Surg. 2011;127:60S–70S.
49. Moiemen NS, Vlachou E, Staiano JJ, Thawy Y, Frame JD. Reconstructive surgery with Integra dermal regeneration template: histologic study, clinical evaluation, and current practice. Plast Reconstr Surg. 2006;117:160S–74S.
50. Engrav LH, Heimbach DM, Reus JL, Harnar TJ, Marvin JA. Early excision and grafting vs. nonoperative treatment of burns of indeterminant depth: a randomized prospective study. J Trauma. 1983;23:1001–4.
51. Deitch EA, Wheelahan TM, Rose MP, Clothier J, Cotter J. Hypertrophic burn scars: analysis of variables. J Trauma. 1983;23:895–8.
52. Bloemen MCT, van der Veer WM, Ulrich MMW, van Zuijlen PPM, Niessen FB, Middelkoop E. Prevention and curative management of hypertrophic scar formation. Burns. 2009;35:463–75.
53. Burke JF. Early excision of the burn wound. J Burn Care Rehabil. 1981;2:266.
54. Lorenz C, Petracic A, Hohl HP, Wessel L, Waag KL. Early wound closure and early reconstruction. Experience with a dermal substitute in a child with 60 per cent surface area burn. Burns. 1997;23:505–8.
55. Yim H, Cho YS, Seo CH, Lee BC, Ko JH, Kim D, Hur J, Chun W, Kim JH. The use of AlloDerm on major burn patients: AlloDerm prevents post-burn joint contracture. Burns. 2010;36:322–8.
56. Fang T, Lineaweaver WC, Sailes FC, Kisner C, Zhang F. Clinical application of cultured epithelial autografts on acellular dermal matrices in the treatment of extended burn injuries. Ann Plast Surg. 2014;73:509–15.
57. Cuadra A, Correa G, Roa R, Piñeros JL, Norambuena H, Searle S, Heras RL, Calderón W. Functional results of burned hands treated with Integra®. J Plast Reconstr Aesthet Surg. 2012;65:228–34.
58. Dantzer E, Queruel P, Salinier L, Palmier B, Quinot JF. Dermal regeneration template for deep hand burns: clinical utility for both early grafting and reconstructive surgery. Br J Plast Surg. 2003;56:764–74.
59. Friedstat JS, Klein MB. Acute management of facial burns. Clin Plast Surg. 2009;36:653–60.
60. Tang B, Zhu B, Liang Y-Y, Bi L-K, Chen B, Hu Z-C, Zhang K, Zhu J-Y. Early escharectomy and concurrent composite skin grafting over human acellular dermal matrix scaffold for covering deep facial burns. Plast Reconstr Surg. 2011;127:1533–8.
61. Atherton DD, Tang R, Jones I, Jawad M. Early excision and application of matriderm with simultaneous autologous skin grafting in facial burns. Plast Reconstr Surg. 2010;125:60e–1e.
62. Demircan M, Cicek T, Yetis MI. Preliminary results in single-step wound closure procedure of full-thickness facial burns in children by using the collagen-elastin matrix and review of pediatric facial burns. Burns. 2015;41:1268–74.
63. Molnar JA, DeFranzo AJ, Marks MW. Single-stage approach to skin grafting the exposed skull. Plast Reconstr Surg. 2000;105:174–7.
64. van der Wal MBA, Vloemans JFPM, Tuinebreijer WE, van de Ven P, van Unen E, van Zuijlen PPM, Middelkoop E. Outcome after burns: an observational study on burn scar maturation and predictors for severe scarring. Wound Repair Regen. 2012;20:676–87.
65. Kwan P, Desmoulière A, Tredget EE. Molecular and cellular basis of hypertrophic scarring. Total Burn Care. 2012:495–505.e5.
66. Ladak A, Tredget EE. Pathophysiology and management of the burn scar. Clin Plast Surg. 2009;36:661–74.
67. Wainwright DJ. Burn reconstruction: the problems, the techniques, and the applications. Clin Plast Surg. 2009;36:687–700.
68. van Zuijlen PP, van Trier AJ, Vloemans JF, Groenevelt F, Kreis RW, Middelkoop E. Graft survival and effectiveness of dermal substitution in burns and reconstructive surgery in a one-stage grafting model. Plast Reconstr Surg. 2000;106:615–23.
69. Dantzer E. Burn contractures: surgical management with integra—long term results. J Burn Care Rehabil. 2003;24:S100.
70. Clayman MA, Clayman SM, Mozingo DW. The use of collagen-glycosaminoglycan copolymer (Integra) for the repair of hypertrophic scars and keloids. J Burn Care Res. 2006;27:404–9.
71. Yeong E-K, Yu Y-C, Chan Z-H, Roan T-L. Is artificial dermis an effective tool in the treatment of tendon-exposed wounds? J Burn Care Res. 2013;34:161–7.
72. Askari M, Cohen MJ, Grossman PH, Kulber DA. The use of acellular dermal matrix in release of burn contracture scars in the hand. Plast Reconstr Surg. 2011;127:1593–9.
73. Kamolz L-P, Frey M, Meissl G, Nathschlaeger G, Haslik W. Use of collagen-elastin matrix (matriderm) for dermal reparation: 12 months experiences in the treatment of severe hand burn injuries. Burns. 2007;33:S19.
74. Gronovich Y, Maisel Lotan A, Retchkiman M. Post-burn breast reconstruction using an artificial dermis-a long-term follow-up. Burns Trauma. 2016;4:12.
75. Palao R, Gómez P, Huguet P. Burned breast reconstructive surgery with Integra dermal regeneration template. Br J Plast Surg. 2003;56:252–9.
76. Fujimori Y, Ueda K, Fumimoto H, Kubo K, Kuroyanagi Y. Skin regeneration for children with burn scar contracture using autologous cultured dermal substitutes and superthin auto-skin grafts: preliminary clinical study. Ann Plast Surg. 2006;57:408–14.
77. Stiefel D, Schiestl C, Meuli M. Integra Artificial Skin® for burn scar revision in adolescents and children. Burns. 2010;36:114–20.
78. Argenta LC, Morykwas MJ, Marks MW, Defranzo AJ, Molnar JA, David LR. Vacuum-assisted closure: state of clinic art. Plast Reconstr Surg. 2006;117:127S–42S.
79. Orgill DP, Bayer LR. Update on negative-pressure wound therapy. Plast Reconstr Surg. 2011;127(Suppl 1):105S–15S.
80. DeFranzo AJ, Argenta LC, Marks MW, Molnar JA, David LR, Webb LX, Ward WG, Teasdall RG. The use of vacuum-assisted closure therapy for the treatment of lower-extremity wounds with exposed bone. Plast Reconstr Surg. 2001;108:1184–91.
81. DeFranzo AJ, Marks MW, Argenta LC, Genecov DG. Vacuum-assisted closure for the treatment of degloving injuries. Plast Reconstr Surg. 1999;104:2145–8.
82. Barnett TM, Shilt JS. Use of vacuum-assisted closure and a dermal regeneration template as an alternative to flap reconstruction in pediatric grade IIIB open lower-extremity injuries. Am J Orthop. 2009;38:301–5.
83. Mooney JF, Argenta LC, Marks MW, Morykwas MJ, DeFranzo AJ. Treatment of soft tissue defects in pediatric patients using the V.A.C. system. Clin Orthop Relat Res. 2000:26–31.
84. Schlatterer D, Hirshorn K. Negative pressure wound therapy with reticulated open cell foam-adjunctive treatment in the management of traumatic wounds of the leg: a review of the literature. J Orthop Trauma. 2008;22:S152–60.
85. Janis JE, Steinberg JS. Discussion. Template for skin regeneration. Plast Reconstr Surg. 2011;127(Suppl 1):71S–4S.
86. Iorio ML, Shuck J, Attinger CE. Wound healing in the upper and lower extremities. Plast Reconstr Surg. 2012;130:232S–41S.
87. Rehim SA, Singhal M, Chung KC. Dermal skin substitutes for upper limb reconstruction: current status, indications, and contraindications. Hand Clin. 2014;30:239–52–vii.
88. Helgeson MD, Potter BK, Evans KN, Shawen SB. Bioartificial dermal substitute: a preliminary report on its use for the management of complex combat-related soft tissue wounds. J Orthop Trauma. 2007;21:394–9.

89. Seavey JG, Masters ZA, Balazs GC, Tintle SM, Sabino J, Fleming ME, Valerio IL. Use of a bioartificial dermal regeneration template for skin restoration in combat casualty injuries. Regen Med. 2016;11:81–90.
90. Butler PD, Longaker MT, Yang GP. Current progress in keloid research and treatment. J Am Coll Surg. 2008;206:731–41.
91. Ogawa R. The most current algorithms for the treatment and prevention of hypertrophic scars and keloids. Plast Reconstr Surg. 2010;125:557–68.
92. Monstrey S, Middelkoop E, Vranckx JJ, Bassetto F, Ziegler UE, Meaume S, Téot L. Updated scar management practical guidelines: non-invasive and invasive measures. Br J Plast Surg. 2014;67:1017–25.
93. Davison SP, Sobanko JF, Clemens MW. Use of a collagen-glycosaminoglycan copolymer (Integra) in combination with adjuvant treatments for reconstruction of severe chest keloids. J Drugs Dermatol. 2010;9:542–8.
94. Bidic SM, Dauwe PB, Heller J, Brown S, Rohrich RJ. Reconstructing large keloids with neodermis: a systematic review. Plast Reconstr Surg. 2012;129:380e–2e.
95. Nguyen KT, Shikowitz L, Kasabian AK, Bastidas N. A novel approach to keloid reconstruction with bilaminar dermal substitute and epidermal skin grafting. Plast Reconstr Surg. 2016;138:235–9.
96. Patel NP, Lawrence Cervino A. Keloid treatment: is there a role for acellular human dermis (Alloderm)? J Plast Reconstr Aesthet Surg. 2010;63:1344–8.
97. Cunningham T, Marks M. Vacuum-assisted closure device and skin substitutes for complex Mohs defects. Dermatol Surg. 2014;40(Suppl 9):S120–6.
98. Schiavon M, Francescon M, Drigo D, Salloum G, Baraziol R, Tesei J, Fraccalanza E, Barbone F. The use of integra dermal regeneration template versus flaps for reconstruction of full-thickness scalp defects involving the calvaria: a cost–benefit analysis. Aesthetic Plast Surg. 2016;40:901–7.
99. Greenwood JE. The evolution of acute burn care—retiring the split skin graft. Ann R Coll Surg Engl. 2017;99:432–8.
100. Rowe NM, Morris L, Delacure MD. Acellular dermal composite allografts for reconstruction of the radial forearm donor site. Ann Plast Surg. 2006;57:305–11.
101. Murray RC, Gordin EA, Saigal K, Leventhal D, Krein H, Heffelfinger RN. Reconstruction of the radial forearm free flap donor site using integra artificial dermis. Microsurgery. 2011;31:104–8.
102. Wagstaff MJD, Schmitt BJ, Coghlan P, Finkemeyer JP, Caplash Y, Greenwood JE. A biodegradable polyurethane dermal matrix in reconstruction of free flap donor sites: a pilot study. Eplasty. 2015;15:e13.
103. Integra's Physician Training Website. (Integra Life Sciences, 2017), http://www.ilstraining.com/. Accessed 14 October 2017.
104. Mosier MJ, Gibran NS. Surgical excision of the burn wound. Clin Plast Surg. 2009;36:617–25.
105. Bezuhly M, Fish JS. Acute burn care. Plast Reconstr Surg. 2012;130:349e–58e.
106. Janis J, Harrison B. Wound healing: part II. Clinical applications. Plast Reconstr Surg. 2014;133:383e–92e.
107. Dickinson LE, Gerecht S. Engineered biopolymeric scaffolds for chronic wound healing. Front Physiol. 2016;7:623–12.
108. van der Veen VC, van der Wal MBA, van Leeuwen MCE, Ulrich MMW, Middelkoop E. Biological background of dermal substitutes. Burns. 2010;36:305–21.
109. Chua AWC, Khoo YC, Tan BK, Tan K-C, Foo CL, Chong SJ. Skin tissue engineering advances in severe burns: review and therapeutic applications. Burns Trauma. 2016;4:3.
110. van Zuijlen P, Gardien K, Jaspers M, Bos EJ, Baas DC, van Trier A, Middelkoop E. Tissue engineering in burn scar reconstruction. Burns Trauma. 2015;3:18.
111. Watt AJ, Friedrich JB, Huang JI. Advances in treating skin defects of the hand: skin substitutes and negative-pressure wound therapy. Hand Clin. 2012;28:519–28.
112. McEwan W, Brown TLH, Mills SM, Muller MJ. Suction dressings to secure a dermal substitute. Burns. 2004;30:259–61.
113. Janis JE, Kwon RK, Lalonde DH. A practical guide to wound healing. Plast Reconstr Surg. 2010;125:230e–44e.
114. Malmsjö M, Ingemansson R, Martin R, Huddleston E. Negative-pressure wound therapy using gauze or open-cell polyurethane foam: similar early effects on pressure transduction and tissue contraction in an experimental porcine wound model. Wound Repair Regen. 2009;17:200–5.
115. Malmsjö M, Huddleston E, Martin R. Biological effects of a disposable, canisterless negative pressure wound therapy system. Eplasty. 2014;14:e15.
116. Wiedner M, Tinhofer IE, Kamolz L-P, Seyedian Moghaddam A, Justich I, Liegl-Atzwanger B, Bubalo V, Weninger WJ, Lumenta DB. Simultaneous dermal matrix and autologous split-thickness skin graft transplantation in a porcine wound model: a three-dimensional histological analysis of revascularization. Wound Repair Regen. 2015;22:749–54.
117. Wood FM, Stoner ML, Fowler BV, Fear MW. The use of a non-cultured autologous cell suspension and Integra dermal regeneration template to repair full-thickness skin wounds in a porcine model: a one-step process. Burns. 2007;33:693–700.
118. Reyzelman A, Crews RT, Moore JC, et al. Clinical effectiveness of an acellular dermal regenerative tissue matrix compared to standard wound management in healing diabetic foot ulcers: a prospective, randomised, multicentre study. Int Wound J. 2009;6:196–208.
119. Brigido SA, Boc SF, Lopez RC. Effective management of major lower extremity wounds using an acellular regenerative tissue matrix: a pilot study. Orthopedics. 2004;27:s145–9.
120. Neill J, James K, Lineaweaver W. Utilizing biologic assimilation of bovine fetal collagen in staged skin grafting. Ann Plast Surg. 2012;68:451–6.
121. Haslik W, Kamolz L-P, Nathschläger G, Andel H, Meissl G, Frey M. First experiences with the collagen-elastin matrix Matriderm® as a dermal substitute in severe burn injuries of the hand. Burns. 2007;33:364–8.
122. Ryssel H, Gazyakan E, Germann G, Öhlbauer M. The use of MatriDerm® in early excision and simultaneous autologous skin grafting in burns—a pilot study. Burns. 2008;34:93–7.
123. Haslik W, Kamolz L-P, Manna F, Hladik M, Rath T, Frey M. Management of full-thickness skin defects in the hand and wrist region: first long-term experiences with the dermal matrix Matriderm. J Plast Reconstr Aesthet Surg. 2010;63:360–4.
124. Min JH, Yun IS, Lew DH, Roh TS, Lee WJ. The use of matriderm and autologous skin graft in the treatment of full thickness skin defects. Arch Plast Surg. 2014;41:330–6.
125. Suzuki S, Kawai K, Ashoori F, Morimoto N, Nishimura Y, Ikada Y. Long-term follow-up study of artificial dermis composed of outer silicone layer and inner collagen sponge. Br J Plast Surg. 2000;53:659–66.
126. Widjaja W, Maitz P. The use of dermal regeneration template (Pelnac®) in acute full-thickness wound closure: a case series. Eur J Plast Surg. 2015;39:125–32.
127. Lee J-W, Jang Y-C, Oh SJ. Use of the artificial dermis for free radial forearm flap donor site. Ann Plast Surg. 2005;55:500–2.
128. Greenwood JE, Dearman BL. Comparison of a sealed, polymer foam biodegradable temporizing matrix against Integra® dermal regeneration template in a porcine wound model. J Burn Care Res. 2012;33:163–73.
129. Wagstaff MJD, Driver S, Coghlan P, Greenwood JE. A randomized, controlled trial of negative pressure wound therapy of pressure ulcers via a novel polyurethane foam. Wound Repair Regen. 2014;22:205–11.

Surgery and Radiation Therapy for Keloids and Hypertrophic Scars

11

Rei Ogawa

11.1 Introduction

Over the past 10 years, our understanding of the pathogenesis of pathological scars, including keloids and hypertrophic scars, has increased markedly [1, 2]. Consequently, keloids and hypertrophic scars are now regarded as treatable diseases [3]. However, the available therapeutic approaches still require improvement. Surgery and radiation therapy should play more prominent roles in current therapeutic strategies for pathological scars [3, 4]. This chapter discusses the reasons for this. Optimal surgical and radiotherapy treatment protocols and the possible side effects of radiotherapy are also discussed.

11.2 Surgical Resection of Keloids and Hypertrophic Scars

The key concept in keloid and hypertrophic scar treatment is that these lesions are driven by inflammation in the reticular dermis [2]. Moreover, in each individual, the degree of inflammation is shaped by interactions between external and internal pathogenic factors [5]. These factors include local skin factors, in particular mechanical tension on the wound/scar. This tension is particularly strong on certain areas of the body such as the anterior chest that show a predilection for pathological scar development [2, 6]. Other factors include systemic factors (such as hypertension, sex hormones, and systemic inflammatory conditions) and/or genetic factors [2, 6]. The degree of inflammation and the pathogenic factors should all be considered before deciding how to treat a pathological scar.

Disclosure: There are no financial disclosures to be made.

R. Ogawa (✉)
Department of Plastic, Reconstructive and Aesthetic Surgery, Nippon Medical School, Tokyo, Japan
e-mail: r.ogawa@nms.ac.jp

Surgical resection essentially removes all or most of the inflamed mass, thus resetting the wound bed inflammation to a more manageable level (I call this the "Reset Concept"). These small amounts of inflammation can be eliminated by postoperative radiation therapy. This in turn should be followed by preventive measures that counter the pathogenic stimuli (e.g., tension on the wound/scar) that could reignite runaway inflammation and lead to recurrence.

If keloids and hypertrophic scars are not resected carefully, the risk of recurrence is high. Worse, the recurrent lesions are often much bigger than the original lesions. While radiation therapy after surgery markedly reduces the risk of recurrence, certain surgical techniques can also strongly limit this risk. There are two basic surgical principles that should be considered carefully when performing any surgery (especially on areas of the body with high skin tension) but particularly when resecting pathological scars: first, the direction of incision, and second, the depth of incision.

In relation to the first principle, if the direction of incision matches the predominant direction of skin tension, the risk of developing pathological scars increases. This is because scars become stiff and are much less inelastic than the surrounding skin after surgery. Thus, when the scar lies in the direction of skin tension, stretching of the skin (by body movements, for example) pulls on the entire length of the scar (top panel in Fig. 11.1). This will hamper the normal progression of wound healing from the inflammatory phase into the skin remodeling phase, thus increasing inflammation and collagen accumulation and resulting in scar growth. However, if the direction of incision does not match the direction of skin tension, the tension imposed by skin movements is dispersed and a high-tension area does not arise (bottom panel in Fig. 11.1).

In terms of surgically removing pathological scars, the scar has often lengthened parallel to the direction of stretch in many cases. In such cases, the surgeon should consider dividing the tension using zig-zag sutures, including z-plasties: these surgical modalities are good for releasing linear scar contractures and tension [7, 8]. Another major benefit is

© Springer Nature Singapore Pte Ltd. 2020

R. Ogawa (ed.), *Total Scar Management*, https://doi.org/10.1007/978-981-32-9791-3_11

that segmented scars mature faster than long linear scars. Z-plasties are particularly suitable for scars that cross a joint: joints are particularly mobile areas of the body, and scars across them readily become hypertrophic as a result of the constant stretching. Zig-zag incision and suturing will help reduce the risk of pathological scar recurrence (Fig. 11.2). Various local flaps are also useful for dividing the tension line of scars [9]. They also prevent contractures because they expand naturally after surgery (Fig. 11.3). Skin grafts are less suitable for dividing the scar tension line because they do not expand. In fact, they tend to generate secondary contractures that result in circular pathological scars around the grafted skin. In terms of flap surgery, skin-pedicled flaps are better than island flaps, including free flaps, because the healthy skin of the skin pedicle can expand after surgery bit by bit; this effectively releases the tension on the flap (top panel of Fig. 11.4) [9]. Free flaps do not have this feature (bottom panel of Fig. 11.4). However, if the scar is large, perforator-pedicled island flaps (propeller flaps) or free flaps can be selected (Fig. 11.5).

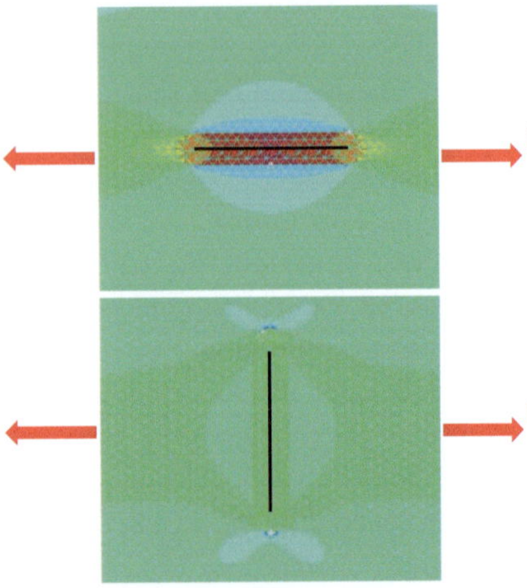

Fig. 11.1 Effect of skin stretch on a scar left by surgical incision if the incision lies parallel to the skin stretch direction. (Top panel) If the incision direction matches the direction of skin tension, there is a high risk of developing pathological scars. This is because scars become stiff in the postoperative course, and any stretching of the skin (by body movements, for example) will stretch the entire scar. This will promote inflammation and growth of the scar. (Bottom panel) If the incision lies perpendicular to the direct of skin tension, the stretching tension will be dispersed along the whole length of the scar. This will reduce inflammation caused by stretching of the scar

In relation to the second surgical principle, namely, the depth of incision, keloids and hypertrophic scars arise from the reticular layer of the dermis [2]. Thus, after any surgical incision, including excision of pathological scars, it is important to limit the tension on the reticular dermis. One way to ensure this is to use dermal sutures only after the much deeper structures (namely, the superficial and deep fascia) have been accessed and sutured (Fig. 11.6) [3, 8]. This type of suturing will elevate the wound edges smoothly, thus allowing them to naturally attach to each other (Fig. 11.7). Only then should the dermal and superficial sutures be placed. Thus, dermal sutures should not be used as “tension-reduction sutures.” This is an important concept for preventing the formation (and recurrence) of pathological scars after surgery.

Special surgical techniques such as wedge excision (Fig. 11.8) and core excision (Fig. 11.9) can be used for pathological scars on specific regions such as the ear.

11.3 Radiation Therapy

Keloids have been treated with radiation for a century. Freund reported in 1898, 3 years after X-rays were first detected by Wilhelm Conrad Röntgen, that hypertrophic scars could be restored to normal skin by Roentgen treatment [10]. Subsequently, in 1901, Harris reported that X-ray exposure could also resolve keloids [10]. In 1909, Freund described the first combination treatment protocol that involved sur-

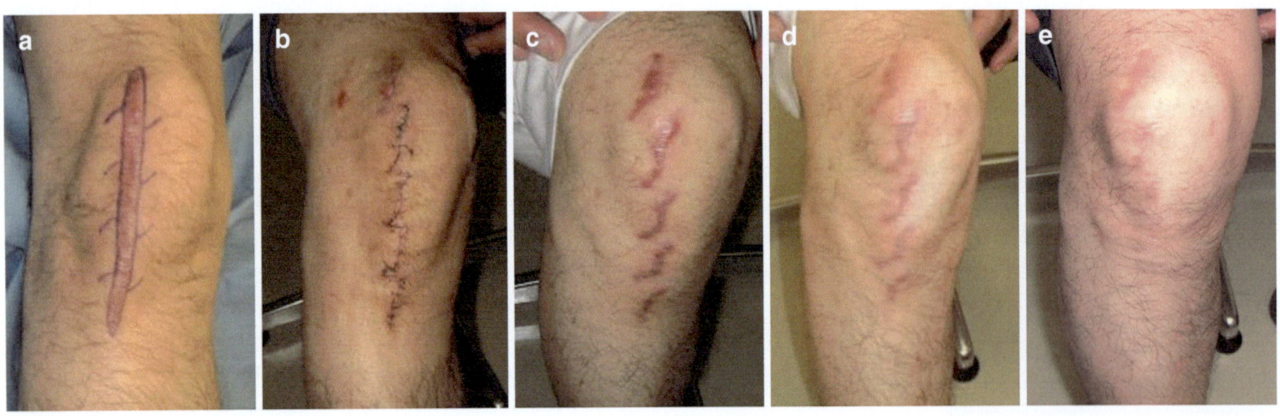

Fig. 11.2 Z-plasty is particularly suitable for hypertrophic scars on the knee. Zig-zag suture approaches such as z-plasty effectively disperse the tension on the contracture line. This slowly decreases inflammation and allows the scars to mature. (**a**) Z-plasty design. (**b**) View immediately after surgery. (**c**) Three months after surgery. (**d**) Six months after surgery. (**e**) Twelve months after surgery

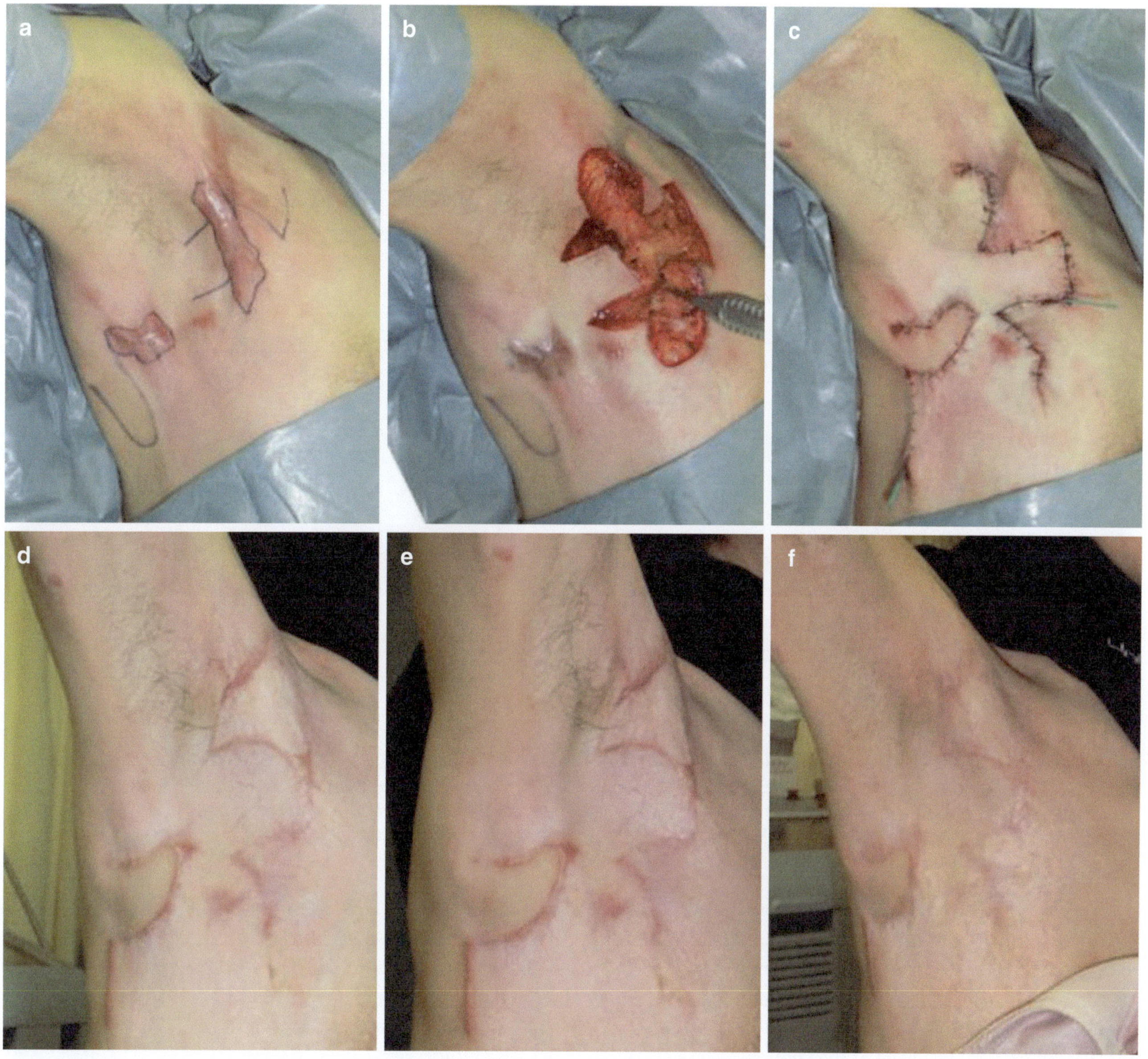

Fig. 11.3 Skin-pedicled flaps are a good choice for releasing axillary scar contracture. Local flaps also disperse the tension on a contracture line because they expand naturally after surgery. This is demonstrated here: a square flap gradually became triangular in shape over time. (**a**) Skin-pedicled flap design. (**b**) Intraoperative view. (**c**) Immediately after surgery. (**d**) Three months after surgery. (**e**) Six months after surgery. (**f**) Twelve months after surgery

gery and postoperative Roentgen treatment [10]. Thereafter, different radiation protocols were developed for keloid treatment. Some involved external irradiation using superficial [11–20] and orthovoltage X-rays (photons) [21–23] and β-rays (electron beams) [24–29]. Others were brachytherapies employing β-rays (32P [30] or 90Sr/90Y [31, 32]) and γ-rays (60Co [33] or 192Ir [3, 34–41]). These radiation therapy protocols have been employed as a monotherapy without surgery, in combination with adjuvant therapy without surgery, and after surgery. However, it is generally believed that keloids are best treated by a combination of surgery and postoperative radiation therapy because relatively little radiation is needed to remove the remaining inflammation after surgery, thereby preventing recurrence [42–44]. By contrast, higher doses seem to be needed when radiotherapy is employed on its own.

Many studies have assessed the effect of postoperative radiation on keloid recurrence. While it is difficult to compare these studies because of study variations in terms of patient ethnicity, age, and sex, keloid area and size, radiation source and dose, result assessment strategies, and the follow-up duration, the reported postoperative radiation response rates (rate of recurrence regardless of patient satisfaction) generally fall between 67% and 98% [28].

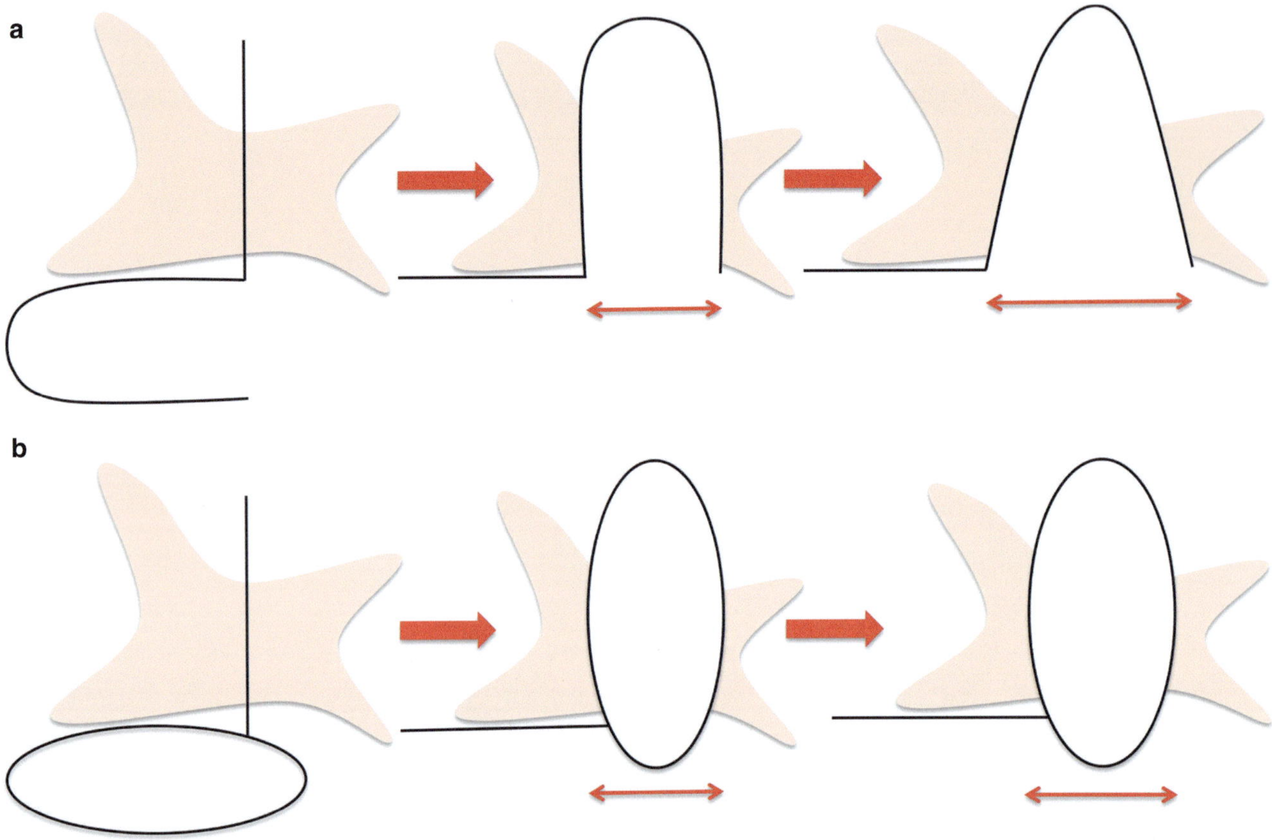

Fig. 11.4 Schematic depiction of the usefulness of skin-pedicled flaps as opposed to island flaps for releasing tension. (Top panel) skin pedicled flap or skin pedicled flap (**a**) effectively release tension on a scar line because the healthy skin of the skin pedicle expands bit by bit after surgery. (Bottom panel) island flap or island flap (**b**), including free flaps, lack that postoperative expansibility

The safety and efficacy of radiation therapy have improved further in recent years. Consequently, radiation in the form of high-dose-rate superficial brachytherapy (HDR-SB) or electron beam therapy is now used routinely as a highly effective postoperative adjuvant therapy (Fig. 11.10) [3, 41]. Depending on the shape of the surgical scar, a HDR-SB applicator can be used to ensure both even and appropriate localization of the radiation to the wound surface. This makes the treatment even more effective. Papers on the effective use of brachytherapy against keloids are increasingly being reported.

Use of the linear-quadratic concept to calculate the biologically effective doses (BEDs) for various radiation regimens for keloid therapy revealed that, when the BEDs exceeded 30 Gy, the recurrence rate was less than 10% [45]. BED is calculated as BED = the total radiation dose multiplied by [1 + one-time dose/(α/β)]. The α/β value of keloids is considered to be 10 since they are inflammatory regions. However, additional studies that determine this value more accurately are needed.

Since the risk of secondary carcinogenesis is reduced when the BED is set to below 30 Gy, we propose that the maximum dose of postoperative radiation therapy for keloids is a BED of 30 Gy. A BED of 30 Gy can be obtained in several ways: a single fraction dose of 13 Gy, two fractions of 8 Gy, three fractions of 6 Gy, or four fractions of 5 Gy.

In terms of the postoperative radiation protocol, we used a 15 Gy unified protocol before 2002 [28]. In this protocol, all keloids, regardless of where they were located, were treated with 15 Gy that was delivered over three consecutive days in daily fractions of 5 Gy. We found that this protocol associated with a recurrence rate of about 30%. Thereafter, we developed a customized dose protocol in which different body sites were treated with different amounts of radiation. Thus, high-risk areas, including the anterior chest wall and the scapular and suprapubic regions, were treated with 20 Gy that was delivered over four consecutive days in daily fractions of 5 Gy. By contrast, the earlobe, which is a low-risk area, was treated with 10 Gy that was delivered over two consecutive days in daily fractions of 5 Gy. Other regions were treated according to the original protocol (i.e., 15 Gy delivered over 3 days in daily fractions of 5 Gy). This change in protocol has reduced the total recurrence rate to 12.3% [29].

We have subsequently further revised this protocol and are currently testing its effect on recurrence. This protocol is

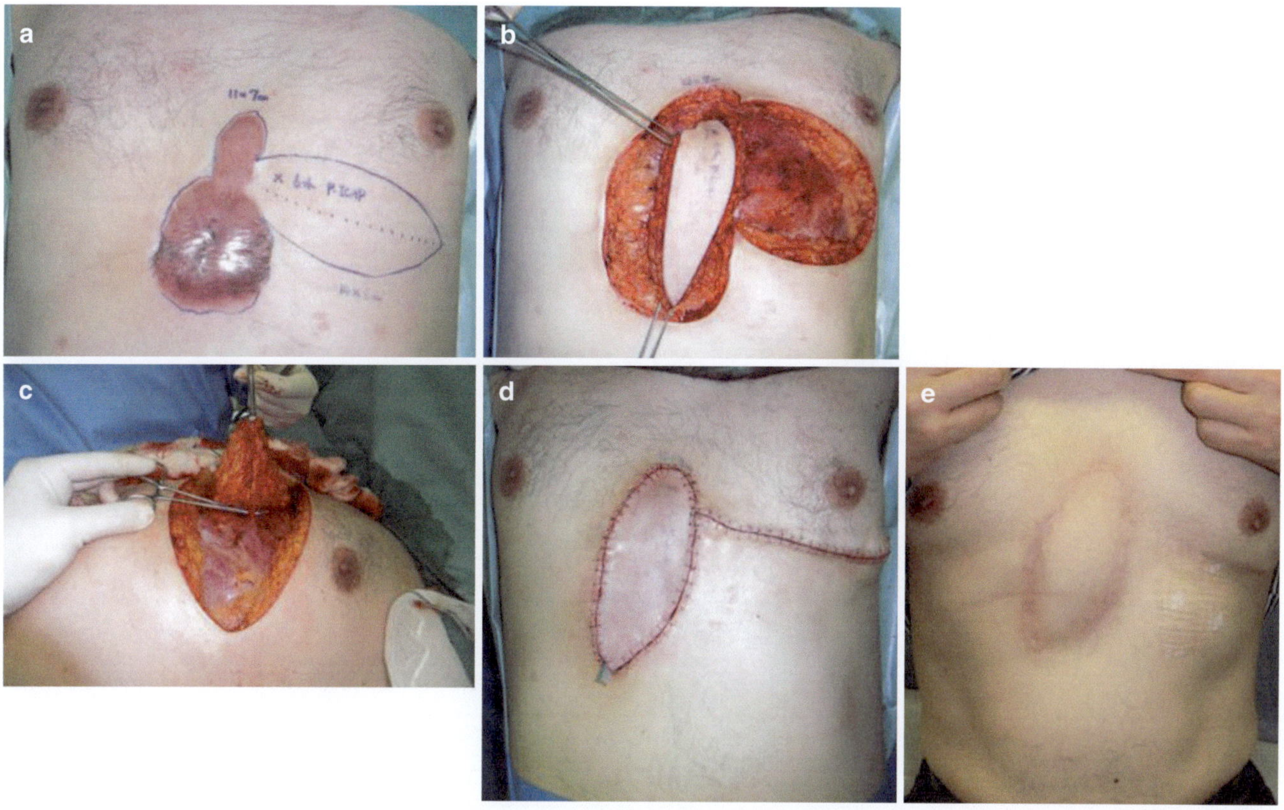

Fig. 11.5 Chest wall keloid reconstruction using a perforator-pedicled propeller flap (an island flap). Perforator-pedicled island flaps (propeller flaps) or free flaps can be selected when the scar size is large. However, they are not as effective as skin-pedicled flap in terms of releasing contractures. (**a**) Propeller flap design. (**b**) Intraoperative view. (**c**) Identification of the perforator. (**d**) View immediately after surgery. (**e**) Three years after surgery

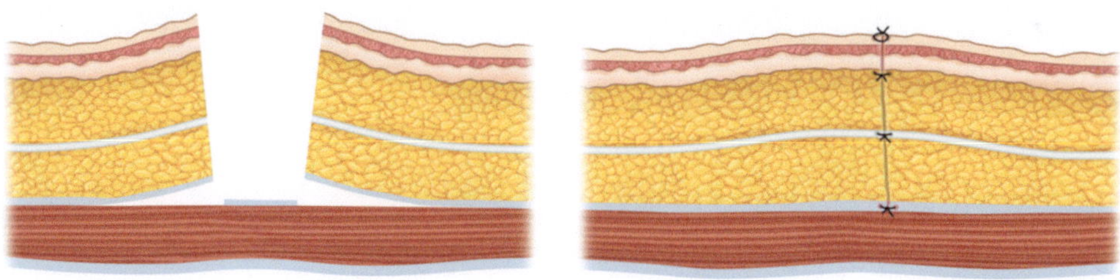

Fig. 11.6 Deep or superficial fascial sutures release tension on the dermis. Since keloids and hypertrophic scars arise from the reticular layer of the dermis, efforts should be made to avoid placing tension on the dermis. Thus, wounds should be closed by accessing the much deeper structures (namely, the superficial and deep fascia) and then suturing them. This will elevate the wound edges smoothly, thus promoting their attachment. Thereafter, dermal and superficial sutures can be placed. This approach will significantly prevent the formation of pathological scars after surgery

as follows: high-risk areas receive 18 Gy/3 fractions/3 days, middle-risk areas receive 15 Gy/2 fractions/2 days, and low-risk areas receive 8 Gy/1 fraction/1 day. To date, we have observed good results (Figs. 11.11 and 11.12) [3].

In terms of radiation side effects, of 10,000 individuals between 18 and 64 years of age, 670 (6.7%) will develop skin cancer if they are subjected to whole body irradiation of 1 Gy [46]. In general, skin cancer kills 1 in 500 patients. Thus, the mortality rate associated with 1 Gy of whole body irradiation would be 6.7% × 1/500 = 0.0134%, namely, 1 in 7500 people. If these sums are applied to earlobe keloid radiotherapy, where 0.05% of the whole body skin is irradiated with 10 Gy, the incidence of cancer associated with this treatment would be 6.7% × 10 Gy × 0.05%/100 = 0.0335%, namely, 1 in 3000 keloid patients. The mortality rate of secondary carcinogenesis of earlobe keloid treatment would be 0.0335/500 = 0.000067%, namely, 1 in 1,500,000 people. We believe that this can be ignored clinically if informed consent is obtained from patients after they have been advised of the benefits and side effects of this type of treatment.

However, it should be remembered that the thyroid and mammary glands are highly sensitive to radiation and lie close to the skin. Thus, efforts must be made to shield these areas from irradiation. Moreover, infants and children under 20 years of age should not be irradiated because their cells are still actively proliferating and they are therefore highly sensitive to radiation as well [47].

We have also used primary radiation therapy (radiation monotherapy) to treat older patients or severe keloid patients in whom surgery is difficult to perform. In these cases, the total

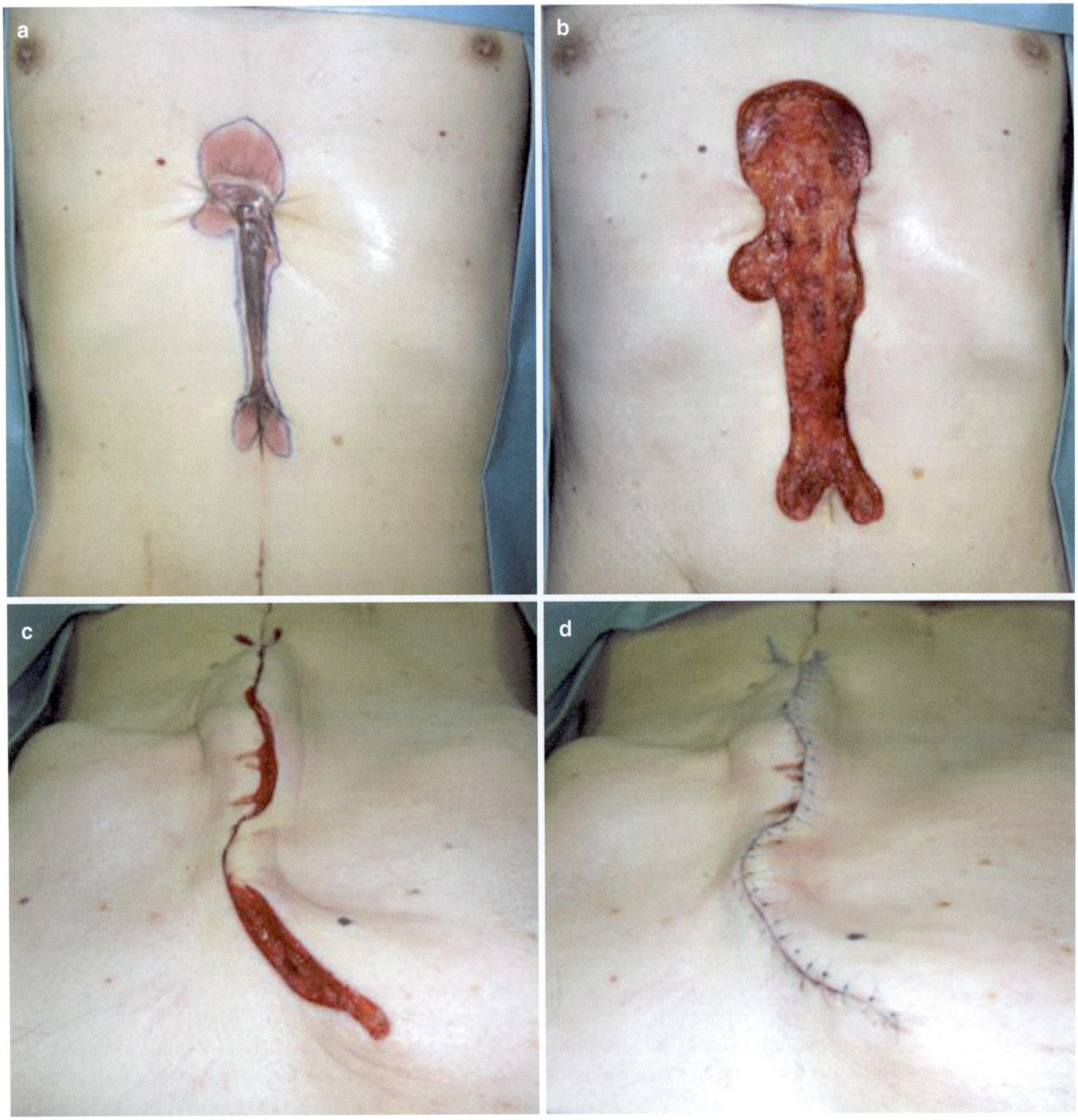

Fig. 11.7 Resection of abdominal keloids followed by closure with fascial sutures and postoperative taping fixation. The abdominal keloid and the fat tissues under the keloid were removed. Subsequently, the deep fascia were sutured with 0 polydioxanone sutures. The superficial fascia were then sutured with 2-0 polydioxanone sutures. Thereafter, dermal and superficial sutures were placed. (**a**) Keloid excision design. (**b**) Intraoperative view. (**c**) Immediately after deep and superficial fascia suturing. (**d**) Immediately after dermal and superficial sutures were placed. (**e**) Postoperative taping fixation of the scar. (**f**) Six months after surgery. (**g**) Two years after surgery

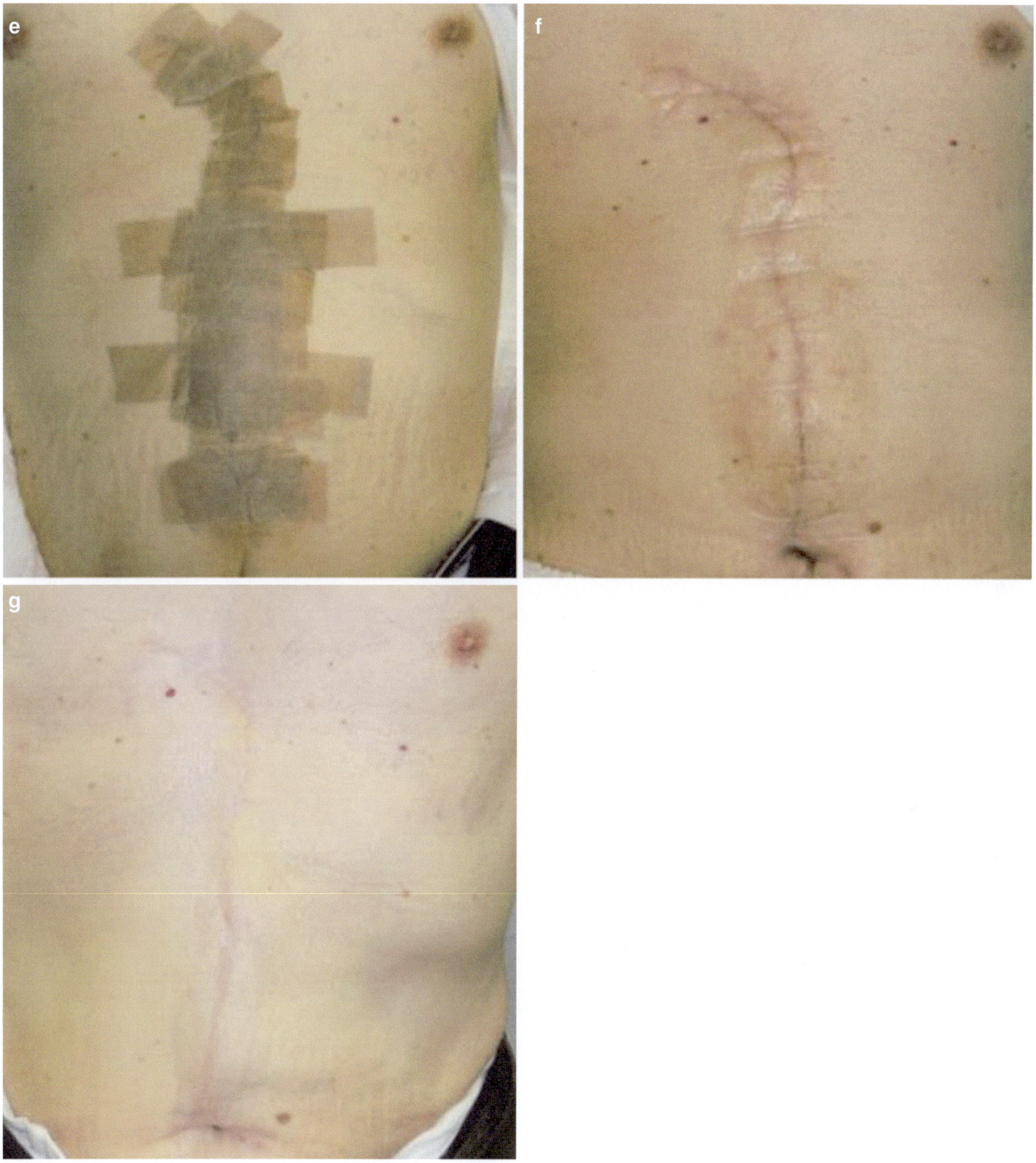

Fig. 11.7 (continued)

radiation dose should be higher than that used for postoperative radiation therapy because the keloid is thick. Therefore, to prevent secondary radiation carcinogenesis, it is necessary to apply the radiation carefully. It is also important to obtain informed consent. However, the benefit of primary radiation therapy is tremendous: subjective symptoms such as pain and itching decrease immediately, and the color and thickness of the scars normalize progressively over a year (Fig. 11.13).

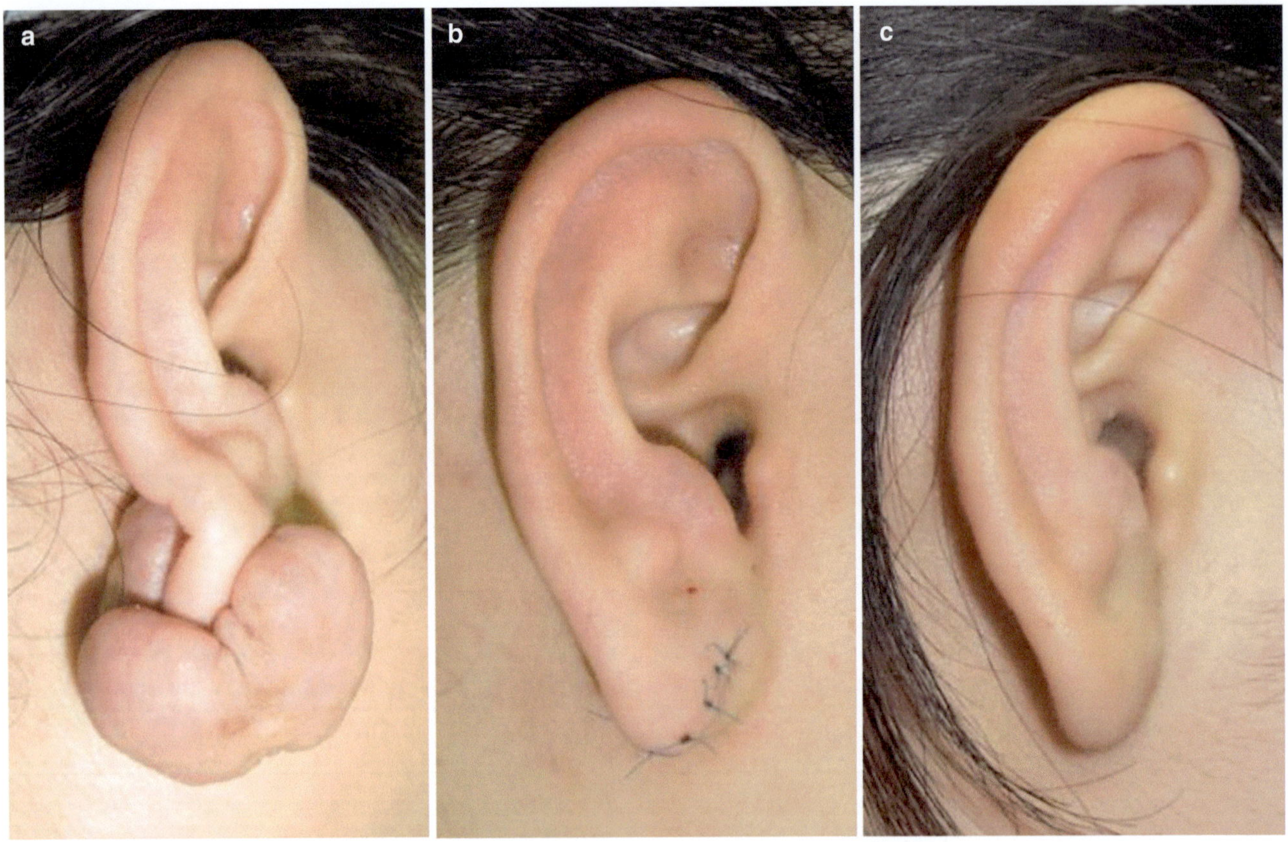

Fig. 11.8 Typical case of wedge excision of earlobe keloid followed by postoperative radiation therapy. The keloid was resected by wedge shape excision, and the wound was sutured directly using 6-0 polypropylene sutures. The earlobe was then subjected to electron beam irradiation (10 Gy/2 fractions/2 days). There was no recurrence 18 months after surgery. (**a**) Preoperative view. (**b**) Immediately after surgery. (**c**) Eighteen months after surgery

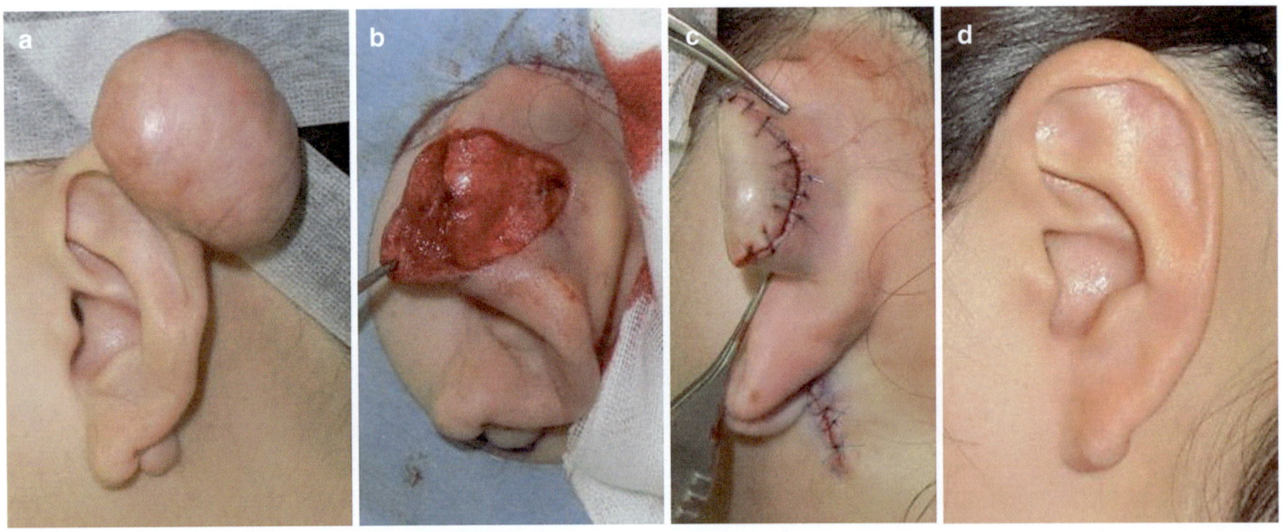

Fig. 11.9 Typical case of core excision of a keloid on the cartilagenous part of the auricle followed by postoperative radiation therapy. The core of the keloid was resected using the core excision method. Since the epidermis and papillary layer of the dermis of the keloid were almost normal, they were used as a flap. After the flap on the keloid was made, it was sutured on the back of the ear using 6-0 polypropylene sutures. The top of the ear was then subjected to electron beam irradiation (15 Gy/3 fractions/3 days). There was no recurrence 18 months after surgery. (**a**) Preoperative view. (**b**) A flap was made on the keloid surface after core excision. (**c**) Immediately after surgery. (**d**) Eighteen months after surgery

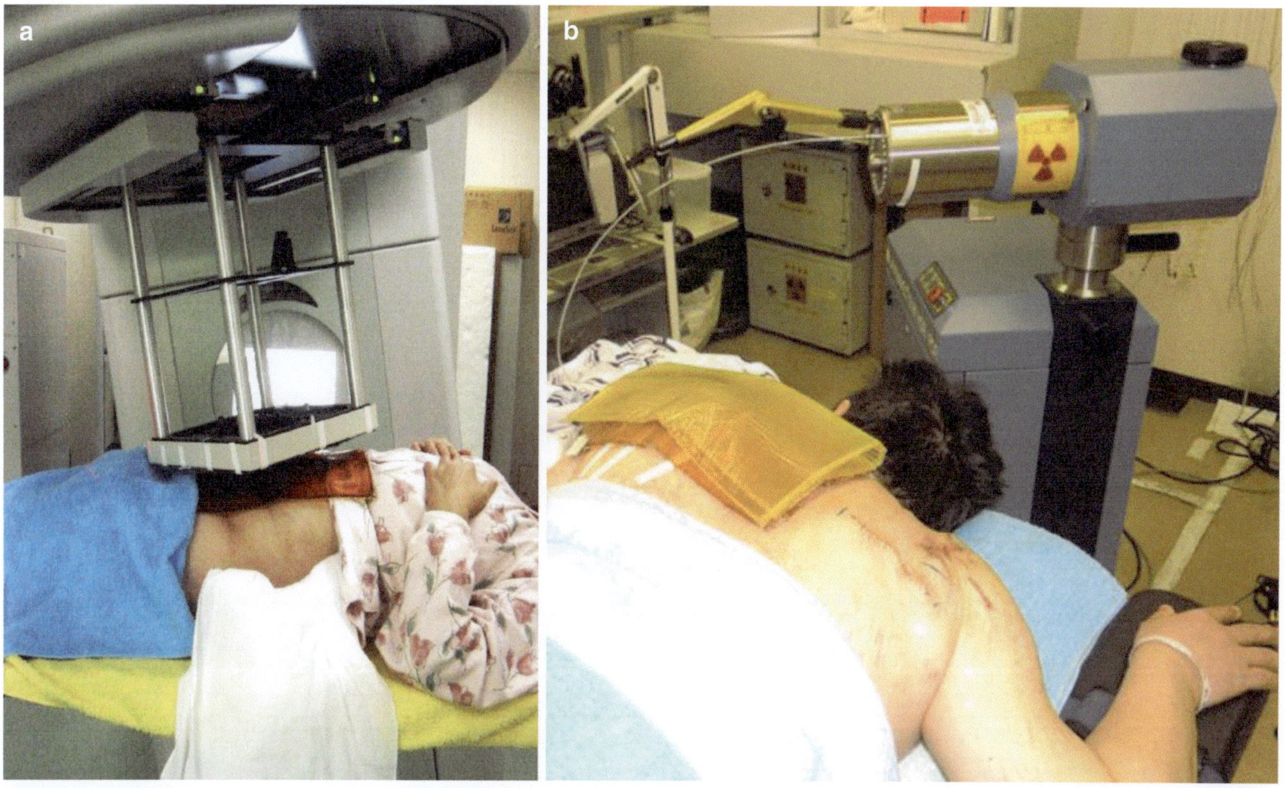

Fig. 11.10 Electron beam (**a**) brachytherapy (**b**). The safety and efficacy of radiation therapy have improved in recent years, and radiation with high-dose-rate superficial brachytherapy (HDR-SB) or electron beam radiation is now used routinely as a highly effective postoperative adjuvant therapy after keloid resection

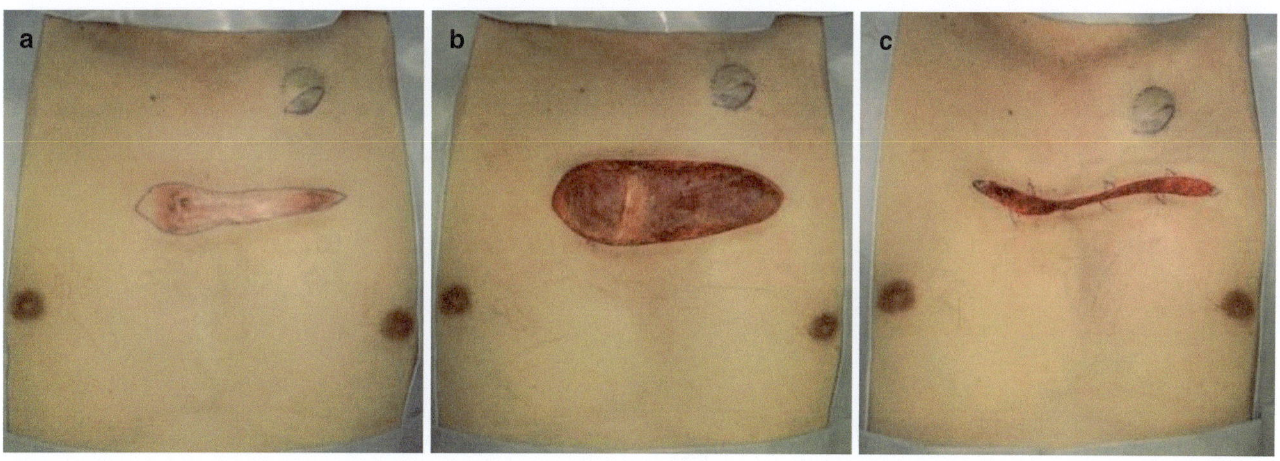

Fig. 11.11 Chest wall keloid resection followed by z-plasty after deep and superficial fascia suturing and postoperative radiotherapy consisting of 18 Gy/3 fractions/3 days. The chest keloid was removed completely, after which the deep and superficial fascia of the pectoralis major muscle were sutured. This allowed the wound edges to attach naturally to each other. Z-plasties were then designed, and the resulting incisions were closed with dermal and superficial sutures using 4-0 polydioxanone and 6-0 polypropylene, respectively. There was no recurrence 18 months after surgery. (**a**) Keloid removal design. (**b**) Intraoperative view after keloid resection. (**c**) Z-plasty design after deep and superficial fascia suturing. (**d**) View immediately after transposition of the z-flaps. (**e**) View immediately after surgery. (**f**) Eighteen months after surgery

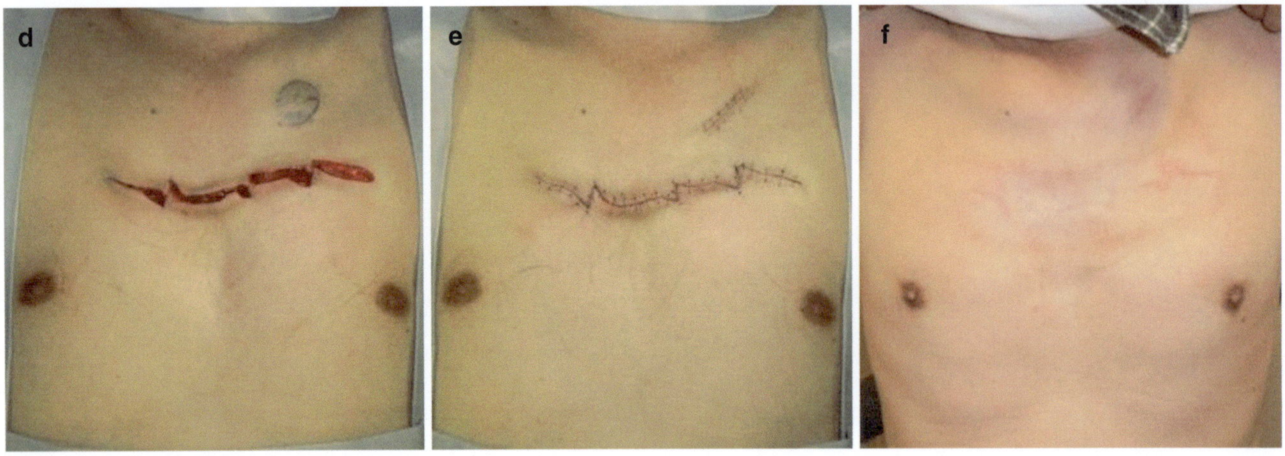

Fig. 11.11 (continued)

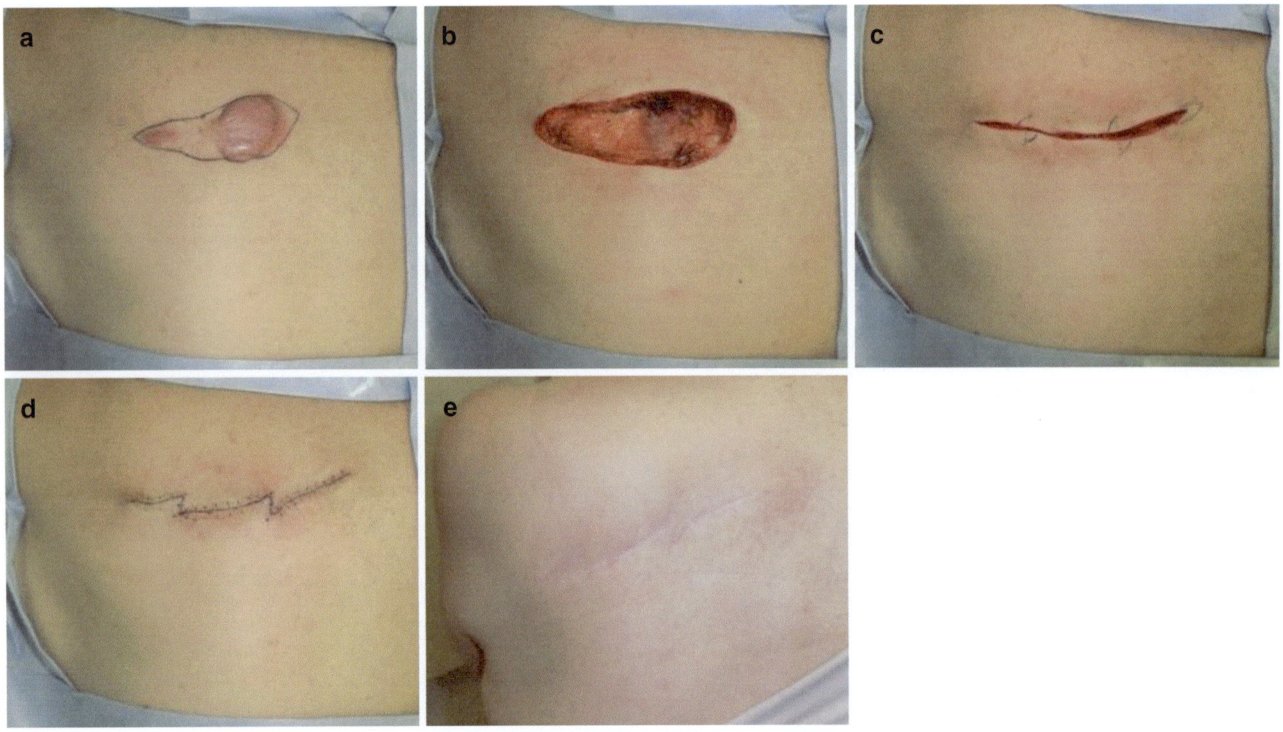

Fig. 11.12 Scapular keloid resection followed by z-plasty after deep and superficial fascia suturing and postoperative radiotherapy consisting of 18 Gy/3 fractions/3 days. The scapular keloid was removed completely, after which the deep and superficial fascia were sutured. The wound edges thus naturally attached to each other. Z-plasties were designed, and the resulting incisions were sutured with dermal and superficial sutures using 4-0 polydioxanone and 6-0 polypropylene, respectively. There was no recurrence 18 months after surgery. (**a**) Keloid removal design. (**b**) Intraoperative view after keloid resection. (**c**) Design of z-plasties after deep and superficial fascia suturing. (**d**) View immediately after surgery. (**e**) Eighteen months after surgery.

11.4 Long-Term Follow-Up and Education

It is important that sequentially treated keloid and hypertrophic scar patients are followed up over the long term, and that they are appropriately educated about scar management. This is because, if patients have a tendency to develop pathological scars, they may be prone to scar recurrence or the ready development of new scars in response to minor stimulation. If such patients can be educated in self-management (including the application of steroid tape/plasters during the early stages of scar development), their scars tend to improve quite rapidly.

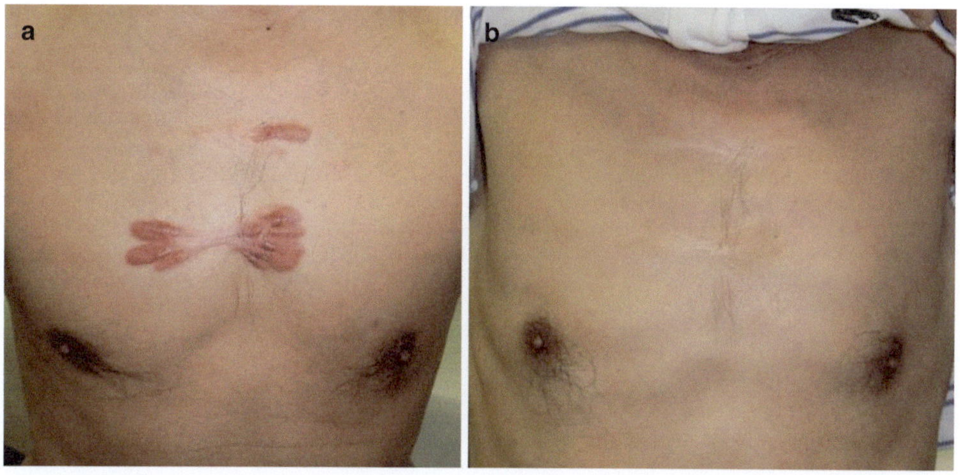

Fig. 11.13 The patient had a chest keloid (**a**) After 1 year of treatment (**b**). Treatment of chest wall keloid with radiation monotherapy using 25 Gy/5 fractions/5 days. The patient had a chest wall keloid that was treated by high-dose-rate superficial brachytherapy. In total, 25 Gy was administered in five fractions over 5 days. The inflammation resolved completely. After 1 year of treatment, both the subjective and objective symptoms had improved dramatically. Pretreatment view. A year after the treatment

11.5 Conclusions

Due to fear of recurrence after keloid resection (which often led to even worse scars), plastic surgeons and dermatologists have been fearful about actively treating keloids. However, there is substantial evidence now that surgery followed by radiation therapy can successfully manage keloids and hypertrophic scars with low levels of recurrence. The development of a standard international algorithm for treating pathological scars on the basis of this evidence is warranted.

References

1. Huang C, Murphy GF, Akaishi S, Ogawa R. Keloids and hypertrophic scars: update and future directions. Plast Reconstr Surg Glob Open. 2013;1(4):e25.
2. Ogawa R. Keloid and hypertrophic scars are the result of chronic inflammation in the reticular dermis. Int J Mol Sci. 2017;18(3):E606.
3. Ogawa R, Akaishi S, Kuribayashi S, Miyashita T. Keloids and hypertrophic scars can now be cured completely: recent progress in our understanding of the pathogenesis of keloids and hypertrophic scars and the most promising current therapeutic strategy. J Nippon Med Sch. 2016;83(2):46–53.
4. Ogawa R. The most current algorithms for the treatment and prevention of hypertrophic scars and keloids. Plast Reconstr Surg. 2010;125(2):557–68.
5. Ogawa R, Akaishi S. Endothelial dysfunction may play a key role in keloid and hypertrophic scar pathogenesis—keloids and hypertrophic scars may be vascular disorders. Med Hypotheses. 2016;96:51–60.
6. Ogawa R. Mechanobiology of scarring. Wound Repair Regen. 2011;19(Suppl 1):s2–9.
7. Mandy SH. The practical use of Z-plasty. J Dermatol Surg. 1975;1(4):57–60.
8. Ogawa R, Akaishi S, Huang C, Dohi T, Aoki M, Omori Y, Koike S, Kobe K, Akimoto M, Hyakusoku H. Clinical applications of basic research that shows reducing skin tension could prevent and treat abnormal scarring: the importance of fascial/subcutaneous tensile reduction sutures and flap surgery for keloid and hypertrophic scar reconstruction. J Nihon Med Sch. 2011;78(2):68–76.
9. Yoshino Y, Kubomura K, Ueda H, Tsuge T, Ogawa R. Extension of flaps associated with burn scar reconstruction: a key difference between island and skin-pedicled flaps. Burns. 2018;44:683–91.
10. Jacobsson F. The treatment of keloids at Radium-hemmet, 1921–1941. Acta Radiol. 1948;29(3):251–67.
11. Levy DS, Salter MM, Roth RE. Postoperative irradiation in the prevention of keloids. AJR Am J Roentgenol. 1976;127(3):509–10.
12. Enhamre A, Hammar H. Keloids with excision and postoperative X-ray irradiation. Dermatologica. 1983;167(2):90–3.
13. Borok TL, Bray M, Sinclair I, Plafker J, LaBirth L, Rollins C. Role of ionizing irradiation for 393 keloids. Int J Radiat Oncol Biol Phys. 1988;15(4):865–70.
14. Kovalic JJ, Perez CA. Radiation therapy following keloidectomy: a 20-year experience. Int J Radiat Oncol Biol Phys. 1989;17(1):77–80.
15. Doornbos JF, Stoffel TJ, Hass AC, Hussey DH, Vigliotti AP, Wen BC, Zahra MK, Sundeen V. The role of kilovoltage irradiation in the treatment of keloids. Int J Radiat Oncol Biol Phys. 1990;18(4):833–9.
16. Chaudhry MR, Akhtar S, Duvalsaint F, Garner L, Lucente FE. Ear lobe keloids, surgical excision followed by radiation therapy: a 10-year experience. Ear Nose Throat J. 1994;73(10):779–81.
17. Norris JE. Superficial X-ray therapy in keloid management: a retrospective study of 24 cases and literature review. Plast Reconstr Surg. 1995;95(6):1051–5.
18. Sclafani AP, Gordon L, Chadha M, Romo T 3rd. Prevention of earlobe keloid recurrence with postoperative corticosteroid injections versus radiation therapy: a randomized, prospective study and review of the literature. Dermatol Surg. 1996;22(6):569–74.
19. Ragoowansi R, Cornes PG, Glees JP, Powell BW, Moss AL. Earlobe keloids: treatment by a protocol of surgical excision and immediate postoperative adjuvant radiotherapy. Br J Plast Surg. 2001;54(6):504–8.
20. Malaker K, Vijayraghavan K, Hodson I, Al Yafi T. Retrospective analysis of treatment of unresectable keloids with primary radiation over 25 years. Clin Oncol (R Coll Radiol). 2004;16(4):290–8.
21. Klumpar DI, Murray JC, Anscher M. Keloids treated with excision followed by radiation therapy. J Am Acad Dermatol. 1994;31(2 Pt 1):225–31.
22. Caccialanza M, Piccinno R, Schiera A. Postoperative radiotherapy of keloids: a twenty-year experience. Eur J Dermatol. 2002;12(1):58–62.
23. Speranza G, Sultanem K, Muanza T. Descriptive study of patients receiving excision and radiotherapy for keloids. Int J Radiat Oncol Biol Phys. 2008;71(5):1465–9.
24. Lo TC, Seckel BR, Salzman FA, Wright KA. Single-dose electron beam irradiation in treatment and prevention of keloids and hypertrophic scars. Radiother Oncol. 1990;19(3):267–72.

25. Chen HC, Ou SY, Lai YL. Combined surgery and irradiation for treatment of hypertrophic scars and keloids. Zhonghua Yi Xue Za Zhi (Taipei). 1991;47(4):249–5.
26. Maarouf M, Schleicher U, Schmachtenberg A, Ammon J. Radiotherapy in the management of keloids. Clinical experience with electron beam irradiation and comparison with X-ray therapy. Strahlenther Onkol. 2002;178(6):330–5.
27. Bischof M, Krempien R, Debus J, Treiber M. Postoperative electron beam radiotherapy for keloids: objective findings and patient satisfaction in self-assessment. Int J Dermatol. 2007;46(9):971–5.
28. Ogawa R, Mitsuhashi K, Hyakusoku H, Miyashita T. Postoperative electron-beam irradiation therapy for keloids and hypertrophic scars: retrospective study of 147 cases followed for more than 18 months. Plast Reconstr Surg. 2003;111(2):547–53. discussion 554–5.
29. Ogawa R, Miyashita T, Hyakusoku H, Akaishi S, Kuribayashi S, Tateno A. Postoperative radiation protocol for keloids and hypertrophic scars: statistical analysis of 370 sites followed for over 18 months. Ann Plast Surg. 2007;59(6):688–91.
30. Vivante H, Salgueiro MJ, Ughetti R, Nicolini J, Zubillaga M. 32P-patch contact brachyradiotherapy in the management of recalcitrant keloids and hypertrophic scars. Indian J Dermatol Venereol Leprol. 2007;73(5):336–9.
31. Supe SS, Supe SJ, Rao SM, Deka AC, Deka BC. Treatment of keloids by 90Sr-90Y beta-rays. Strahlenther Onkol. 1991;167(7):397–402.
32. Fraunholz IB, Gerstenhauer A, Böttcher HD. Results of postoperative (90)Sr radiotherapy of keloids in view of patients' subjective assessment. Strahlenther Onkol. 2005;181(11):724–9.
33. Malaker K, Zaidi M, Franka MR. Treatment of earlobe keloids using the cobalt 60 teletherapy unit. Ann Plast Surg. 2004;52(6):602–4.
34. Malaker A, Ellis F, Paine CH. Keloid scars: a new method of treatment combining surgery with interstitial radiotherapy. Clin Radiol. 1976;27(2):179–83.
35. Escarmant P, Zimmermann S, Amar A, Ratoanina JL, Moris A, Azaloux H, Francois H, Gosserez O, Michel M, G'Baguidi R. The treatment of 783 keloid scars by iridium 192 interstitial irradiation after surgical excision. Int J Radiat Oncol Biol Phys. 1993;26(2):245–51.
36. Clavere P, Bedane C, Bonnetblanc JM, Bonnafoux-Clavere A, Rousseau J. Postoperative interstitial radiotherapy of keloids by iridium 192: a retrospective study of 46 treated scars. Dermatology. 1997;195(4):349–52.
37. Guix B, Henríquez I, Andrés A, Finestres F, Tello JI, Martínez A. Treatment of keloids by high-dose-rate brachytherapy: a seven-year study. Int J Radiat Oncol Biol Phys. 2001;50(1):167–72.
38. Garg MK, Weiss P, Sharma AK, Gorla GR, Jaggernauth W, Yaparpalvi R, Delrowe J, Beitler JJ. Adjuvant high dose rate brachytherapy (Ir-192) in the management of keloids which have recurred after surgical excision and external radiation. Radiother Oncol. 2004;73(2):233–6.
39. Narkwong L, Thirakhupt P. Postoperative radiotherapy with high dose rate iridium 192 mould for prevention of earlobe keloids. J Med Assoc Thai. 2006;89(4):428–33.
40. Veen RE, Kal HB. Postoperative high-dose-rate brachytherapy in the prevention of keloids. Int J Radiat Oncol Biol Phys. 2007;69(4):1205–8.
41. Kuribayashi S, Miyashita T, Ozawa Y, Iwano M, Ogawa R, Akaishi S, Dohi T, Hyakusoku H, Kumita S. Post-keloidectomy irradiation using high-dose-rate superficial brachytherapy. J Radiat Res. 2011;52(3):365–8.
42. Ogawa R, Huang C, Akaishi S, Dohi T, Sugimoto A, Kuribayashi S, Miyashita T, Hyakusoku H. Analysis of surgical treatments for earlobe keloids: analysis of 174 lesions in 145 patients. Plast Reconstr Surg. 2013;132(5):818e–25e.
43. Ogawa R, Akaishi S, Dohi T, Kuribayashi S, Miyashita T, Hyakusoku H. Analysis of the surgical treatments of 63 keloids on the cartilaginous part of the auricle: effectiveness of the core excision method. Plast Reconstr Surg. 2015;135(3):868–75.
44. Ogawa R, Ono S, Akaishi S, Dohi T, Iimura T, Nakao J. Reconstruction after anterior chest wall keloid resection using internal mammary artery perforator propeller flaps. Plast Reconstr Surg Glob Open. 2016;4(9):e1049.
45. Kal HB, Veen RE. Biologically effective doses of postoperative radiotherapy in the prevention of keloids. Dose-effect relationship. Strahlenther Onkol. 2005;181:717–23.
46. Preston DL, Ron E, Tokuoka S, Funamoto S, Nishi N, Soda M, Mabuchi K, Kodama K. Solid cancer incidence in atomic bomb survivors: 1958–1998. Radiat Res. 2007;168(1):1–64.
47. Ogawa R, Yoshitatsu S, Yoshida K, Miyashita T. Is radiation therapy for keloids acceptable? The risk of radiation-induced carcinogenesis. Plast Reconstr Surg. 2009;124(4):1196–201.

12 Steroids for Scars

Ioannis Goutos

12.1 History of Steroid Administration in Scar Management

The first report of steroid use in the international scar literature dates back to 1950 with Behrmann and Goodwin noting improvement of keloid scars in patients receiving a combination of adrenocorticotropic hormone (ACTH) and cortisone [1]. During the same year, Baker and Whitaker demonstrated that topical application of steroids over a prolonged period of time produces dermal thinning in an animal model [2].

A year later, in 1951, Polson, Pattee and Woolhouse published a case report in which they used intramuscular cortisone preoperatively coupled with oral and intramuscular administration in association with surgical keloid excision; nevertheless they identified that this approach was not successful in preventing recurrence [3].

Conway and Stark in 1951 trialled the combination of surgery and postoperative parenteral ACTH for the treatment of two keloid scars and noted no recurrence at 5 and 8 months. Additionally, four cases were treated with intralesional injections of ACTH and hyaluronidase; symptomatic relief (pain and itch) was observed, nevertheless a significant change in the physical appearance was noted in only one of the treated lesions [4].

Goldman, Thompson and Trice were the first authors to investigate the value of cortisone cream for keloids with disappointing results [5]. Coste, Degos et al. reported beneficial effects of local injections of hydrocortisone acetate into keloids [6], while De Kleine noted that local injections of cortisone (0.25 mg/cc) following excision of keloids in two patients resulted in delayed recurrence in one and by a lesser degree of recurrence in the other [7].

Table 12.1 Summary of the key milestones related to the use of corticosteroid preparations in scar management

Author	Year	Description
Berhman	1950	First use of oral/parenteral steroid in keloid scar treatment
Polson et al. and Goodwin	1951	Use of steroids as adjunct in surgical treatment
Goldman and Trice	1952	First report of cortisone cream application to keloids
Coste and Degos	1953	Local injections of hydrocortisone acetate as monotherapy
Hollander	1961	Fluorinated derivative triamcinolone showed successful scar regression as well as symptomatic relief
Murray	1963	The injection of steroids into the edges of excised scars to prevent recurrence
Maguire HC Griffith BH Minkowitz F	1965 1966 1967	The successful intralesional treatment of scars with triamcinolone as a mainstay in keloid management

In 1961, Hollander used the fluorinated steroid derivative triamcinolone for keloid management and showed successful regression in the cohort as well as the achievement of significant symptomatic relief [8]. Murray in 1963 proposed the injection of steroids into the edges of the excised scar to prevent recurrence [9] heralding the use of injectable steroids as a perioperative adjunct. In the late 1960s, Maguire HC, Griffith BH and Minkowitz F reported the successful intralesional treatment of scars with triamcinolone and placed this agent as the most popular steroid agent in keloid management [10–12]. Table 12.1 illustrates the key milestones pertinent to the use of corticosteroids in the scar management field.

12.2 Chemical Structure and Mechanism of Action of Steroids

Steroids are cholesterol derivatives and divided into two classes, namely mineralocorticoids and glucocorticoids. The main endogenous corticosteroid (hydrocortisone) influences

I. Goutos (✉)
Royal London Hospital, Barts Health NHS Trust, Whitechapel, UK

Centre for Cutaneous Research, Blizard Institute, Queen Mary University of London, London, UK
e-mail: i.goutos@qmul.ac.uk

© Springer Nature Singapore Pte Ltd. 2020
R. Ogawa (ed.), *Total Scar Management*, https://doi.org/10.1007/978-981-32-9791-3_12

carbohydrate and protein metabolism and has significant anti-inflammatory and immunosuppressive effects; the latter biological actions are exploited in clinical practice in relation to scar management [13]. Glucocorticoid receptors are present in all cell types, which explains the potential for steroids to cause a spectrum of both local and systemic side effects in patients undergoing treatment for hypertrophic and keloid scars [14].

Steroids suppress inflammation via/scar formation the following main mechanisms [15, 16]:

(a) Inhibition of leukocyte/monocyte migration and phagocytosis.
(b) Vasoconstriction, which reduces the delivery of oxygen and nutrients to the wound bed.
(c) Antimitotic effect through inhibition of fibroblast proliferation (by decreasing mitogenic factors such as TGF-beta 1, VEGF and IGF-1) and induction of cellular degeneration.
(d) Decrease of collagen synthesis and enhancement of collagen degradation via reduction of levels of alpha-2 macroglobulin and alpha-1 antitrypsin (potent collagenase inhibitors).

Steroids can be administered in a variety of ways to hypertrophic and keloid scars, including injectable, ointment and tape form. This chapter does not explicitly differentiate between the administration of steroids for hypertrophic and keloid scars; this relates to the fact that current theories support the notion that they both lie on the spectrum of unfavourable scar formation with keloids being the extreme end of hypertrophic scarring diathesis [17]. Furthermore, the majority of literature reports lack a clear histological or objective clinical differentiation of keloid vs. hypertrophic scars making it challenging to accurately subcategorise the available evidence.

12.3 Methods of Steroid Administration

12.3.1 Injectable Steroids

12.3.1.1 Popular Steroid Preparations and Dosing Regimens

A variety of injectable steroids have been used over a number of decades, including hydrocortisone acetate (25 mg/mL), dexamethasone (4 mg/mL) and methylprednisolone (4 mg/mL) [13, 18].

By far, the most commonly used preparation is triamcinolone acetonide (TAC), which is commercially available in 10 and 40 mg/mL preparations in the UK and the USA. This fluorinated derivative of prednisolone is four times as potent as hydrocortisone; this is by virtue of its reduced solubility and resulting capacity to remain biologically active at the injection site for longer periods of time [19–21].

Although injectable steroids, especially triamcinolone, represent the most popular steroid for the treatment of keloid and hypertrophic scars, little objective evidence exists to support definitive recommendations with regard to treatment protocols. The frequency of administration varies widely in the literature and ranges from twice weekly [7] to 6 week intervals between each treatment session [22, 23].

A survey among over one hundred international plastic surgeons revealed that the most popular steroid preparation for scar management is TAC (40 mg/mL) and the most frequent time interval advised between injections is 3 and 4 weeks (31%) closely followed by 4–5 weeks (26%) [24]. Darzi proposed a dosing schedule according to the volume of scar tissue per course as follows: 20–40 mg of triamcinolone for lesions with surface area of 1–2 cm^2, 40–80 mg for those with 2–6 cm^2 and 80–120 mg for scars with surface area of 6–12 cm^2 with an interval between injections of 1 and 2 weeks [25]. Jalali suggested a similar protocol based on the length of linear scar, i.e. 0.1 mL of 10 mg TAC per linear centimetre of scar repeated every 4–6 weeks until the scar is successfully reduced [13]. A maximum dose of 5 mg triamcinolone per session has been suggested by a different group in an attempt to avoid menstrual irregularities as well as hypopigmentation and skin atrophy to the treatment area [26]. An international panel of experts in 2010 recommended triamcinolone injections of 2.5–20 mg per mL for the face and 20–40 mg per mL for the rest of the body repeated every month; most interestingly, no specific doses for children have been established as yet [27].

12.3.1.2 Injection Techniques

Intralesional Technique

The intralesional injection of corticosteroids represents mainstay treatment for hypertrophic and keloid scars. One of the most well-designed studies proving the efficacy of this modality employed a validated three-dimensional speckle pattern stereophotogrammetry to assess objective scar volume quantification. In a cohort of 12 adults with keloid scars, TAC (0.5–4 mL depending on lesion size) was administered intralesionally and scar assessment was undertaken before and after a minimum of 8 weeks steroid therapy. Results showed that the mean scar volume of reduction was statistically significant [change from 0.73 ± 0.701 cm^3 to 0.14 ± 0.302 cm^3 ($p < 0.001$)], with the majority of patients achieving a greater than 50% response within 8 weeks [28].

A variety of technical tips have been described in the literature to increase the efficacy of administration and minimise discomfort to the patient.

Small diameter needles (ranges between 25 and 30 gauge) in conjunction with a Luer lock syringe or insulin syringes with an integrated needle have been advocated for intralesional injection in order to withstand the pressure encountered during injection into stiff scars [22, 29]. In terms of recommendations with regard to injection technique, a number of authors have advised that the needle should be inserted into the papillary dermis (where collagenase is produced) and the substance administered while withdrawing [29, 30]. Other authors have supported the injection at mid-dermis level in order to avoid irreversible epidermal atrophy, which is more likely with superficial injections [31]. Blanching/complete distension of the scar during the injection is widely considered as a sufficient procedural endpoint; clinical experience suggests that younger more compliant scars respond better compared to more long-standing lesions [7, 30]. The principle of inserting the needle within the keloidal lesion (as opposed to the adjacent healthy skin) in order to avoid the development of an iatrogenic keloid has been reported but not substantiated with solid evidence in the literature [32]. A variety of techniques have been described to ease the discomfort associated with steroid injection, including:

(a) Use of topical anaesthetic cream before the procedure or incorporation of a local anaesthetic solution with the steroid in the same syringe. Although the latter does not ease the initial pain of injection, it theoretically allows the performance of serial injections within the lesion and eases post procedural pain [29].
(b) Use of pressure jet apparatus [23, 33] or an electric pump (at an injection speed of 3–6 mL per h) has been shown to be effective in minimising discomfort [34].
(c) Liquid nitrogen administration (with 10–15 s freeze cycle duration) [35] has been reported to ease injection-related discomfort and improve the retention of steroid; this is thought to occur via the induction of cellular damage and oedema within the scar [36].

Injectable steroids have been proven to be particularly effective in relieving symptoms of itch and pain as well as reducing the bulk of scars. Repeated administration is required in cycles and treatment stops on the grounds of:

- Significant scar regression/satisfactory symptomatic relief.
- Development of local or systemic adverse effects during treatment.
- Failure to induce significant scar regression. It is widely recognized in clinical practice that a subset of scars fail to respond to injectable steroids and recent work has indicated that this might relate to a different expression pattern of tissue glucocorticoid receptors rendering a subset of scars steroid resistant [30].
- Poor patient compliance. A descriptive study in Asian patients with keloid scars treated with four weekly triamcinolone injections (1–10 mg of 10 mg/mL) identified that 33% patients abandoned treatment within ten injections due to a combination of procedural pain and lack of clinical improvement [37].

Sublesional Technique

The literature review findings on the intralesional injectable approach reveals a number of shortcomings including the development of local side effects as well as procedure-associated pain impacting on patient compliance. The sublesional technique involves delivering steroids to the deepest part of the dermis in an attempt to overcome the shortcomings of the intralesional approach.

This technique using 20–40 mg/mL Kenacort has been reported in a single publication of long-standing burn-related keloids (at the end of their second year of development) [38]. The authors employed light and electron microscope examination of the treated scars and showed that that the positive changes in histology appeared earlier compared to those achieved with the intralesional approach with a most interestingly similar pattern of side effects, including atrophy, depigmentation and telangiectasia. The adoption of this approach has been supported in a very recent publication [26] and also represents the author's preferred approach, especially in non-compliant, long-standing scars.

12.3.1.3 Intralesional Steroid Administration as an Adjunct to Surgical Scar Excision

Steroid administration is commonly used as an adjunct to surgical scar management and a variety of practices have been described in relation to timing of administration (i.e. pre-, intra- as well as postoperatively) as well as the exact site of delivery (i.e. intra- vs. extra-lesional injection).

Preoperative Use of Steroid

The use of preoperative steroid injections has been described; the underlying principle is to produce scar atrophy until no further regression is feasibly noted before surgical excision removes the scar remnant in a field with reduced inflammatory potential. Different authors have suggested varying regimens starting injections 1–3 months preoperatively and continuing for a variable amount of time with injections following scar excision [22, 39]. The only study investigating the preoperative use of corticosteroids in the management of keloids comprised a randomized prospective trial; one arm included patients receiving two preoperative and three postoperative doses of triamcinolone and the other surgery plus colchicine orally (1.2 mg/day). The authors concluded that there was no significant difference in the rate of recurrence between the two groups but commented on the limited acceptance of the study protocol, which makes any valid conclusions about the value of preoperative steroid administration challenging [18].

Intralesional Excision and Postoperative Injection

The principle behind this technique relies on excising the bulk of the lesion and leaving a rim of keloid in the periphery, which allows closure of the resulting keloidal flaps with preservation of the peripheral scar scaffolding. This practice is particularly popular in the UK and permits easier postoperative administration of steroid into the peripheral scar remnants.

Steroid injection has been reported at different time intervals after the operation, varying from immediately after skin closure [40] to the time of suture removal (10–14 days); follow-up injections have been timed at variable (2–4 week) intervals in a number of reports [41, 42]. Tang proposed the combination of intralesional scar excision, tension relieving undermining, 10–30 mg TAC administration at the wound margins intraoperatively and follow-up injections postoperatively for up to 5 months. In his published case series of 11 keloids and hypertrophic scars treated with this protocol at a median follow-up of 15 months (range: 12–36), the rate of recurrence was reported as 8.2% [42].

Extralesional Excision and Postoperative Injection

The rationale for this approach is to excise the entirety of the scar lesion and minimise the recurrence at the surgical excision site by dampening down the inflammatory response using steroid preparations delivered in the wound margins. Variable practices have been described regarding dosing of steroid preparations as well as administration timing. Some reports support the injection of perilesional skin before extralesional excision [43], while others commence steroids immediately at the time of closure [44–47] with a variable number of monthly follow-up injections. A single report in the literature supports the notion of starting injections at least 10 days following the extralesional scar excision in an attempt to decrease the risk of infection/dehiscence [48]. A study investigated the histological appearance of scars following keloid excision and immediate vs. delayed (at 2 weeks) injection of triamcinolone. It was shown that downregulation of collagen type 1 is elicited by immediate TA injection after keloid excision and wound healing is not compromised as a result. Furthermore, examination of the immediately treated fields showed that the collagen bundles were thinner and less dense compared to the delayed injection group [49]. The findings of this study provide some supporting evidence in favour of immediate wound edge injection accompanying extralesional keloid excision. Chowdhury et al. performed a study of 58 patients with hypertrophic and keloid scars who underwent surgical excision and triamcinolone acetonide injection at the time of surgery as well as postoperatively (2–5 weekly injections initially followed by monthly injections for 4–6 months). All patients achieved some degree of symptomatic relief and no recurrence at mean follow-up for 30 months was observed in 92% of the keloid and 95% of the hypertrophic scar patients [45].

12.3.1.4 Side Effects of Corticosteroids

Local Side Effects

Up to 63% patients experience side effects following corticosteroid therapy for hypertrophic and keloid scars; these are more likely to occur if the injected material spills into surrounding dermis or subcutaneous tissue or is wrongly placed close to the epidermal layer [50–52]. The most common reported side effects include [29, 53–55]:

1. Hypopigmentation (this may be permanent or resolve over 6–12 months).
2. Cutaneous atrophy.
3. Telangiectasia.
4. Plaque/yellow deposit formation.
5. Ulceration/local skin necrosis.
6. Linear perilymphatic atrophy has been reported in patients following triamcinolone injection, which regresses over a period of months.

Figure 12.1 [(a) pretreatment and (b) posttreatment view] show the clinical response as well as localised side effects of injectable corticosteroids to a traumatic periauricular hypertrophic scar. The patient received two cycles of triamcinolone acetonide (40 mg/mL).

Systemic Side Effects

Aside the risk of local side effects with steroid administration, the development of excessive systemic levels of steroids exists; this can lead to adrenal suppression and the development of Cushing's syndrome (Table 12.2) [14, 24]. High doses of triamcinolone appear to reduce its total body clearance via saturation of physiological elimination mechanisms; this combined with the slow release formulation of TAC may explain the resulting adrenal suppression in patients receiving multiple injections [56].

A systematic review of the literature from 1950 to 2012 has confirmed 18 cases of Cushing's syndrome after intralesional TAC administration [24]. Objective indicators for the establishment of safe dosing regimens do not exist given the lack of absorption studies for intralesionally injected glucocorticoids. Nevertheless it appears that intrinsic factors like the individual sensitivity to steroids may play a role in the propensity towards the development of Cushing's syndrome [57].

The most discriminating features of Cushing's syndrome (systemic accumulation of glucocorticoids) are facial plethora, easy bruising, proximal myopathy and broad purple striae [58]. The median time for the development of initial symptoms of Cushing's syndrome appear to be 6.5 weeks (range: 2 weeks–9 months), and a follow-up assessment within 2 weeks has been recommended to ensure early detection and management of possible systemic side effects fol-

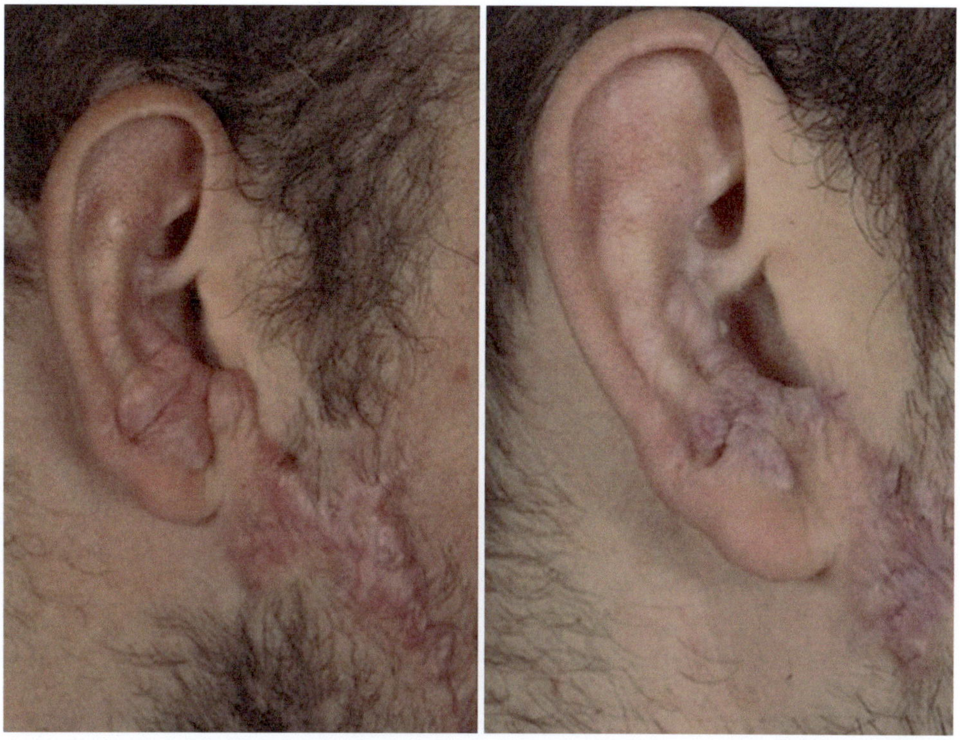

Fig. 12.1 (**a**) Pre- and (**b**) post-treatment views showing the clinical response as well as localised side effects of injectable corticosteroids for a traumatic periauricular hypertrophic scar following two cycles of triamcinolone acetonide (40 mg/mL) injections

Table 12.2 Summary of the systemic side effects of steroid administration

System	Side effects
Ocular	Increased intraocular pressure resulting in glaucoma
Musculoskeletal	Calcium resorption resulting in osteoporosis, muscle weakness, growth stunting in children
Immune	Immune suppression, susceptibility to infection
Cardiovascular	Increase in cardiac output and decrease in total peripheral resistance
Neurological	From minor sleep disorders to psychosis, seizures, headaches and decreased libido
Skin	Acne, purple striae and bruising diathesis
Metabolism	Weight gain, hyperglycaemia and diabetes, redistribution of fat (buffalo hump, facial plethora, supraclavicular fat pad)

lowing the commencement of corticosteroid administration [24]. Table 12.2 summarises the systemic manifestations of Cushing's syndrome.

Literature review reveals that 80% of Cushing's syndrome reports concern paediatric patients with the majority of those having received more than 40 mg of corticosteroid within a period of a month. It remains unclear whether children are physiologically more prone to systemic side effects from intralesional corticosteroids irrespective of strict pharmacological dose per kilogram considerations; nevertheless given the reported trend in the literature, increased caution must be advertised when administering steroids in paediatric scars (recommended maximum dose of 30 mg TAC per month) [24]. With regard to adult dosage guidance, the international panel of experts in 2010 recommended triamcinolone injections of 2.5–20 mg per mL for facial scars and 20–40 mg per mL (for the rest of the bodily sites) repeated every month [28].

12.3.2 Steroid Ointment Preparations

A small number of publications have studied the efficacy of steroid ointments in the treatment of hypertrophic and keloid scars. Marsden et al. investigated the use of 0.25% fluocinolone acetonide cream applied three times/day in 192 patients with a variety of dermatological conditions, including lichen planus, psoriasis as well as 12 cases of keloids. Results suggested a significant response or clearance in 9 out of 12 cases; nevertheless the longevity of this response cannot be assessed given that the study follow-up period was not specified [59].

A prospective observational study investigated the effectiveness of a triamcinolone emulsion in 32 hypertrophic and 9 keloid patients. The product was applied twice a day on the scars with an adjacent part of the lesion left untreated to act as the comparison area. Assessment was done using a five-point scale parameter (colour, elevation, texture, itch and pain) and a beneficial result was considered if the scars improved in at least 3/5. In the hypertrophic scar group, 84.4% showed improvement, whereas in the keloid group the response rate was 44.5%. However, all patients achieved pain and itch symptomatic relief [60]. One of the main limitations of the study is the very short duration (maximum 7 months), which makes any valid conclusions about the value of this preparation very challenging.

Another literature report investigated the efficacy of a combined regimen of surgical excision, intralesional steroid (20 mg/mL of triamcinolone acetonide) injection and steroid ointment [61]. Following complete scar excision, the first steroid injection was given at the time of suture removal (7 days postoperatively) and subsequently every 2 weeks for five sessions. A range of steroid ointment products were applied twice weekly for 6 months after suture removal (diflorasone diacetate: first 2 months, difluprednate: third and fourth month, betamethasone valerate: fifth and sixth month).

At a median follow-up of 32 months, 14.3% keloids and 16.7% hypertrophic scars had recurred (defined as observable dermal elevation at the excision site). It becomes clear from the literature review that the evidence behind the use of steroid ointments for hypertrophic and keloid scars is very weak; this relates to small cohort sizes, the non-randomised nature of existing reports as well as the short follow-up periods employed.

12.3.3 Steroid Tape Preparations

The transdermal route for steroid administration using a tape carrier was introduced in 1960s [62] and currently has a number of clinical indications in the field of scar management, including [26, 63]:

- First-line treatment of small-sized/thin keloids and hypertrophic scars.
- Secondary management adjunct following induction of scar regression with steroid injections, radiotherapy or surgery.
- Prophylaxis for patients at high risk for hypertrophy commencing shortly after completion of wound re-epithelialisation.

Steroid tapes consist of a pharmacologically inactive carrier (adhesive tape) and a steroid component, which varies in different parts of the world.

In Japan, a 4 μg/cm² fludroxycortide (medium potency) and a 20 μg/cm² deprodone propionate (high potency) product is available, whereas in the USA and the UK only medium strength—4 μg/cm² flurandrenolide (USA) and fludroxycortide (UK)—formulations exist. Steroid tape is applied to the scar with minimum overlap onto normal skin. Patients can perform personal hygiene as normal and simply pat the area dry over the tape, which should be changed within 48 h in order to maintain its biological efficacy [26].

The mechanism of action of tape formulations relates alongside the well-described pharmacological effects of steroids on scar tissue, on the non-pharmacological effects of the carrier tape, including:

(a) *Occlusion.* It is widely recognised that occlusion increases the percutaneous absorption of steroids. Proposed mechanisms for the therapeutic effect of occlusion include maintenance of stratum corneum hydration as well as the retention of heat underneath the tape [64, 65]. Interestingly, studies have confirmed that total occlusion is not necessary for this physiological effect to materialise; semiocclusive tape carriers can mediate this effect and have the advantage of preventing certain side effects, including maceration and skin irritation [66, 67].
(b) *Vasoconstriction.* One of the main mechanisms of action of steroids relates to a strong vasoactive effect, which appears to be augmented by occlusion. Vasoconstriction is thought to be mediated via glucocorticoid receptors affecting a number of possible pathways, including local norepinephrine release, cutaneous mast cell function and phospholipase A activity [23–27].
(c) *Scar support.* It is widely accepted that tension across the scar can be a contributing factor towards hypertrophy; hence mechanical support effected by the tape carrier material may contribute to the involution of keloid and hypertrophic scars acting on the complex mechanotransduction pathways within the scar tissue [68].

Tape formulations were introduced based on a number of advantageous properties in comparison to steroid injections/ointments, including [69]:

(a) Ease of application.
(b) Noninvasive nature compared to injectable formulations.
(c) Enhanced absorption relating to occlusion.
(d) Protection from mechanical irritation.
(e) Controlled medication release; one of the theoretical advantages of tape formulations is avoidance of peaks and troughs of steroid concentration as applied to the periodical administration of injectables. The constant influx of medication delivery might be critical in controlling the inflammatory milieu of the scar central to the keloid and hypertrophic pathophysiology [70, 71].

12.3.3.1 Evidence Base for the Adoption of Steroid Tape in Scar Management

The use of steroid tape on keloid and hypertrophic scars was first reported in the English literature in 1967 in a mixed cohort of 285 patients with dermatological disorders [61]. Subsequently, a number of additional reports have provided preliminary evidence supporting the use of steroid tape in the scar management field.

A study of 74 patients with various skin diseases including hypertrophic/keloid scars investigated the effect of flurandrenolide tape (4 μg/cm^2). The duration of the tape application for each episode varied between 12 h and 7 days. Nineteen patients had hypertrophic scarring (defined as scars present for less than 12 months) and were treated for a period between 2 and 120 days (average of 51 days). Excellent response (complete disappearance of excessive scarring) was seen in eight patients, whereas a good response was seen in ten and partial in four. In the keloid group (defined as scar duration of more than 12 months) consisted of 12 patients treated for a period between 7 and 288 days (average 77 days). Two patients had excellent and four had good results, while partial improvement was observed in four patients. The author of this report concluded that 'individuals with partial and good improvement in the hypertrophic scar group could be possibly converted to the excellent category by greater persistence in the regularity of tape application and by increasing the period of treatment'. Furthermore, for well-established cases of keloid scarring, long treatment periods were needed [72].

Another clinical trial at Glasgow Western Infirmary, UK, investigated the use of steroid tape in 11 keloid scars within a cohort of 40 patients with a variety of dermatoses. The age range for the keloid group was between 2 and 76 years and the tape was applied for 12–24 h a day over the 18 month period of the trial. The area of the tape application was in most of the cases less than 0.5% of total body surface area (TBSA) and only two children had up to 5% TBSA treated with steroid tape. The author of this work stated that 'the most gratifying response to the application of the tape was in the cases of keloids, notably children'. The majority of the scars improved by becoming flatter and paler than the surrounding skin and the redness and irritation disappeared in the most severely affected patients [73].

The use of steroid tape has also been investigated in more recent years in the Japanese literature. An open trial employed deprodone propionate plaster to a large cohort of patients with dermatological diseases including 24 hypertrophic and 30 keloid scars age range between 10 and 70 years. (The tape was applied for 15 h a day over 6 weeks and the outcomes were assessed based on subjective reports by the physician). The tape was found to be very effective in three patients, effective in 21, whereas a minor response was seen in 18 and no response in 12 patients [74].

Another observational report assessed the use of fludroxycortide tape in 60 hypertrophic and keloid scars in 30 adult (mean age: 37 years, range: 23–67) and 30 paediatric (mean age: 7.2 years, range: 2–15 years) patients. The scars were over 1 year old and the tape was applied for at least 1 year for 24 h/day; the exact TBSA of application was not specified in the study.

In terms of outcome measures, the Japan Scar Workshop scale was used; this is based on risk factors as well as symptoms in scars to assign a score between 0 and 25 (the higher the score the more scars are considered to be in the hypertrophic/keloid group). 20% of adults and 80% of paediatric patients improved with fludroxycortide tape from 18 to less than 2 points on the scale (almost mature scar). The non-responsive adult subgroup was started on deprodone proprionate after 12 months of the medium strength tape application, and as a result, 17 out of 24 cases improved to less than two points (70.8%). The evidence stemming from this report suggests that adult patients benefit from the stronger formulation of tape to attain a satisfactory treatment response, while the medium strength tape (fludroxycortide) appears to be sufficient for children; this finding may relate to the decreased thickness of the skin in childhood [26].

Side effects. The five most commonly reported local side effects of steroid tape include in order of mean decreasing frequency [33]:

(a) Burning/stinging sensation: 12.21%.
(b) Contact dermatitis: 11%.

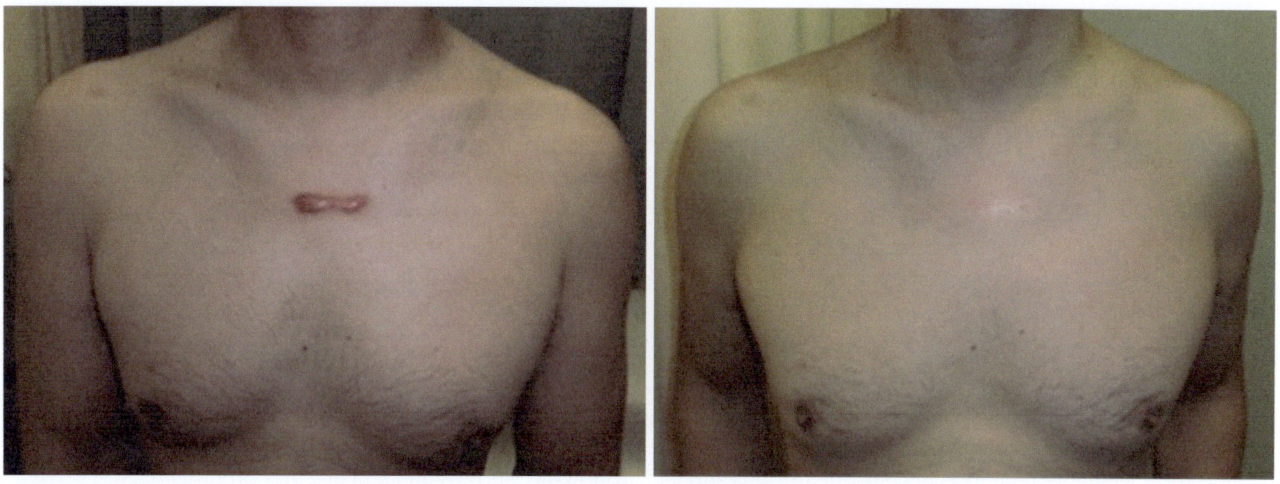

Fig. 12.2 A 45 year old male, whose presternal keloid scar was treated with tape application for 36 months

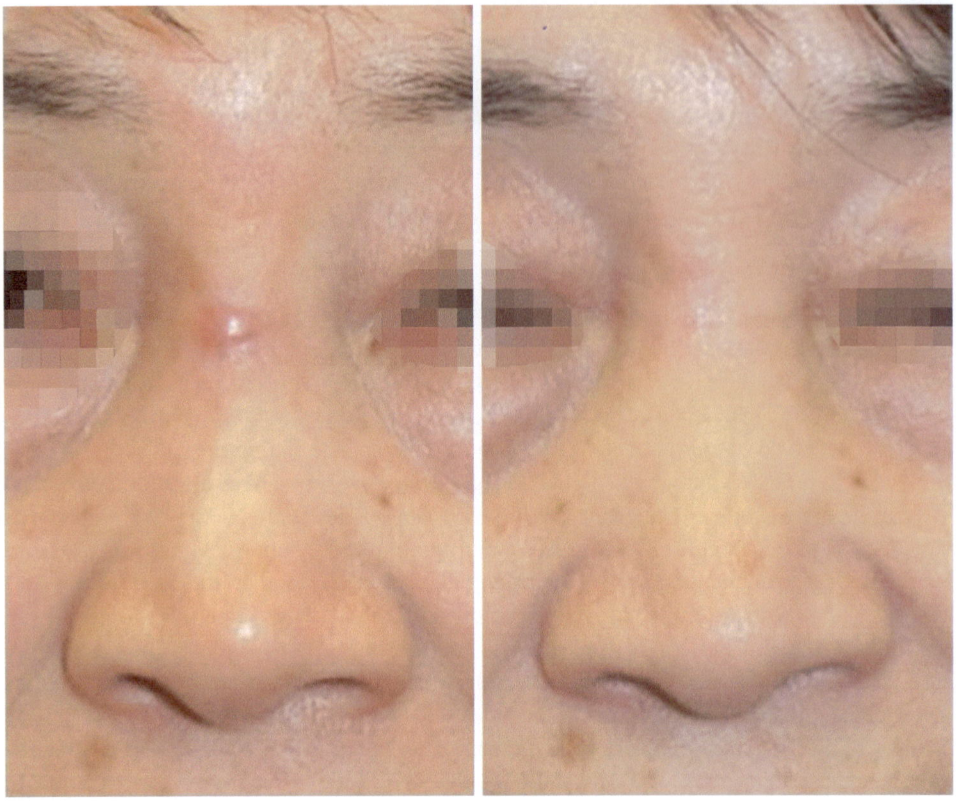

Fig. 12.3 The results of a 2-month long application on a hypertrophic scar on the nose of a 73-year old female patient

(c) Local skin irritation: 10.6%.
(d) Folliculitis: 8.79%.
(e) Erosion formation: 4.9%.

One of the questions in terms of steroid tape administration to scars relates to the maximum total body surface area and duration of use before systemic side effects may develop. A general dermatological (non-scar cohort) database search to date has revealed that there is a single level-one study in psoriasis patients, which suggests that a 2-week treatment of 24-h long application of the medium strength flurandrenolide tape (4 microgram/cm^2) is effective without any reported systemic side effects [75].

Based on available data from scar-specific studies, it appears that daily application of a medium strength tape (e.g. 4 micrograms/cm^2) to small hypertrophic and keloid scars up to 5% TBSA for at least 6–8 weeks is associated with no reported systemic side effects; most interestingly the most recent Japanese publication reported the use of fludroxycortide tape for at least 1 year in a mixed adult and paediatric cohort with no associated reports of toxicity [26].

In conclusion, the literature review reveals that following the peak of research activity in 1960s and 1970s, there is currently renewed interest for the use of steroid tape in scar management, especially in the Orient (Japan) where steroid tape represents mainstay standard of care [26]. The studies currently available comprise uncontrolled observational studies with either physician- or patient-reported outcomes and one of the limiting factors for widespread adoption of tape is the lack of absorption data for adult and paediatric patients. Nevertheless, the preliminary evidence suggests that steroid tape is a patient friendly and low-risk adjunct for scar management in appropriately selected cases of hypertrophic and keloid scars.

12.4 Evolution of the Role of Steroids in Scar Management Protocols

Steroids have been an integral part of a number of scar management protocols over the last decades; nevertheless their role has evolved with regard to whether they represent first- or second-line options and their use as either an isolated or combination modality in scar management.

In 2002, a consensus statement from the international advisory panel on scar management was published and recommended the use of intralesional steroid injections for prophylaxis against hypertrophic scar formation; these can be employed concurrently with first-line agents (hypoallergenic taping/silicone sheets) in severe cases of established linear hypertrophic scars. Regarding keloids, a combination of silicone gel sheeting and intralesional steroids was recommended; in cases of no clinical resolution, surgery with follow-up steroids and silicone was proposed [28].

In 2013, separate guidelines for Asian patients were published and these concurred on the use of steroids as a second-line therapy for hypertrophic scars, following a trial of silicone-based products. In terms of keloids, steroids were proposed as first line (either as monotherapy for symptom management or as an adjunct to surgical excision) [76].

In 2014, a protocol re-evaluation was undertaken by the advisory panel on scar management; the work reinforced the prominent position of steroids in scar management nevertheless modified various aspects of previous recommendations as described below [77, 78]:

- For severe hypertrophic scars, surgical excision with concurrent triamcinolone injection, and subsequent monthly follow-up injections was recommended. An additional proposed strategy for this subset of scars, was the combination of TAC with 5-fluorouracil (5-FU) repeated monthly.
- Regarding minor keloids, the first-line recommendation was steroids along with silicone sheets/gel and in resistant cases the combined approach with 5-FU was put forward.
- For major keloids, intralesional steroids with or without adjuvant cryotherapy were recommended as first-line and a combination of steroid and 5FU as second-line strategy.

The authors of this work emphasised the need to employ a combination of agents in order to provide maximum potential for successful scar management and proposed the additional adoption of ablating fractional laser technology in conjunction with triamcinolone as an efficient, safe and effective therapy for scar management. They also supported the use of low doses of steroids in an attempt to help minimize side effects, including atrophy, telangiectasia and hypopigmentation.

In 2014, the European consensus guidelines for keloid and hypertrophic scar management embraced the use of steroids as second line for linear scar hypertrophy (following 6 months of treatment with silicone products and compression) and recommended a dose of 40 mg/mL of TAC at 2–4 week intervals. For widespread hypertrophic scars, the use of corticosteroid injection is advised to commence earlier (6 weeks following trauma) and combined with other agents like 5-FU for refractory scars. Regarding keloids, intralesional injections of steroids have been recommended to start at 4 weeks combined with other agents like 5-FU in addition to first-line treatment (silicone and compression) [79]. It becomes clear that steroid administration holds a central position in scar management protocols internationally and the current trends focus on maximising the benefits of steroid administration and minimising side effects through a combined approach with other adjuncts including lasers and chemotherapeutic agents.

12.5 Comparative Evidence for the Use of Steroids in Scar Management

It is evident from the current state of knowledge that steroids represent a valid adjunct to scar management. It would be particularly interesting to review how steroids compare to other widely adopted modalities in the field focusing on the highest level of evidence available in the literature.

12.5.1 Steroids and Radiation

A randomised controlled trial investigated the recurrence rates following earlobe keloid ($N = 31$) excision with corticosteroid injections (1–4 postoperative injections of 0.4 mL of 40 mg/mL triamcinolone) versus radiation therapy (7–10 Gy superficial X-rays or electron beam as single fraction). At a minimum follow-up of 12 months, the recurrence following surgery and radiotherapy was 12.5% compared to 33% after surgery and steroid injections. Although a statistically significant difference was not observed in the study, radiotherapy appeared to be more effective than steroid injections in preventing keloid recurrence. Additionally, the radiotherapy cohort showed better compliance compared to the corticosteroid injection group [80].

In another randomised controlled trial involving 58 keloids and 42 hypertrophic scars, a number of treatment arms were appraised as follows:

- Beta radiation alone (16 Gy over 4 fractions) ($N = 58$).
- Intralesional triamcinolone alone administered as four injections at 1–2 week intervals (20–120 mg depending on size per course) ($N = 17$).
- Excision with pre- and postoperative radiation ($N = 15$).
- Excision with postoperative radiation only (15KS).

Comparison between the first two subgroups showed that steroids contributed to better symptomatic relief albeit in a non-statistically significant manner; the response in terms of scar thickness reduction was significantly more prominent in the steroid group [25]. The study has a number of shortcomings including the small sample size and lack of allocation blinding among others, which make valid conclusions challenging.

12.5.2 Steroids and Cryotherapy

Cryotherapy employs the use of either a spray apparatus or a probe inserted into the lesion to produce cold-induced necrosis in the scar tissue. This modality has been combined with steroid injections in a small number of studies; the rationale of this approach rests on cryotherapy producing oedema and cellular breakdown, hence facilitating the subsequent administration of steroid.

A small (n = 11) RCT with short follow-up (8 weeks) showed that cryotherapy was more effective than triamcinolone in terms of flattening 'early' vascular scars [81]. Another study concurred towards the synergistic effect of cryotherapy and 10–20 mg/mL TAC injection; nevertheless the authors reported that several injections were necessary to achieve a therapeutic effect, which becomes evident at 8 weeks following the treatment course [35].

12.5.3 Steroids and 5FU

Five-fluorouracil (5-FU) is a pyrimidine analogue, which inhibits the synthesis of deoxyribonucleic acids through the inhibition of thymidine synthase. Additionally, type I collagen gene expression and the effects of tumour growth factor beta are believed to be hindered, and as a result rapidly dividing cells are halted and scar breakdown is promoted [82].

A RCT compared weekly intralesional 50 mg/mL 5-FU to 40 mg/mL triamcinolone injections in 44 patients with keloid scars. Both regimens were found to be equally effective in reducing keloid volume but the side effects in the 5-FU group (pain and superficial ulceration) were noticeably worse [83]. Similar results were obtained in another comparative trial of weekly 50 mg/mL 5-FU injections versus 40 mg/mL TAC in 30 patients with keloids for 4 weeks. A statistically significant difference was seen in terms of flattening in favour of 5-FU (87% vs. 64%) at the expense of a higher rate of complications (however in a non-statistically significant manner) [84].

A number of studies have investigated the therapeutic benefits and side effect profile of combined steroid and 5FU administration. A trial involving 150 patients appraised the outcomes of either 0.25 mL of 40 mg/mL TAC diluted with 0.75 mL normal saline or 0.9 mL 50 mg/mL 5-FU mixed with 0.1 mL of 40 mg/mL TAC. A significant improvement was seen in the 5-FU/TAC patients compared to the TAC monotherapy (84% vs. 68%) with no reports of scar recurrence at 6 months follow-up. The rate of complications in the combination group was nevertheless higher (24% vs. 8%) [85].

In a 12-week double-blind clinical trial of 40 keloid and hypertrophic scars, patients were randomised into either receiving weekly injections of 10 mg TAC or a mixture of 4 mg TAC and 45 mg 5-FU for overall eight treatments. The reductions in length, width, height, erythema and induration were statistically significant in favour of the combination group. Both patient and trained observer assessments were higher for the TAC/5-FU group, with only the patient-reported outcomes reaching statistical significance (20% vs. 55%, p = 0.02) [86]. The superiority of the combination of 5-fluorouracil and triamcinolone in the treatment of scars has been demonstrated in further studies in terms of higher efficacy and better side effect profile, namely erythema and inflammatory changes (92% average reduction in lesion size with combination compared to 73% with steroid monotherapy) in a number of other studies [82, 87].

12.5.4 Steroids and Laser

A prospective RCT compared the following treatments for median sternotomy hypertrophic and keloid scars:

- Pulse dye laser (585 nm 5 J/cm^2).
- Intralesional triamcinolone (20 mg/mL every 4 weeks for 6 treatments), intralesional 5-FU (50 mg/mL for ten treatments).
- Mixture (1 mg/mL triamcinolone mixed with 45 mg/mL 5-FU for 10 treatments).

As part of the study, one segment of the scar received no treatment to serve as control. There was a statistically significant clinical improvement in all treated segments but no significant differences in outcome (scar height/erythema) were noted with regard to a particular modality [88]. Adverse effects (hypopigmentation, telangiectasias and skin atrophy) were observed in 50% of the segments treated with steroid injections alone. Limitations of the study included small sample size, limited follow-up of 32 weeks, no report of randomization technique or on whether outcome assessments were blinded.

In a 12-week single-blinded trial, 69 patients (keloid and hypertrophic scars) were randomly assigned into three study groups:

(a) Group 1 (10 mg/mL TAC at weekly intervals for 8 weeks).
(b) Group 2 (0.1 mL TAC and 0.9 mL 50 mg/mL 5-FU at weekly intervals for 8 weeks).
(c) Group 3 (as group 2 and 585 nm pulsed dye laser: 5–7 J/cm^2 at the 1st, 4th and 8th weeks).

At the end of the study (12 weeks), improvement in groups 2 and 3 was found to be statistically significant by blinded observers in contrast to group 1 (40% and 70% vs. 25%, respectively). Both patient and blinded observer reports for good to excellent improvements (>50% improvement) were in favour of group 2 and 3 in a statistically significant manner, suggesting a promising effect of laser in this mixed scar (hypertrophic and keloid) cohort [89].

Another literature report compared scars treated with pulsed dye laser with and without intralesional steroid in a total of 22 female patients with bilateral hypertrophic breast reduction scars (mean scar duration of 18.5 months, range:

4–72). Patients had one inframammary scar treated with laser alone, while the contralateral was additionally treated with corticosteroids (10–20 mg) at 6-weekly treatment intervals for two sessions only. Assessments were carried out before and 6 weeks after their second and final treatment by two blinded independent assessors as well as a blinded dermatopathologist. Results suggested that the treatment of scars with lasers produced significant clinical and histological improvement in all operations, whereas the use of corticosteroids did not significantly improve the clinical outcomes apart from decreasing itch in symptomatic scars. These results might reflect the low dose of steroids used in the study [90].

Numerous strategies have been adopted to enhance topical delivery of steroids into the fibrotic scar tissue including laser assisted delivery (L.A.D.) techniques, which take advantage of the temporary barrier impairment induced by the various ablative and non-ablative fractional photothermolytic modalities. One prospective case series involving 15 patients with hypertrophic scars employed the combined use of an ablative fractional laser and subsequent topical application of the triamcinolone (10–20 mg/mL) in the same treatment session. Results indicated that after 3–5 treatment sessions at 2–3 month intervals, there was an overall improvement in scar parameters, with texture showing the most significant level of improvement and dyschromia the least amount of change [91].

Martin et al. combined carbon dioxide fractional laser (10,600 nm), a pulsed dye laser (585 nm) with triamcinolone (40 mg/mL) injections monthly for seven sessions for the treatment of keloid scars reporting good results with minimal flatness, diminished pruritus and lighter pigmentation nevertheless minimal effect on size [92]. Son et al. showed that 42% of patients reported more than 75% improvement after treatment of keloid and hypertrophic scars with a 578 nm copper bromide laser combined with intralesional (10 mg/mL triamcinolone) at 4-week intervals steroid injections [93]. Parameters included erythema, pruritus and telangiectasia. It is clear that the laser-assisted delivery of steroid for scar lesions is a promising modality nevertheless needs further evaluation.

12.6 Conclusion

Steroid administration has remained a mainstay modality for the management of hypertrophic and steroid scars over the last number of decades. The most popular modality internationally is the intralesional injection of scars followed by the transdermal (tape) as well as the laser-assisted modalities, which are gaining momentum. Further high quality comparative studies are needed to delineate the exact value of different steroid preparations as standalone and combination strategies in scar management protocols.

Acknowledgements I would like to acknowledge Dr. Osaid Alser and Miss Ruthann Fanstone for their helpful contributions and input into this piece of work.

References

1. Behrman HT, Goodman JJ. Skin complications of cortisone and ACTH therapy. JAMA. 1950;144(3):218–21.
2. Baker BL, Whitaker WL. Interference with wound healing by the local action of adrenocortical steroids. Endocrinology. 1950;46(6):544–51.
3. Polson JS, et al. Keloid. Can Med Assoc J. 1951;65(5):447–9.
4. Conway H, Stark RB. ACTH in plastic surgery. Plast Reconstr Surg (1946). 1951;8(5):354–77.
5. Goldman L, Thompson RG, Trice ER. Cortisone acetate in skin disease; local effect in the skin from topical application and local injection. AMA Arch Derm Syphilol. 1952;65(2):177–86.
6. Coste F, Piguet B, Civitte J, Degos R, Vial-Weissenbach V, Grupper C. Traitement de Chelloides par Injections Locales d'Hydrocortisone. Trans Soc Franc de Derm et de Syph Presse med. 1953;61:1157.
7. De Kleine EH. Observations on the effect of cortisone on wound healing and scar formation. Plast Reconstr Surg. 1954;88:429.
8. Hollander A. Intralesional injections of triamcinolone acetonide; a therapy for dermatoses. Antibiotic Med Clin Ther (New York). 1961;8:78–83.
9. Murray RD. Kenalog and the treatment of hypertrophied scars and keloids in Negroes and whites. Plast Reconstr Surg. 1963;31:275–80.
10. Maguire HC Jr. Treatment of keloids with triamcinolone acetonide injected intralesionally. JAMA. 1965;192:325–6.
11. Griffith BH. The treatment of keloids with triamcinolone acetonide. Plast Reconstr Surg. 1966;38(3):202–8.
12. Minkowitz F. Regression of massive keloid following partial excision and post-operative intralesional administration of triamcinolone. Br J Plast Surg. 1967;20(4):432–5.
13. Jalali M, Bayat A. Current use of steroids in management of abnormal raised skin scars. Surgeon. 2007;5(3):175–80.
14. McMaster A, Ray DW. Drug insight: selective agonists and antagonists of the glucocorticoid receptor. Nat Clin Pract Endocrinol Metab. 2008;4(2):91–101.
15. Kang N, Sivakumar B, Sanders R, Nduka C, Gault D. Intralesional injections of collagenase are ineffective in the treatment of keloid and hypertrophic scars. J Plast Reconstr Aesthet Surg. 2006;59(7):693–9.
16. McCoy BJ, Diegelmann RF, Cohen IK. In vitro inhibition of cell growth, collagen synthesis, and prolyl hydroxylase activity by triamcinolone acetonide. Proc Soc Exp Biol Med. 1980;163(2):216–22.
17. Ogawa R. Keloid and hypertrophic scars are the result of chronic inflammation in the reticular dermis. Int J Mol Sci. 2017;18(3):E606.
18. Lawrence WT. In search of the optimal treatment of keloids: report of a series and a review of the literature. Ann Plast Surg. 1991;27(2):164–78.
19. Doggrell SA. Triamcinolone: new and old indications. Expert Opin Pharmacother. 2001;2(7):1177–86.
20. Lucky AW. Principles of the use of glucocorticosteroids in the growing child. Pediatr Dermatol. 1984;1:226–35.
21. Grumbine N, Dobrowolski C, Bernstein A. Retrospective evaluation of postoperative intralesional steroid injections on wound healing. J Foot Ankle Surg. 1998;37(2):135–44. discussion 74.
22. Brissett AE, Sherris DA. Scar contractures, hypertrophic scars, and keloids. Facial Plast Surg. 2001;17(4):263–72.

23. Kill J. Kleoids treated with topical injections of triamcinolone acetonide (Kenalog). Scand J Plast Reconsrt Surg. 1977;11:169–72.
24. Fredman R, Tenenhaus M. Cushing's syndrome after intralesional triamcinolone acetonide: a systematic review of the literature and multinational survey. Burns. 2013;39(4):549–57.
25. Darzi MA, Chowdri NA, Kaul SK, Khan M. Evaluation of various methods of treating keloids and hypertrophic scars: a 10-year follow-up study. Br J Plast Surg. 1992;45(5):374–9.
26. Ogawa R, Akaishi S, Kuribayashi S, Miyashita T. Keloids and hypertrophic scars can now be cured completely: recent progress in our understanding of the pathogenesis of keloids and hypertrophic scars and the most promising current therapeutic strategy. J Nippon Med Sch. 2016;83(2):46–53.
27. Mustoe TA, Cooter RD, Gold MH, Hobbs FD, Ramelet AA, Shakespeare PG, et al. International clinical recommendations on scar management. Plast Reconstr Surg. 2002;110(2):560–71.
28. Ardehali B, Nouraei SA, Van Dam H, Dex E, Wood S, Nduka C. Objective assessment of keloid scars with three-dimensional imaging: quantifying response to intralesional steroid therapy. Plast Reconstr Surg. 2007;119(2):556–61.
29. Kelly AP. Update on the management of keloids. Semin Cutan Med Surg. 2009;28(2):71–6.
30. Rutkowski D, Syed F, Matthews LC, Ray DW, McGrouther DA, Watson RE, et al. An abnormality in glucocorticoid receptor expression differentiates steroid responders from nonresponders in keloid disease. Br J Dermatol. 2015;173(3):690–700.
31. Gupta S, Sharma VK. Standard guidelines of care: keloids and hypertrophic scars. Indian J Dermatol Venereol Leprol. 2011;77(1):94–100.
32. Mandal A, Imran D. Painless steroid injections for hypertrophic scars and keloids. Br J Plast Surg. 2003;56(1):79.
33. Vallis CP. Intralesional injection of keloids and hypertrophic scars with the Dermo-Jet. Plast Reconstr Surg. 1967;40(3):255–62.
34. Ono N. Pain-free intralesional injection of triamcinolone for the treatment of keloid. Scand J Plast Reconstr Surg Hand Surg. 1999;33(1):89–91.
35. Ceilley RI, Babin RW. The combined use of cryosurgery and intralesional injections of suspensions of fluorinated adrenocorticosteroids for reducing keloids and hypertrophic scars. J Dermatol Surg Oncol. 1979;5(1):54–6.
36. Zuber TJ, DeWitt DE. Earlobe keloids. Am Fam Physician. 1994;49(8):1835–41.
37. Muneuchi G, Suzuki S, Onodera M, Ito O, Hata Y, Igawa HH. Long-term outcome of intralesional injection of triamcinolone acetonide for the treatment of keloid scars in Asian patients. Scand J Plast Reconstr Surg Hand Surg. 2006;40(2):111–6.
38. Boyadjiev C, Popchristova E, Mazgalova J. Histomorphologic changes in keloids treated with Kenacort. J Trauma. 1995;38(2):299–302.
39. Brown LA Jr, Pierce HE. Keloids: scar revision. J Dermatol Surg Oncol. 1986;12(1):51–6.
40. Barton RP. Auricular keloids: a simple method of management. Ann R Coll Surg Engl. 1978;60(4):324–5.
41. Donkor P. Head and neck keloid: treatment by core excision and delayed intralesional injection of steroid. J Oral Maxillofac Surg. 2007;65(7):1292–6.
42. Tang YW. Intra- and postoperative steroid injections for keloids and hypertrophic scars. Br J Plast Surg. 1992;45(5):371–3.
43. Golladay ES. Treatment of keloids by single intraoperative perilesional injection of repository steroid. South Med J. 1988;81(6):736–8.
44. Tripoli M, Cordova A, Melloni C, Zabbia G, Maggì F, Moschella F. The use of triamcinolone combined with surgery in major ear keloid treatment: a personal two stages approach. Eur J Plast Surg. 2015;38(3):205–10.
45. Chowdri NA, Masarat M, Mattoo A, Darzi MA. Keloids and hypertrophic scars: results with intraoperative and serial postoperative corticosteroid injection therapy. Aust N Z J Surg. 1999;69(9):655–9.
46. Park TH, Seo SW, Kim JK, Chang CH. Clinical characteristics of facial keloids treated with surgical excision followed by intra- and postoperative intralesional steroid injections. Aesthetic Plast Surg. 2012;36(1):169–73.
47. Rosen DJ, Patel MK, Freeman K, Weiss PR. A primary protocol for the management of ear keloids: results of excision combined with intraoperative and postoperative steroid injections. Plast Reconstr Surg. 2007;120(5):1395–400.
48. Moustafa MFH, Abdel-Fattah AMA. Keloids of the ear lobes in Egypt: their rarity in childhood and their treatment. Br J Plast Surg. 1976;29:59.
49. Kauh YC, Rouda S, Mondragon G, Tokarek R, di Leonardo M, Tuan RS, et al. Major suppression of pro-alpha1(I) type I collagen gene expression in the dermis after keloid excision and immediate intrawound injection of triamcinolone acetonide. J Am Acad Dermatol. 1997;37(4):586–9.
50. Sproat JE, Dalcin A, Weitauer N, Roberts RS. Hypertrophic sternal scars: silicone gel sheet versus Kenalog injection treatment. Plast Reconstr Surg. 1992;90(6):988–92.
51. Al-Attar A, Mess S, Thomassen JM, Kauffman CL, Davison SP. Keloid pathogenesis and treatment. Plast Reconstr Surg. 2006;117(1):286–300.
52. Murray JC. Scars and keloids. Dermatol Clin. 1993;11(4):697–708.
53. Ledon JA, Savas J, Franca K, Chacon A, Nouri K. Intralesional treatment for keloids and hypertrophic scars: a review. Dermatol Surg. 2013;39(12):1745–57.
54. Shaffer JJ, Taylor SC, Cook-Bolden F. Keloidal scars: a review with a critical look at therapeutic options. J Am Acad Dermatol. 2002;46(2 Suppl Understanding):S63–97.
55. Jemec GB. Linear atrophy following intralesional steroid injections. J Dermatol Surg Oncol. 1988;14(1):88–9.
56. Mollmann H, Rohdewald P, Schmidt EW, Salomon V, Derendorf H. Pharmacokinetics of triamcinolone acetonide and its phosphate ester. Eur J Clin Pharmacol. 1985;29:85–9.
57. Meikle AW, Clarke DH, Tyler FH. Cushing syndrome form low doses of dexamethasone a result of slow plasma clearance. JAMA. 1976;235:1592–3.
58. Ross EJ, Linch DC. Cushing's syndrome—killing disease: discriminatory value of signs and symptoms aiding early diagnosis. Lancet (London, England). 1982;2(8299):646–9.
59. Marsden CW. Fluocinolone acetonide 0.25 cream-a co-operative clinical trial. Br J Dermatol. 1968;80:614–7.
60. Yi NW, Frame JD. Evaluation of cynthaskin and topical steroid in the treatment of hypertrophic scars and keloids. Eur J Plast Surg. 1996;19:162–5.
61. Hayashi T, Furukawa H, Oyama A, Funayama E, Saito A, Murao N, Yamamoto Y. A new uniform protocol of combined corticosteroid injections and ointment application reduces recurrence rates after surgical keloid/hypertrophic scar excision. Dermatol Surg. 2012;38:893–7.
62. Goldman L, Igelman JM, Kitzmiller KW. Clinical investigative studies with flurandrenolone tape. Cutis. 1967;3:367–71.
63. Rauscher GE, Kolmer WL. Treatment of recurrent earlobe keloids. Cutis. 1986;37:67–8.
64. Tillman WJ, Higuchi T. Quantitative evaluation of the interaction of callus strips with some hydroxylic solvents. J Invest Dermatol. 1961;27:87.
65. Frank L, Rapp Y. Occlusive topical corticosteroids and heat in psoriasis. Arch Dermatol. 1963;87:32.
66. Riley K. Flurandrenolone (Cordran) tape as occlusive therapy. JSC Med Assoc. 1969;65:171–2.
67. Fisher LB, Maibach HI, Trancik RJ. Effects of occlusive tape systems on the mitotic activity of epidermis with and without corticosteroids. Arch Dermatol. 1978;114:384–6.
68. Widgerow AD, Chait LA, Stals R, et al. New innovations in scar management. Aesthetic Plast Surg. 2000;24:227–34.

69. Goutos I, Ogawa R. Steroid tape: a promising adjunct to scar management. Scars, Burn Heal. 2017;3:2059513117690937.
70. Huang C, Akaishi S, Hyakusoku H, Ogawa R. Are keloid and hypertrophic scar different forms of the same disorder? A fibroproliferative skin disorder hypothesis based on keloid findings. Int Wound J. 2014;11(5):517–22.
71. Huang C, Murphy GF, Akaishi S, Ogawa R. Keloids and hypertrophic scars: update and future directions. Plast Reconstr Surg Glob Open. 2013;1(4):e25.
72. Goldblatt S. The use of Cordran tape in dermatology. Ohio State Med J. 1969;65(11):1118–21.
73. Ratzer MA. A clinical trial of flurandrenolone tape. Br J Clin Pract. 1970;24:185–9.
74. DP Study Group. Analysis of clinical outcomes of deprodone propionate plaster for various skin diseases. Rinsholyaku. 1989;5:2177–85. (in Japanese).
75. Labow TA, Eisert J, Sanders SL. Flurandrenolide tape in the treatment of psoriasis. NY State J Med. 1969;69:3138–40.
76. Kim S, Choi TH, Liu W, Ogawa R, Suh JS, Mustoe TA. Update on scar management: guidelines for treating Asian patients. Plast Reconstr Surg. 2013;132:1580.
77. Gold MH, Berman B, Clementoni MT, Gauglitz GG, Nahai F, Murcia C. Updated international clinical recommendations on scar management: part 1—evaluating the evidence. Dermatol Surg. 2014;40(8):817–24.
78. Gold MH, McGuire M, Mustoe TA, Pusic A, Sachdev M, Waibel J, et al. Updated international clinical recommendations on scar management: part 2—algorithms for scar prevention and treatment. Dermatol Surg. 2014;40(8):825–31.
79. Meaume S, Le Pillouer-Prost A, Richert B, Roseeuw D, Vadoud J. Management of scars: updated practical guidelines and use of silicones. Eur J Dermatol. 2014;24(4):435–43.
80. Sclafani AP, Gordon L, Chadha M, Romo T 3rd. Prevention of earlobe keloid recurrence with postoperative corticosteroid injections versus radiation therapy: a randomized, prospective study and review of the literature. Dermatol Surg. 1996;22(6):569–74.
81. Layton AM, Yip J, Cunliffe WJ. A comparison of intralesional triamcinolone and cryosurgery in the treatment of acne keloids. Br J Dermatol. 1994;130:498–501.
82. Shah VV, Aldahan AS, Mlacker S, Alsaidan M, Samarkendy S, Nouri K. 5_Fluorouracil in the treatment of keloids and hypertrophic scars: a comprehensive review of the literature. Dermatol Ther. 2016;6:169–83.
83. Saha AK, Mukhopadhyay M. A comparative clinical study on role of 5-fluorouracil versus triamcinolone in the treatment of keloids. Indian J Surg. 2012;74(4):326–9.
84. Prabhu A, et al. A randomized controlled trial comparing the efficacy of intralesional 5-fluorouracil versus triamcinolone acetonide in the treatment of keloids. J Sci Soc. 2012;39(1):19.
85. Khan MA, Bashir MM, Khan FA. Intralesional triamcinolone alone and in combination with 5-fluorouracil for the treatment of keloid and hypertrophic scars. J Pak Med Assoc. 2014;64(9):1003–7.
86. Darougheh A, Asilian A, Shariati F. Intralesional triamcinolone alone or in combination with 5-fluorouracil for the treatment of keloid and hypertrophic scars. Clin Exp Dermatol. 2009;34(2):219–23.
87. Davison SP, Dayan JH, Clemens MW, Sonni S, Wang A, Crane A. Efficacy of intralesional 5-fluorouracil and triamcinolone in the treatment of keloids. Aesthet Surg J. 2009;29:40–6.
88. Manuskiatti W, Fitzpatrick RE. Treatment response of keloidal and hypertrophic sternotomy scars: comparison among intralesional corticosteroid, 5-fluorouracil, and 585 nm flashlamp-pumped pulsed-dye laser treatments. Arch Dermatol. 2002;138:1149–55.
89. Asilian A, Darougheh A, Shariati F. New combination of triamcinolone, 5-Fluorouracil, and pulsed-dye laser for treatment of keloid and hypertrophic scars. Dermatol Surg. 2006;32(7):907–15.
90. Alster T. Laser scar revision: comparison study of 585-nm pulsed dye laser with and without intralesional corticosteroids. Dermatol Surg. 2003;29:25–9.
91. Waibel JS, Wulkan AJ, Shumaker PR. Treatment of hypertrophic scars using laser and laser assisted corticosteroid delivery. Lasers Surg Med. 2013;45(3):135–40.
92. Martin MS, Collawn SS. Combination treatment of CO2 fractional laser, pulse dye laser and triamcinolone acetonide injection for refractory keloid scars on the upper back. J Cosmet Laser Ther. 2013;15(3):166–70.
93. Son IP, Park KY, Kim B, et al. Pilot study of the efficacy of 578 nm copper bromide corporate laser combined with intralesional corticosteroid injection for treatment of keloids and hypertrophic scars. Ann Dermatol. 2014;26:156–61.

Intralesional Cryosurgery for the Treatment of Hypertrophic Scars and Keloids

13

Yaron Har-Shai and Lior Har-Shai

13.1 Background

Cryosurgery is an effective and safe therapeutic regimen in the treatment of hypertrophic scars and keloids [1]. Because of its major advantage of a low relapse rate, the technique, either as monotherapy or in combination, has been established as the treatment of choice for keloids and hypertrophic scars.

Zouboulis and Orfanos [2], Zouboulis et al. [3, 4], and Zouboulis and Orfanos (1999, [5]) have shown that repeated contact cryosurgical sessions can exhibit a beneficial effect on keloids and hypertrophic scars and additionally prevent relapses. However, 1–20 treatment sessions were required to achieve these results using the contact cryosurgery method. Thus, the need for new, more potent, and quickly effective cryosurgical methods and instrumentation has been recognized.

13.2 Intralesional Cryosurgery

Intralesional cryosurgery using cryoneedles was initially described by Weshahy [6] for the treatment of epidermal and dermal skin lesions. A first intralesional cryosurgery method for the treatment of keloids was introduced by Zouboulis [7] (also in Zouboulis and Orfanos [5], Zouboulis et al. [8], and Gupta and Kumar [9]) and was improved and further developed by Har-Shai et al. [10–12]. This technique exhibits an increased efficacy in the treatment of hypertrophic scars and keloids when compared with the contact method, due to the enhanced freezing area of deeply located scar tissue. In addition, fewer cryosurgical sessions are required and less hypopigmentation is evident following the application of intralesional cryosurgery.

13.3 Intralesional Cryoneedle

Weshahy [6] was the first to describe a cryoneedle probe which consisted of a curved hypodermal needle with an open tip which was inserted underneath the skin lesion/tumor. Zouboulis et al. [5, 8] further developed this method by freezing hypertrophic scars and keloids using a hypodermal needle (long G20). Later, Gupta and Kumar [9] have published their experience with intralesional approach by employing simultaneously several hypodermal needles (G21) to treat hypertrophic scars and keloids. The results which have been obtained using these open-ended and thin hypodermal cryoneedles demonstrated suboptimal results which necessitated up to 10 cryosurgical sessions for scar flattening. In 2003, Har-Shai et al. have refined the technique by developing a novel intralesional cryoneedle (CryoShape, FDA and CE approved, Etgar Group International Ltd., Rannana) (Fig. 13.1). This probe consists of an elongated double-lumen un-insulated needle with a safety vent and a sharp-cutting, sealed, distal tip which enhances the penetration of the often hard, rubbery, and dense hypertrophic scars and keloids. The proximal end of the cryoprobe is connected via an elongation tube to a cryogen source. By forcing liquid nitrogen to circulate through the needle, an

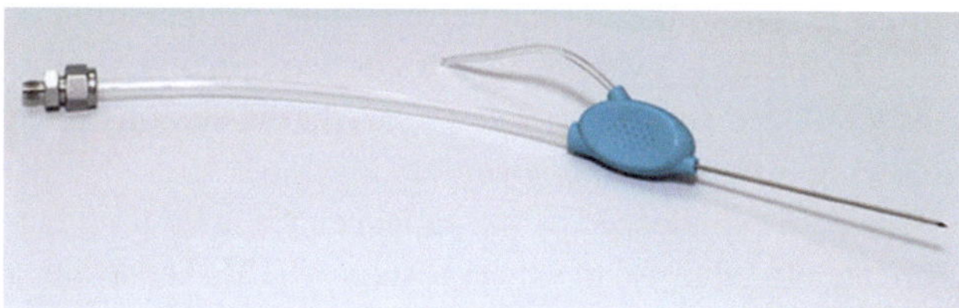

Fig. 13.1 The CryoShape cryoprobe

Y. Har-Shai (✉) · L. Har-Shai
The Unit of Plastic Surgery, Carmel Medical Center, The Bruce Rappaport Faculty of Medicine, Technion Israel of Technology, Haifa, Israel

The Department of Plastic and Reconstructive Surgery, Rabin Medical Center, Petach Tikva, Israel

© Springer Nature Singapore Pte Ltd. 2020
R. Ogawa (ed.), *Total Scar Management*, https://doi.org/10.1007/978-981-32-9791-3_13

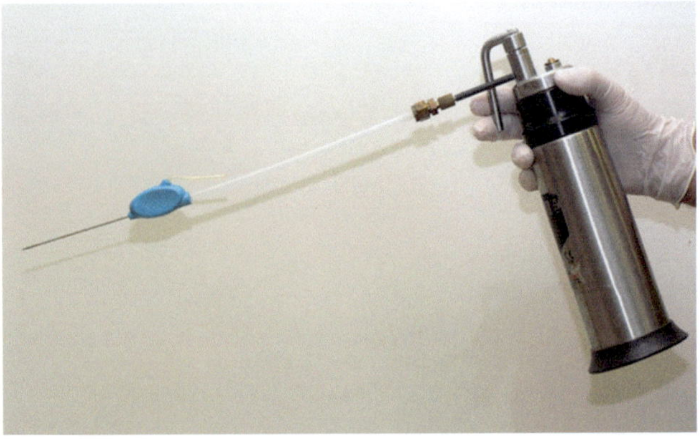

Fig. 13.2 The intralesional cryosurgery system composed of the CryoShape cryoprobe which is connected to the cryogen

ice ball around the cryoneedle developed causing the abutted scar tissue to be completely frozen while the generated gas is dispersed to the atmosphere away from the patient via a safety vent (Fig. 13.2).

13.4 Experimental Studies

Experimental studies conducted by Har-Shai et al. [11] have demonstrated that the intralesional cryoprobe showed a slower cooling rate (20 °C/min) with an end temperature of −30 °C. However, the thawing rate was faster (35 °C/min). The hold time, i.e., the time in which the freezing process retained its lowest temperature, was found to be significantly long (minutes to hours). In addition, the skin surface of the keloids treated by the intralesional method did not exhibit marked hypopigmentation. It has been assumed that the end temperature during intralesional cryosurgery and the moderate cooling and thawing rates, which are measured on the keloid skin surface, are more "friendly" for melanocyte survival. Thus, intralesional cryosurgery destroys the core of the keloid, while at the surface, cells including melanocytes are much less affected and therefore less hypopigmentation is evident (Fig. 13.3).

Har-Shai et al. [10, 11] have studied the histomorphometrical changes occurring in the scar tissue following intralesional cryosurgery. It has been demonstrated that following intralesional cryosurgery, the architectural pattern of the collagen is more organized, i.e., the parallel organization of the collagen fibers in the treated scar is similar to that in the normal dermis; thus, rejuvenation of the scar tissue is evident, which can explain the significantly reduced recurrence rate (<3%) that is demonstrated following intralesional cryosurgery.

The pain experienced by the patient can be a limiting factor in the effective use of skin cryosurgery [13]. Therefore, a pain control protocol has been developed which has showed an effective reduction in pain and discomfort during and following the procedure [14, 15]. It accounts of taking a pain reliever tablet 1 h prior to cryotreatment. Thereafter, a translesional approach for local anesthesia with ½% bupivacaine, in which a 23G hypodermal needle is inserted perpendicular and through the entire thickness of the scar tissue in order to infiltrate the subcutaneous fat tissue beneath the scar, is executed (Fig. 13.4).This method enables to infiltrate easily into the loose subcutaneous fatty tissue, thus causing a significant reduction in pain when compared with the intralesional anesthesia which generates increased pain due to the limited availability of the often dense and hard scar tissue to expand. The level of pain reported by the patients using this regimen had been reduced significantly, i.e., ≤3 in the VAS scale.

13.5 Technical Approach

With the patient lying at a supine position, the skin surface of the scar is cleansed with disinfecting solution and draped. The area of penetration into the scar and the underlying subcutaneous tissue is anesthetized locally, by a translesional approach, with bupivacaine hydrochloride ½% (Marcaine) (Fig. 13.3a). Thereafter, the sterile cryoprobe is forced into the long axis of the scar in a forward rotary movement, which is parallel to the skin surface. The cryoneedle is inserted into the core of the scar, which is approximately the mid height of the scar. The scar itself is grasped between the index and thumb of the other hand, until the sharp tip of the needle penetrated the opposite distal edge of the scar, thus maximizing the volume of scar tissue to be frozen. Attention is taken to prevent any penetration of the cryoneedle into uninvolved healthy surrounding skin. Sterile gauzes are placed under the proximal and distal parts of the cryoprobe and care is taken to assure that the vent nostril is positioned away from the patient to prevent accidental freezing of adjacent skin or tissue (Fig. 13.3a).

The proximal part of the probe is connected via an elongation tube to the cryogun (CryoPro Maxi 500cc, Cortex Technology, Hadsund, Denmark), which is filled with liquid nitrogen to 3/4 of the cryogen volume and about 30 min beforehand in order to allow a sufficient pressure to build-up inside it [about 0.7 atm (10 psi)]. It is advisable to label on the cryogen the filling time with liquid nitrogen in order to make sure that 30 min have elapsed prior to the cryotreatment and prevent confusion and possible malfunction. A full pressurized cryogen can operate continuously for 1 h, thus 2–3 medium-size keloids can be treated without the need to refill.

The cryogun is grasped or placed on a steady surface which is located higher than the scar to facilitate the liquid nitrogen flow with no direct contact with the patient body. By activating the cryogun trigger, the pressure valve is opened and the cryogen enters the cryoneedle, thereby freezing the

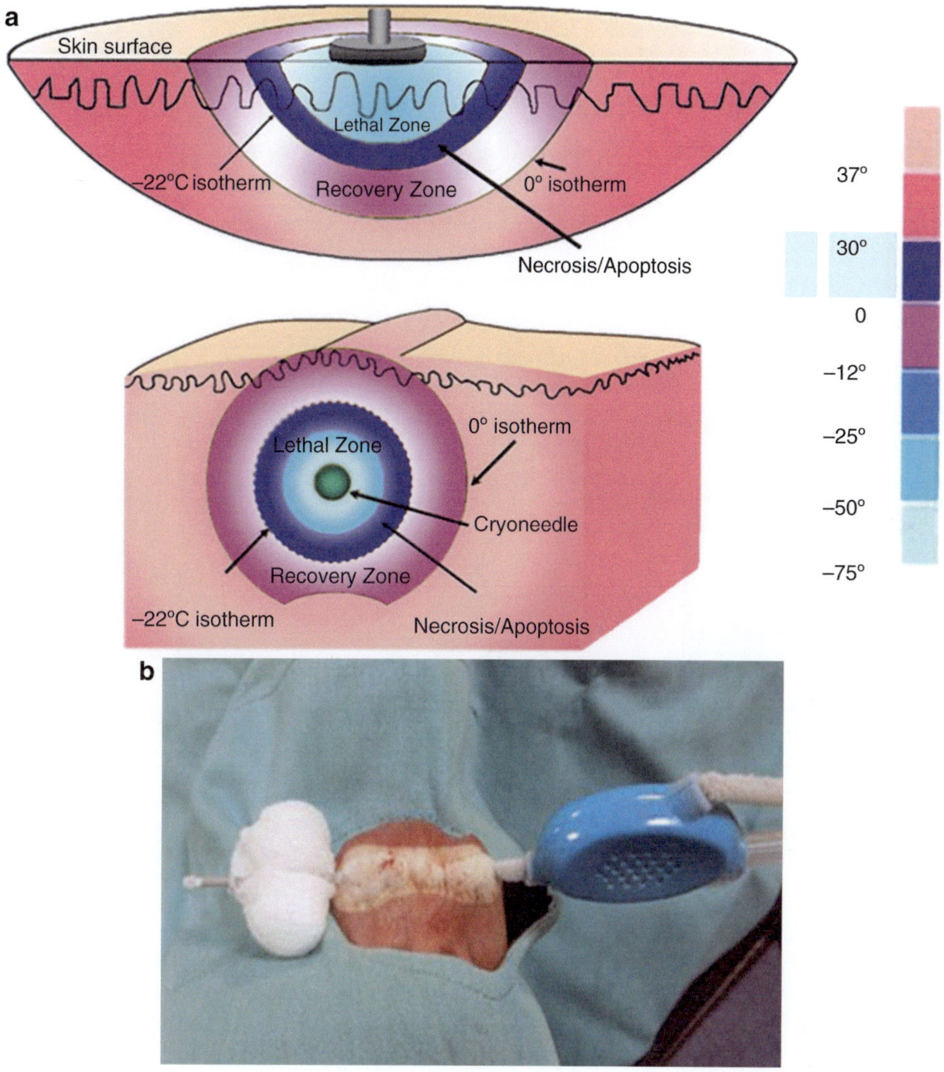

Fig. 13.3 Upper: Ice ball induced by the contact cryoprobe. The interface between the ice ball and unfrozen tissue represents the 0 °C isotherm. The volume of tissue located between the −22 °C isotherm and contact probe is the lethal zone in which cells undergo cryonecrosis. Cells situated in the warmer region between −22 °C isotherm and the 0 °C isotherm (recovery zone) generally survive the freeze. The melanocytes are located within the lethal zone. Bottom: Ice ball induced by the intralesional cryoneedle. The interface between the ice ball and unfrozen tissue represents the 0 °C isotherm. The volume of tissue located between the −22 °C isotherm and contact probe is the lethal zone in which cells undergo cryonecrosis. Cells situated in the warmer region between −22 °C isotherm and the 0 °C isotherm (recovery zone) generally survive the freeze. The melanocytes are located within the recovery zone. (**a**) Intraoperative view of the intralesional cryosurgery technique employing the cryoneedle for the treatment of a keloid. The exposed parts of the cryoneedle are protected by sterile gauzes to prevent possible cryoinjury to the surrounding skin

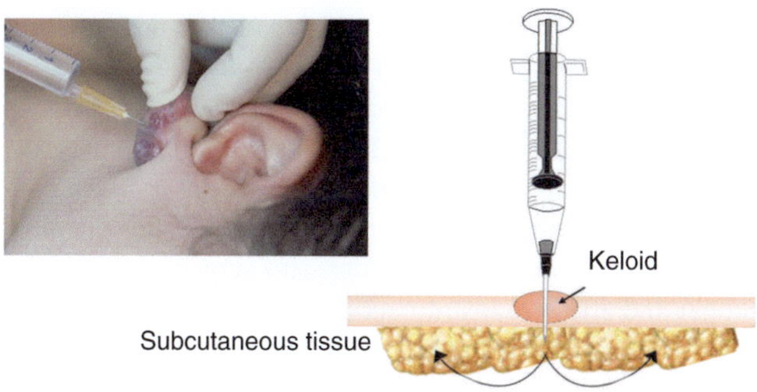

Fig. 13.4 A schematic diagram and a clinical photo demonstrating the translesional technique to achieve local anesthesia prior to inserting the cryoneedle probe into the scar

scar. A forced steam of the liquid nitrogen gas flows out from the vent nostril during the entire freezing process. The strength of the steam flow, which is observed by the naked eye during the entire freezing procedure, indicated an appropriate working pressure. Two ice balls appear shortly at the two cryoprobe penetration sites and with time they gradually spread towards each other until a complete freezing of the scar is achieved clinically. Following the complete freezing of the scar which is evident clinically, regardless of the duration of the cryosurgery process (without the necessity of time taking), the cryogun trigger is released to stop the freezing process and the cryoneedle is left to thaw for 1–2 min and is then withdrawn in a reverse rotary movement. The length of the intralesional cryosurgery process depends upon the scar volume and ranges between 5 min and two and a half hours (Fig. 13.5). After a complete thawing of the scar is clinically noticed, slight bleeding from the penetration points of the needle requires the application of a sterile dressing. The patients were instructed to wash daily the treated scar and to apply an antibiotic ointment until full healing was accomplished.

In cases where the scar was longer than the cryoneedle length or very wide, two or three parallel needles or

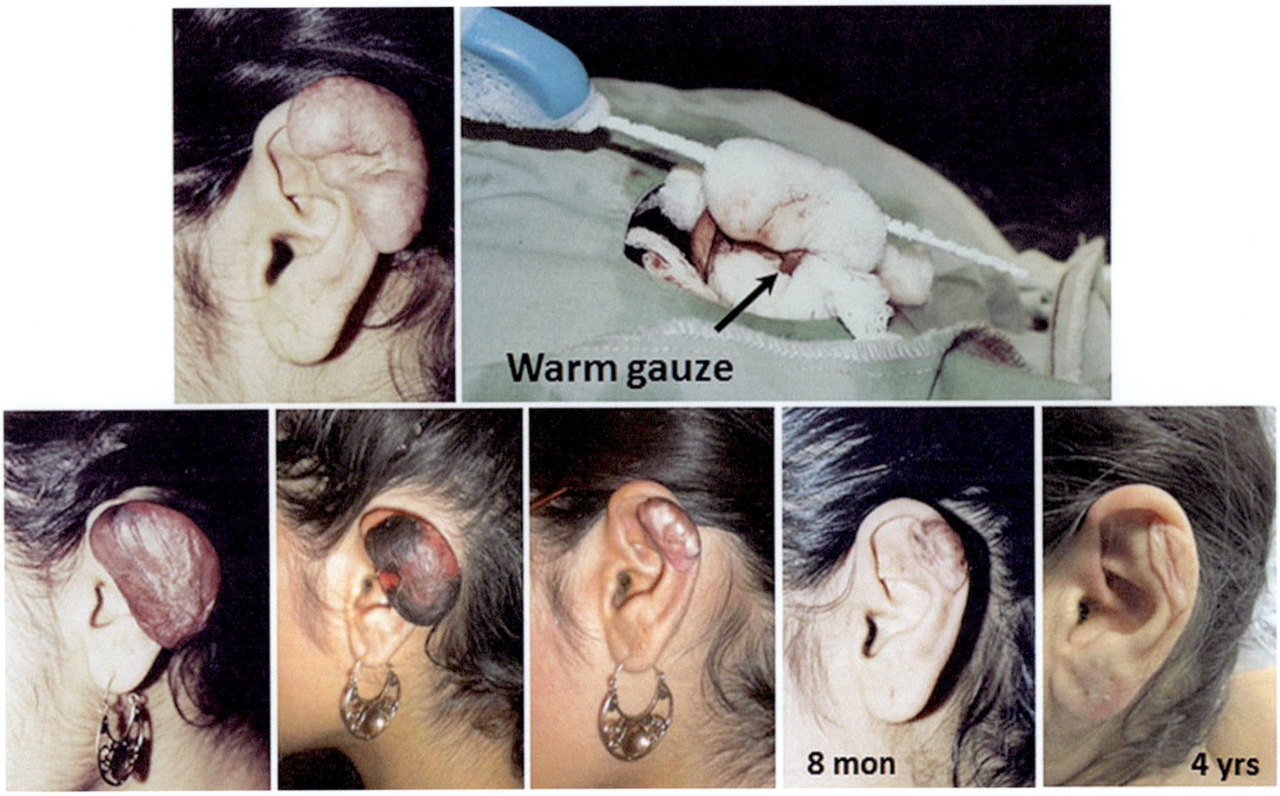

Fig. 13.5 Sequential steps of the intralesional cryosurgery procedure and final result. Upper Left: Preoperative view of a large keloid of the left upper helix following piercing. Upper Right: Following penetration of the cryoneedle into the keloid, two ice balls are formed at the two penetration points of the scar. Warm gauzes are placed opposite to the treated scar (posterior aspect of the auricle) in order to prevent cryoinjury to the auricular cartilage. Lower Left to Lower Right: One week following the cryotreatment, a blister is evident. Three weeks following treatment, scar necrosis is evident. Six months following the treatment, the helical keloid has reduced significantly without distortion of the lobule and with almost no hypopigmentation. Four years following a single cryosession, the scars are flat with some extra pliable skin above them, which can be excised via an intralesional approach. No recurrence is evident

successive insertions of the same needle were necessary to freeze the entire keloid in one session (Fig. 13.5).

Recently, a new combined method to treat oversized and therapy-resistant keloids has been published which consists of intralesional excision and intralesional cryosurgery [16].

13.6 Clinical Results

It has been reported by Har-Shai et al. ([10, 11], 2007, 2016) that a total average of 51.4% of scar volume reduction was achieved following one session of intralesional cryosurgery treatment. In the auricular area the scar volume reduction of 70% was achieved, on the back and shoulder 60% and on the chest 50% scar volume reduction has been attained (Figs. 13.6, 13.7, 13.8, 13.9, 13.10, 13.11). Similar clinical results were published by Stromps et al. [17], Chopinaud et al. [18], O'boyle et al. [19], and others.

Six months after a single session of intralesional cryosurgery, a significant alleviation of objective (hardness and color) and subjective clinical symptoms (pain/tenderness and itchiness/discomfort) were documented.

In order to evaluate the patient degree of concern and deformity from their keloid or hypertrophic scars prior and after the intralesional cryosurgery treatment, a modified "Gorney Gram" scale [20, 21], which had been designed and employed by Har-Shai et al. [12], was applied.

The obtained results demonstrate a significant and relative quick reduction in dissatisfaction among individuals suffering from unsightly and bothering scars.

The intralesional cryosurgery technique enables the plastic surgeon, dermatologist, or dermato-surgeon to have the proper and effective instrument to reduce, in a relative short time, the dissatisfaction of those patients who developed hypertrophic scars and keloids following aesthetic surgery. Thus, the patient confidence in the plastic surgeon is maintained which creates a positive attitude for a successful solution for those challenging scars.

Mild pain or discomfort during and after the procedure was easily managed (see pain relief protocol). Significant local edema and epidermolysis, followed by a relatively short re-epithelialization period depending on the pretreatment scar volume, were evident. Very rare local hypo-/hyperesthesia were documented, with no impact on the quality of life of the patient.

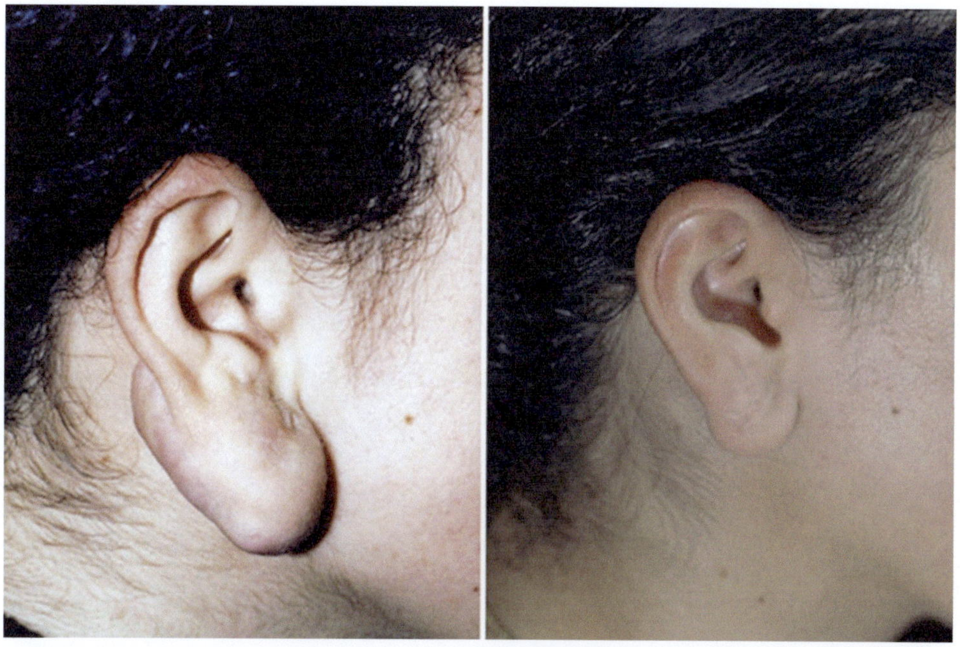

Fig. 13.6 Left: Preoperative view of a lobular keloid following piercing with a complete recurrence following two surgical excisions. Right: Postoperative view 6 years following a single session of intralesional cryosurgery demonstrates a complete involution of the scar with no hypopigmentation or recurrence

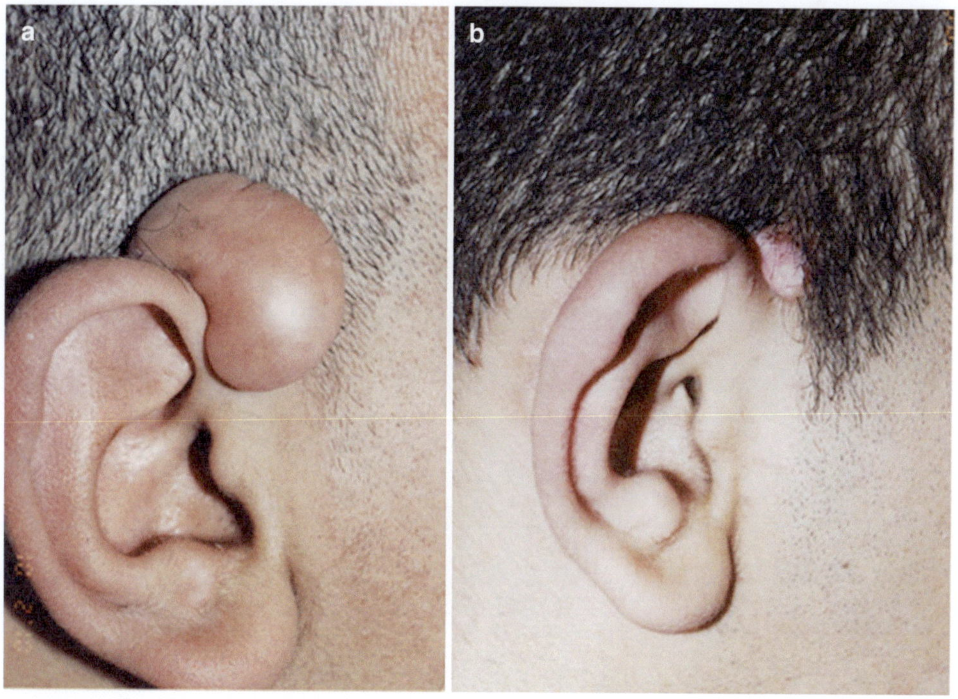

Fig. 13.7 Preoperative view of a keloid on the left radix helix following an excision of cholesteatoma (third attempt) in a 16-year-old male patient. (**a**) Preoperative view. (**b**) Postoperative view demonstrating a complete flattening of the scar 30 months following a single cryosession with no recurrence

During the 18-month follow-up period there was no evidence of bleeding, infection, or other adverse effects. The nonresponse rate was less than 3%. No worsening of the scars was evident and hypopigmentation was minimal.

The absolute contraindications are [22]: cold-inducible urticaria, cryoglubulinemia, cryofibrinogenemia, and Raynaud's disease. The relative contraindications are: collagen diseases and wound healing problems, pregnancy and scars which are adjacent to vital organs should be treated with caution. If the total tissue to be frozen accedes is more than 7% of total body weight, hypothermia might occur.

13.7 Discussion

It has been noticed that hypertrophic scars and keloids of black/darker colored skin exhibits less depigmentation following intralesional cryosurgery when compared with the contact method [11]. These findings may encourage the use

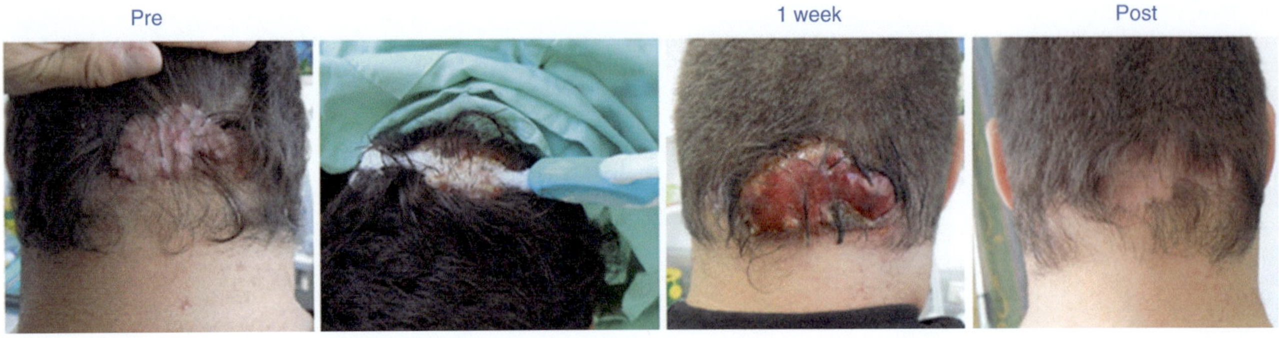

Fig. 13.8 Left: Preoperative view of a large acne keloidalis nucha on the right upper nape. Following intralesional cryosurgery a blister develops which drained after 7 days. Right: Postoperative view demonstrating a complete flattening of the scar 24 months following a single cryosession

Fig. 13.9 Left: Preoperative view of a large keloid scar on the left axilla following a second degree burn. Right: Postoperative view demonstrating a complete flattening of the scar 24 months following a single cryosession with no recurrence

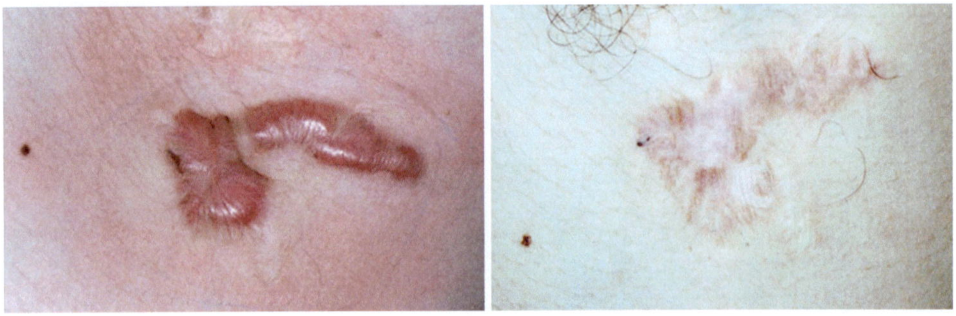

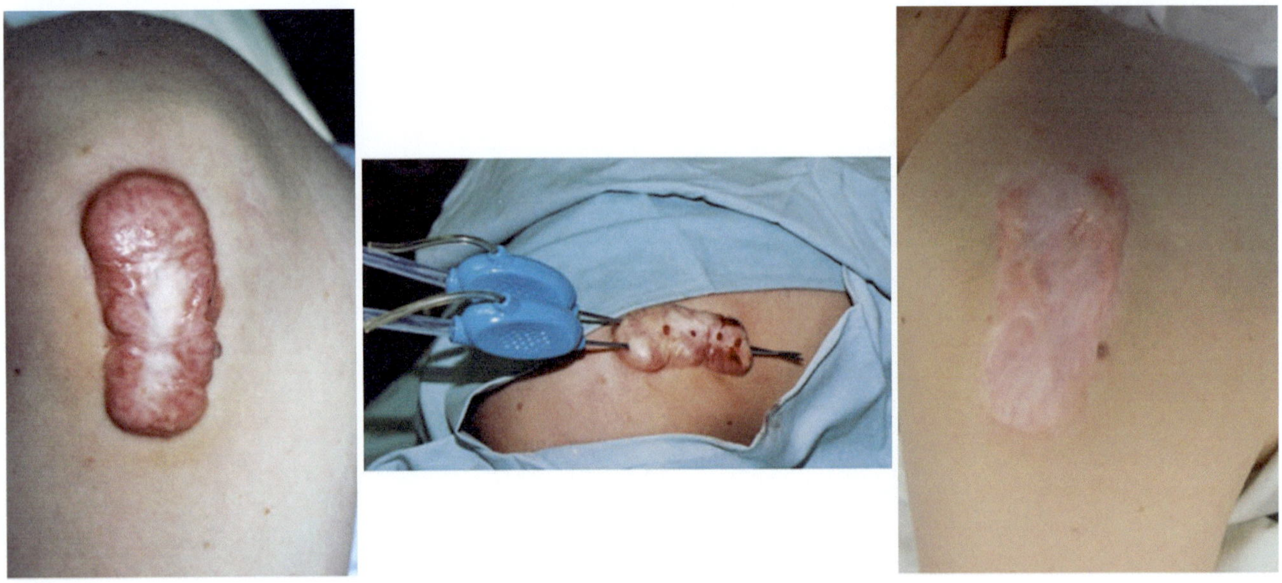

Fig. 13.10 Left: Preoperative view of a large keloid on the left upper arm following an excision of a congenital pigmented nevus. Middle: Two cryoneedles are inserted in parallel in order to facilitate the cryotreatment. Left: Postoperative view demonstrating a complete flattening of the scar 24 months following a single cryosession with no recurrence

of intralesional cryosurgery for dark-skinned individuals [20, 23] suffering from such scars or following aesthetic surgery, thus minimizing the depigmentation problem.

The trend for a longer hold time demonstrated during the intralesional cryosurgery process when compared with the contact method, which is solely related to the scar volume, i.e., a larger scar volume needs a longer freezing/hold time, may explain the superior efficacy of the intralesional technique in the treatment of keloids [11, 15]. Lower temperatures are present around the needle, which increase the freezing area of the core of the keloid tissue, which is abutting the cryoneedle, causing cryonecrosis. The long hold

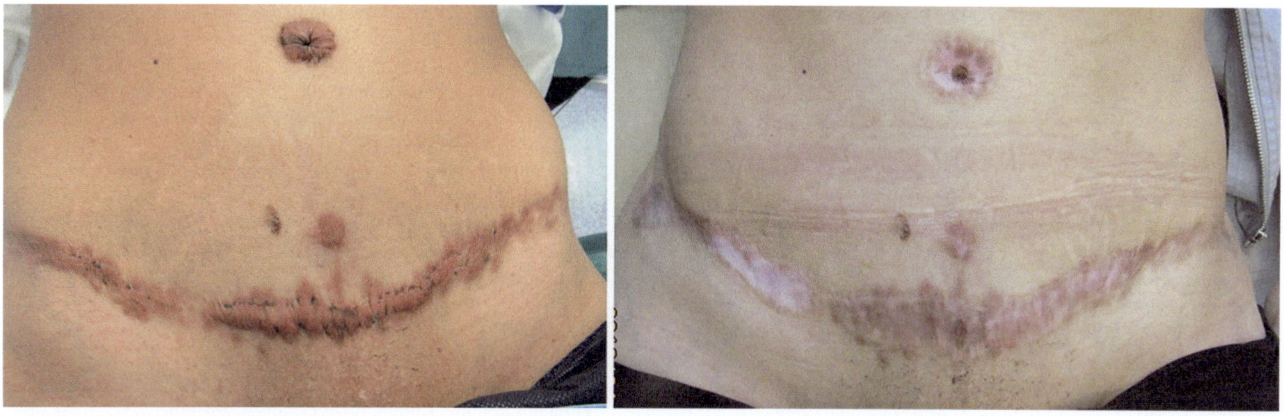

Fig. 13.11 Left: Preoperative view of large keloids on the umbilicus and lower abdomen following an abdominoplasty surgery for aesthetic reasons. Right: Postoperative view 18 months following a single session of intralesional cryosurgery demonstrating a complete involution of the scars on the umbilicus and lower abdomen with no recurrence

time, which was found significantly longer, when compared with the contact method, allows time for solute effects, ice crystal formation, and recrystallization. Furthermore, in a long duration of freezing, the biochemical changes and the growth of ice crystals are enhanced, increasing the rate of cell death [24]. Therefore, the intralesional technique is more effective than the contact method. On the other hand, the contact method causes a severe superficial cryodestruction harming mainly the epidermis, including the melanocytes, and upper dermis; thus, significantly less cryosurgical sessions (mainly 1–2 cryotreatments) are required to obtain keloid flattening.

It has been reported by Massalha and Shitzer [25] in an experimental study that the freezing process was retarded in an area in which a heat source was situated simulating a blood vessel. The ambient body temperature might act as such a heat source, thus preventing the injury of vital deep organs or implants underneath the cryoprocess.

The absence of infection following the intralesional cryosurgery might be explained by an immune response involving interplay of humoral and cellular factors, which occur locally and systemically. Following cryosurgery, a very rapid response of neutrophils to injury as well as activity of natural killer cells is demonstrated.

The low recurrence rates demonstrated following intralesional cryosurgery (<3%) could be explained by the long-term suppression effect of the cryotreatment on the abnormal fibroblasts [26, 27], or the destruction of all pathological fibroblasts in the scar by cryosurgery which are replaced by the recruitment of the neighboring normal fibroblasts, which produce normal collagen [10, 11]. Therefore, if a second cryosession in indicated, it is recommended to wait for at least 6 months prior to the next cryotreatment in order to enable the scar to complete its humoral and cellular events and reach its final volume and appearance, including pigmentation.

This simple-to-operate intralesional cryosurgery technology can be applied, as an office procedure, to every shape or contour of hypertrophic scar and keloid with a sufficient volume into which the cryoneedle can be introduced. In addition, it is safe to use, causes significant less hypopigmentation, is not time consuming, requires less cryogen fluid, necessitates less postoperative care of the wound, possesses a short learning curve, and can easily be added to a preexisting cryosurgical cryogun or unit.

The final goal of the treatment of hypertrophic scars and keloids is a complete and entire flattening of the scar in addition to significant reduction of objective and subjective clinical complaints. Therefore, if some residual scar volume is remaining after intralesional cryosurgery, it can be further dealt with a repeated intralesional cryosurgery session, only if there is sufficient scar volume to be penetrated or applying other appropriate therapies such as surface contact cryosurgery, silicone sheets, intralesional corticosteroids, and pressure garments.

References

1. Butler PD, Longaker MT, Yang GP. Current progress in keloid research and treatment. J Am Coll Surg. 2008;206:731–41.
2. Zouboulis CC, Orfanos CE. Kryochirurgische Behandlung Von Hypertropten Narben Und Keloiden. Hautarzt. 1990;41:683–8.
3. Zouboulis CC, Zouridaki E, Rosenberger A, Dalkowski A. Current developments and uses of cryosurgery in the treatment of keloids and hypertrophic scars. Wound Repair Regen. 2002;10:98–102.
4. Zouboulis CC, Blume V, Buttner P, Orfanos CE. Outcomes of cryosurgery in keloids and hypertrophic scars. A prospective consecutive trial of case series. Arch Dermatol. 1993;129:1146–51.
5. Zouboulis CC, Orfanos CE. Cryosurgical treatment. In: Harahap M, editor. Surgical techniques for cutaneous scar revision. New York: Marcel Delcker, Inc.; 2000. p. 185–234.
6. Weshahy AH. Intralesional cryosurgery, a new technique using cryoneedles. J Dermatol Surg Oncol. 1993;19:123–6.

7. Zouboulis CC. Principles of cutaneous cryosurgery: an update. Dermatology. 1999;198:111–7.
8. Zouboulis CC, Rosenberger AD, Forster T, Beller G, Kratzsch M, Felsenberg D. Modification of a device and its application for intralesional cryosurgery of old recalcitrant keloids. Arch Dermatol. 2004;140:1293–4.
9. Gupta S, Kumar B. Intralesional cryosurgery using lumbar puncture and/or hypodermic needles for large, bulky, recalcitrant keloids. Int J Dermatol. 2001;40:349–53.
10. Har-Shai Y, Amar M, Sabo E. Intralesional cryotherapy for enhancing the involution of hypertrophic scars and keloids. Plast Reconstr Surg. 2003;111:1841–52.
11. Har-Shai Y, Dujovny E, Rohde E, Zouboulis CC. Effect of skin surface temperature on skin pigmentation during contact and intralesional cryosurgery of keloids. J Eur Acad Dermatol Venereol. 2007;21:191–8. Erratum in: J Eur Acad Dermatol Venereol. 21:292, 2007.
12. Har-Shai Y, Brown W, Labbê D, Dompmartin A, Goldine I, Gil T, Mettanes I, Pallua N. Intralesional cryosurgery for the treatment of hypertrophic scars and keloid following aesthetic surgery: the results of a prospective observational study. Int J Low Extrem Wounds. 2008;6:169.
13. Fikrle T, Pizinger K. Cryosurgery in the treatment of earlobe keloids: report of seven cases. Dermatol Surg. 2005;31:1728–31.
14. Mirmovich O, Gil T, Goldin I, Lavi I, Mettanes I, Har-Shai Y. Pain evaluation and control during and following the treatment of hypertrophic scars and keloids by contact and intralesional cryosurgery—a preliminary study. J Eur Acad Dermatol Venereol. 2012;26:440–7.
15. Har-Shai Y, Zouboulis CC. Intralesional cryosurgery for the treatment of hypertrophic scars and keloids. Chapter 86. In: Abramovich W, Graham G, Har-Shai Y, Strumia R, editors. Dermatological cryosurgery and cryotherapy. London: Springer; 2016. p. 453–74.
16. Har-Shai L, Pallua N, Grasys I, Metanes I, Har-Shai Y. Intralesional excision combined with intralesional cryosurgery for the treatment of oversized and therapy-resistant keloids of the neck and ears. Eur J Plast Surg. 2018;41:233–8.
17. Stromps JP, Dunda S, Eppstein RJ, Babic D, Har-Shai Y, Pallua N. Intralesional cryosurgery combined with topical silicone gel sheeting for the treatment of refractory keloids. Dermatol Surg. 2014;40:996–1003.
18. Chopinaud M, Pham A-D, Labbe D, Verneuil L, Gourio C, Benateau H, Dompmartin A. Intralesional cryosurgery to treat keloid scars: results from a retrospective study. Dermatology. 2014;229:263–70.
19. O'boyle CP, Shayan-Arani H, Hamada MW. Intralesional cryotherapy for hypertrophic scars and keloids: a review. Scars Burns Heal. 2017;3:1–9.
20. Gorney M. Medical malpractice and plastic surgery: the carrier's point of view, Chapter 5. In: Goldwyn RM, Cohen MN, editors. The unfavorable results in plastic surgery: avoidance and treatment. Philadelphia, PA: Lippincott Williams & Wilkins; 2001. p. 38–43.
21. Gorney M. Recognition of the patient unsuitable for aesthetic surgery. Aesthetic Surg. 2007;27:626–7.
22. Har-Shai Y. Special indications and contraindications. Chapter 54. In: Abramovich W, Graham G, Har-Shai Y, Strumia R, editors. Dermatological cryosurgery and cryotherapy. London: Springer; 2016. p. 265–8.
23. Grimes PE, Hunt SG. Considerations for cosmetic surgery in the black population. Clin Plast Surg. 1993;20:27–34.
24. Baust JG, Gage AA. The molecular basis of cryosurgery. BJU Int. 2005;95:1187–91.
25. Massalha L, Shitzer A. Freezing by flat, circular surface cryoprobe of a tissue phantom with an embedded cylindric heat source simulating a blood vessel. J Biomech Eng. 2004;126:736–44.
26. Dalkowski A, Schuppan D, Orfanos CE, Zouboulis CC. Increased expression of tenascin-C by keloids in vivo and in vitro. Br J Dermatol. 1999;141:50–6.
27. Dalkowski A, Fimmel S, Beutler C, Zouboulis CC. Cryotherapy modifies synthetic activity and differentiation of keloidal fibroblasts in vitro. Exp Dermatol. 2003;12:673–81.

Laser Therapy for Scars

14

Timothy A. Durso, Nathanial R. Miletta, Bart O. Iddins, and Matthias B. Donelan

14.1 Introduction

Scars may result from intrinsic (e.g., acne and inflammatory dermatoses) or extrinsic (e.g., burns, trauma, surgery) forces. Regardless of etiology, scars may have a far-reaching and often devastating impact upon the life of the patient. Scar contractures over joints secondary to burn trauma have been shown to severely impair physical function after the recovery from acute injury [1, 2]. Persistent dysesthesias, such as pain and pruritus, are also commonly encountered in traumatic and pathologic scar types [3, 4]. Scars have been shown to contribute to an increased incidence of psychiatric comorbidities such as depression and post-traumatic stress disorder [5, 6]. As a result of these physiologic and psychologic effects, scar patients consistently demonstrate decreased quality of life that transcends a wide spectrum of populations [7–9]. Laser therapy facilitates incremental and long-term improvement in the physical and aesthetic profiles of scars. In combination with tissue-conserving surgical interventions, such as z-plasty and pharmacotherapy, laser therapy has helped usher in a paradigm shift in scar management [10]. Laser therapy and conservative treatments often obviate the need for larger surgical interventions, such as scar excision, skin flaps, and grafts [11–13]. It is therefore critical that surgeons managing scars be familiar with this unique and invaluable scar management modality.

T. A. Durso · N. R. Miletta
Laser Surgery and Scar Center, San Antonio Military Health System, San Antonio, TX, USA

Uniformed Services University of the Health Sciences, Bethesda, MD, USA

B. O. Iddins
Laser Surgery and Scar Center, San Antonio Military Health System, San Antonio, TX, USA

Uniformed Services University of the Health Sciences, Bethesda, MD, USA

Oak Ridge National Laboratory, Oak Ridge, TN, USA

M. B. Donelan (✉)
Shriners Hospital for Children—Boston, Boston, MA, USA

Massachusetts General Hospital, Boston, MA, USA

Harvard Medical School, Boston, MA, USA
e-mail: mdonelan@mgh.harvard.edu

14.2 Basic Laser Principles

LASER is an acronym for light amplification by stimulated emission of radiation. The principles of laser physics were first posited by Albert Einstein in 1917 [14]. At its core, a laser consists of an activatable material, known as a medium, housed within a laser apparatus. The atoms that make up the medium exist in a stable low-energy ground state. These atoms are then stimulated when a secondary energy source is used to "pump," or excite, the atoms of the medium to an unstable state. In spontaneous fashion, one or more of the excited atoms will return to the ground state and thus emit a discrete packet of light, or photon, in the process. If this photon collides with other adjacent atoms, it propagates the reaction resulting in the release of another photon. This chain reaction can be further amplified through the use of reflective mirrors in the optical cavity in order to intensify the laser energy [15].

The laser medium may be gaseous, liquid, or solid, and all three states of matter are utilized in the laser therapy of scars (Table 14.1). Due to the uniformity of the atoms in the lasing medium, the photons emitted are monochromatic, meaning they have an identical and consistently predictable wavelength. Moreover, during the process of amplification described above, photons are released in the same phase and direction of travel as one another through constructive and destructive interference [15]. This synchrony leads to both temporal and spatial coherence, as well as collimation. This means that the laser photons travel in phase and parallel to one another. In sum, the laser apparatus emits a narrow beam of photons traveling at the same wavelength, in the same direction, at the same time, that can be used to effectively treat scars.

© Springer Nature Singapore Pte Ltd. 2020
R. Ogawa (ed.), *Total Scar Management*, https://doi.org/10.1007/978-981-32-9791-3_14

14.3 Laser–Tissue Interactions

14.3.1 Selective Photothermolysis of Discrete Skin Structures

Within the skin, there are several endogenous substances that absorb laser light, including hemoglobin, melanin, and water. Molecules that absorb laser light are referred to as chromophores. Once absorbed, laser light can be converted into thermal energy that can be harnessed to destroy discrete targets within the skin, such as blood vessels, epidermal/dermal pigmentation, and the epidermis and/or dermis. This principle of selective photothermolysis was first described in 1983 by Anderson and Parrish [16]. Targeting of discrete structures relies upon matching the absorption spectrum of the chromophore and the wavelength of the laser selected (Fig. 14.1). Wavelength may also be varied depending upon the depth and concentration of the chromophore, absorption spectrum of adjacent chromophores, and the optical properties of the skin.

Table 14.1 A selection of energy-based devices commonly used in the treatment of scars and their characteristics

Name	Medium type	Wavelength (nm)	Chromophore
PDL	Liquid	585–595	Hemoglobin
KTP	Solid	532	Hemoglobin
IPL	N/A (not a true laser)	515–1200	Hemoglobin[a]
CO_2	Gas	10,600	Water
Er:YAG	Solid	2940	Water
Er:Glass	Solid	1540–1565	Water

PDL Pulsed dye laser, *KTP* Potassium titanyl phosphate, *IPL* Intense pulsed light, *Er:YAG* Erbium-doped yttrium aluminum garnet, *Er:Glass* Erbium-doped glass.

[a]The chromophore target of IPL varies based on the filter used and may include melanin, although for scars the primary chromophore of interest is hemoglobin.

14.3.2 Spatially Selective Fractional Photothermolysis of the Skin

Spatially selective fractional photothermolysis of the skin relies upon the theory of selective photothermolysis as it pertains to the absorption of laser light by the chromophore water. Water is located ubiquitously within the skin and within many discrete skin structures, including blood vessels. Given the global presence of water, wavelengths of laser light absorbed by this chromophore are capable of creating highly specific injury patterns of both ablation and coagulation throughout the skin. Spatially selective

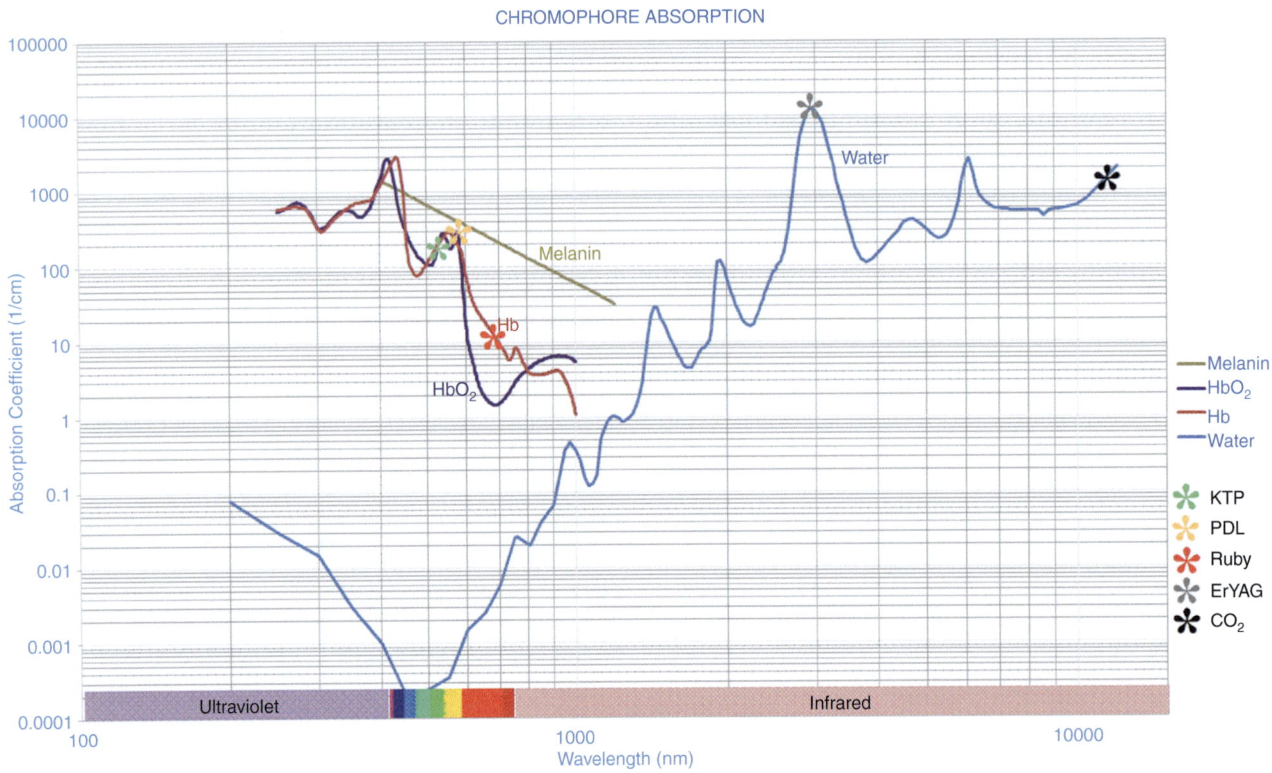

Fig. 14.1 Cutaneous chromophore absorption spectrum with common laser medium wavelengths noted

patterns of injury can be created for specific aims including the stimulation of scar remodeling.

14.4 Scar Treatment Wavelengths

With respect to scars, the most commonly leveraged chromophores include hemoglobin and water. The absorption of laser light by hemoglobin allows for the selective destruction of fine vasculature located within the scar. Major peaks of hemoglobin absorption include 418, 542, and 577 nm [15]. Selective photothermolysis of the vasculature allows the reduction of erythema, reduced delivery of inflammatory cytokines, and, therefore, a reduction in patient symptoms.

As the wavelength of the laser medium increases beyond 1000 nm, water becomes the primary chromophore with the strongest amount of absorption occurring at wavelengths greater than 2000 nm [15]. Thermal heating of water results in ablation and coagulation (non-ablation) that can be leveraged to induce tissue remodeling within the scars. Spatially selective photothermolysis can be accomplished with both ablative fractional lasers (AFLs) and non-ablative fractional lasers (NAFLs).

14.5 Conceptual Approach to Laser Therapy

14.5.1 Selective Photothermolysis of the Vasculature or Pigmentation

For lasers utilizing wavelengths selecting the chromophores of hemoglobin and melanin (as outlined above), the physician must appropriately select the laser pulse width that correlates with the size of the target. While the chromophore absorbs the laser light, it is the target that must be eliminated to achieve the clinical goal. For instance, hemoglobin is the chromophore for the vasculature-selective lasers, but it is the blood vessel that is being targeted. The larger the vessel, the longer the relative pulse width should be. After the pulse width has been selected, the laser surgeon must select the spot size. If treating a large area, a larger spot size is appropriate. Due to laser scatter phenomena, larger spot sizes typically require less fluence to deliver the same clinical endpoint. Additionally, measures to cool the epidermis are needed to protect against unnecessary side effects and tissue breakdown. Different lasers employ various cooling methods, with some engaging direct contact cooling or noncontact methods (e.g., cryogen spray, forced cold air). Lastly, the fluence, or amount of energy delivered per unit area, must be titrated to elicit the desired treatment endpoint, such as transient purpura for erythema in scars. Modern laser platforms have auto-populated fluence settings depending on the selected target structure. The clinician may then titrate the fluence to the desired clinical response at subsequent treatments or in real time based on immediately observable clinical endpoints after each laser pulse.

14.5.2 Spatially Selective Fractional Photothermolysis of the Skin

For AFLs and NAFLs that create individual micro-columns, or microscopic treatment zones (MTZs), of tissue ablation and injury, the energy delivered correlates to the depth of energy penetration. Changing the spot size of the laser allows the clinician to target either small treatment areas with specific shapes or large treatment areas for extensive lesions. Most importantly, the density of these MTZs can be varied within a fixed size or shape. This allows skin recapitulation from both adnexal structures and intervening epidermal stem cells to expedite healing and permit increased scar treatment depth. The frequency at which pulses are delivered, defined by Hertz, allows the experienced clinician to increase the speed of treatment. However, the escalation of pulse frequency may lead to bulk heating of tissue resulting in unwanted side effects, such as dyspigmentation, worsening of the scar, and patient discomfort.

14.6 Initial Scar Assessment

14.6.1 History

Scars develop from a wide variety of causes and vary greatly in their impact upon a patient's quality of life and overall health. Consequently, it is important to understand the mechanism of injury, age of the scar, physical limitations secondary to the scar, scar symptoms (e.g., pain, pruritus), and if the scar impacts the patient's mental or emotional well-being. Additionally, prior interventions such as traditional surgery, laser therapy, intralesional medication injections, occupational therapy, and physical therapy should be noted along with their efficacy in alleviating the patient's symptoms and concerns. Finally, patients must be thoroughly educated regarding expectations. Specifically, laser therapy provides an incremental benefit over several treatment sessions, and maximal improvement may take months due to collagen remodeling. Patience and understanding are key factors to scar treatment success.

14.6.2 Physical Exam

After considering the history of the scar, the physician next needs to determine if the scar is immature or mature. Immature scars are generally considered to be those less than 4 weeks postinciting event. Of note, many scars may demonstrate immature features (e.g., exuberant tissue, bright red erythema, pruritus) well after this period, which represents an arrest in the maturation process. This is important to consider since it impacts the treatment approach and potential outcome. Typically, an acute scar or scar arrested in the immature phase of healing can improve greatly through laser intervention. Mature scars also often demonstrate variations in erythema, pigmentation, thickness, and elasticity, but tend to respond more slowly to treatment. Once the maturation of the scar is assessed, the physician should analyze the scar characteristics and develop a treatment plan based on the clinical appearance in order to optimize outcome. In addition, scars under excessive tension tend not to respond as well as those with less mechanical strain. Often, z-plasty or serial miniature z-plasties are beneficial in releasing excess tension in order to "prepare" the scar for laser treatment [10]. For severe cases, scar release and grafting may still be necessary.

14.7 Scar Characteristics and Evidence-Based Treatment Approaches

14.7.1 Erythema

14.7.1.1 Background

Scars may be erythematous, avascular, or both depending upon the size and mechanism of injury. Scar vascularity manifests as erythema due to imperceptible fine superficial capillaries and discrete telangiectasias (Fig. 14.2). Despite hemoglobin being the common chromophore to both erythema and telangiectasias, the laser settings differ greatly. Recall from above, longer pulse widths target vessels of larger diameters. If the physician selects a short pulse width for a scar with prominent telangiectasias, the desired outcome of selectively destroying relatively large blood vessels will not be achieved. Conversely, if the selected pulse width is relatively too long relative to the blood vessel diameter, dyspigmentation and/or worsening of the scar may occur. This happens due to bulk heating of the surrounding tissue as a result of exceeding the thermal relaxation time of the vessel. Commonly used lasers for targeting vascular structures include pulsed dye laser (PDL), frequency-doubled, neodymium-doped yttrium aluminum garnet (Nd:YAG), potassium titanyl phosphate crystal (referred to as KTP or KTP-Nd:YAG), and intense pulsed light (IPL).

14.7.1.2 Evidence-Based Literature

Pulsed dye laser (PDL) at 595 nm has been utilized for the treatment of scar erythema for over 20 years [17]. PDL is also the laser most frequently utilized by the authors in treating vascular structures within scars. The obvious benefit of PDL-induced vascular destruction is a subsequent decrease in redness of the scar tissue. In addition, decreased pruritus is commonly noted after PDL treatment, due to a decrease in the delivery of inflammatory cytokines [18–20]. At the molecular level, additional benefits in keloids have included decreased fibroblast proliferation and increased fibroblast apoptosis [21].

The PDL system used by the authors is the 595 nm VBeam Perfecta (Syneron Candela, Wayland, MA). Spot sizes on this device range from 3 to 12 mm (including an oval-shaped 3 mm × 10 mm spot size intended for tracing along telangiectasias). The fluence ranges from 40 J/cm^2 at the 3 mm spot size to 7 J/cm^2 at the 12 mm spot size. Pulse widths range from 0.45 to 40 ms. Cooling is achieved by noncontact cryo-

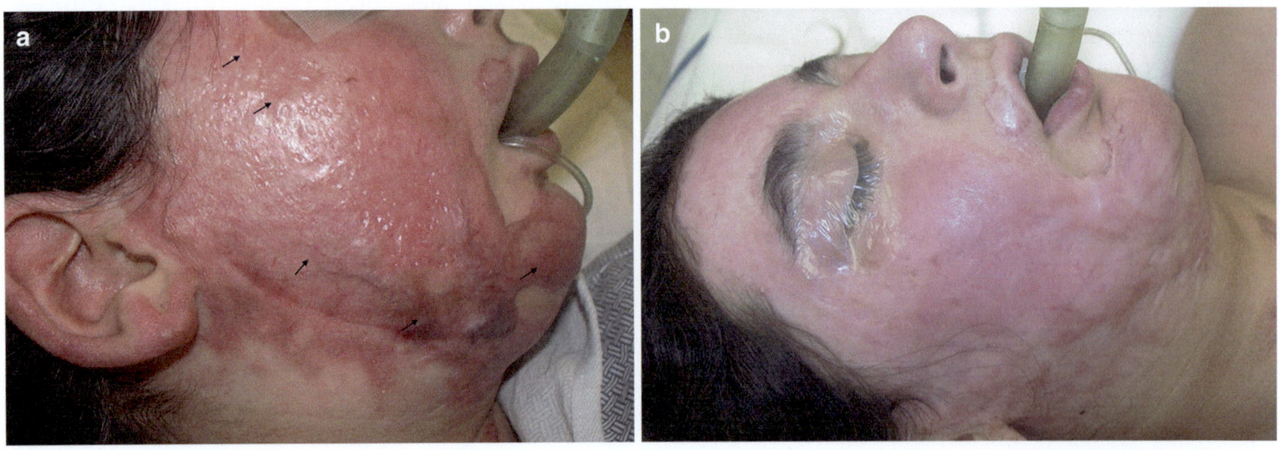

Fig. 14.2 (**a**) Immature burn scar on the face prior to laser therapy with severe erythema, discernable fine telangiectasias (arrows), and symptomatic pruritus. (**b**) Expedited maturation of the immature burn scar 11 months after nine pulsed dye laser treatments. The erythema is markedly less, the telangiectasias is eliminated, and the pruritus has resolved

gen spray with each pulse, which is quite helpful over irregular scar topography. Pulses may be triggered either by finger switch or by foot pedal [22].

Potassium Titanyl Phosphate (KTP) Laser

KTP achieves a wavelength of 532 nm through the frequency-doubling of a 1064 nm Nd:YAG laser beam. The 1064 nm beam is passed through a KTP crystal for this effect. Because wavelength is inversely proportional to frequency, doubling of the frequency leads to a halving of the wavelength [16]. This decrease in wavelength permits targeting of hemoglobin, and thus vasculature. KTP has been shown in both retrospective and prospective analyses to have similar efficacy in treating scar erythema when compared to PDL [23, 24]. KTP utilizes a sapphire contact cooling built into the laser handpiece. The handpiece also requires a gel interface, such as ultrasound jelly, between itself and the skin surface for operation. As a result of these constraints (e.g., contact cooling and necessity for gel interface), expedient treatment of larger surface areas is less feasible in the authors' experience. Treating irregular contours of burn and trauma scars can also be more difficult due to surface irregularities. Settings reported as effective in treating surgical scar erythema for the Excel V platform (Cutera, Brisbane, CA) are as follows: spot size: 7 mm, fluence: 4.6 J/cm^2, and pulse width: 3 ms [23].

Intense Pulsed Light (IPL)

IPL is not technically a laser, as it does not emit a monochromatic wavelength of photons. Instead, IPL emits a broad band of pulsed light ranging from 515 to 1200 nm. With the use of selective filters, the appropriate wavelength for the targeting of vasculature and melanin can be achieved [25]. Commonly used scar erythema filters include 515 and 590 nm. One case series of 20 patients had subjective improvement in overall scar color. In that case series, a mean fluence of 15.4 J/cm^2 was used (pulse width was not reported, although 10–20 ms is generally appropriate) [26]. IPL has also been reported in the literature as being useful as an adjunct with other treatment modalities including lasers and intralesional pharmacotherapy injections [27–29]. Despite this reported success, IPL can lead to significant side effects, such as ulceration, if the contact cooling is not appropriately applied. Given the efficacy and superior safety profile of the PDL for scar erythema, IPL is best reserved for refractory cases of scar erythema, as an adjunct therapy with other treatment modalities, or when specific targeting of hyperpigmentation is desired.

14.7.1.3 Treatment Approach

Pulsed Dye Laser (PDL)

As noted above, for scar erythema, shorter pulse widths are desired in order to target the small-caliber vasculature present. Typical PDL settings used include a pulse width of 0.45–1.5 ms, a spot size of 7 mm, and an initial fluence of approximately 5.0 J/cm^2. The treatment endpoint is transient purpura lasting for a less than 5 s. If the clinical endpoint is not achieved, the fluence may be titrated upward until transient purpura is observed [30].

For larger vessels (e.g., visible telangiectasias), longer pulse widths are needed. Typical pulse widths used range from 6 to 20 ms. The clinical endpoint for telangiectasias is immediate vessel darkening or disappearance [30]. Persistent purpura as a clinical endpoint for the treatment of telangiectasias has shown greater single-treatment efficacy; however, sub-purpuric settings are also efficacious with relatively less downtime for the patient [31]. A spot size of 10 mm with a fluence of 8–12 J/cm^2 at the pulse widths noted above generally achieve the necessary clinical endpoint.

Common technical pitfalls include the use of epinephrine during infiltration with local anesthetics and excess pressure applied by the laser handpiece prior to each pulse. Epinephrine causes localized vasoconstriction, leading to less available chromophore to absorb the laser light. If planning to perform subsequent ablative fractional laser (AFL) requiring numbing, we would suggest numbing after PDL is performed to decrease the risk of blanching. Similarly, excess pressure applied by the physician via the laser handpiece will blanch the vasculature leading to less availability of the local hemoglobin chromophore. For ideal results, the handpiece should be held perpendicular to the skin and in very light contact prior to each pulse.

PDL, in general, leads to very little, if any, downtime for the patient. A transient increase in erythema, swelling, bruising, and dyspigmentation may follow PDL therapy. Post-inflammatory hyperpigmentation is often due to sun exposure in the days immediately following treatment. To minimize this complication, patients should be counseled to avoid the sun for at least 72 h after the procedure. Treatments are spaced 4–6 weeks apart to allow for the full clinical effects of each treatment to be appreciated. Very significant reduction in erythema can be achieved in as little as 3–4 sessions with minimal invasiveness (Figs. 14.1 and 14.2). As with all lasers, prior to the first treatment, patients should be screened for a history of skin conditions that worsen with trauma (e.g., vitiligo), as these conditions may be induced or exacerbated at sites of laser therapy [32].

14.7.2 Scar Projection

14.7.2.1 Background

Scar projection is another key, albeit relatively simple, characteristic to assess. Scars can be atrophic (as is often the case with acne scarring), flush with the surrounding skin but with surface textural irregularities (e.g., skin graft donor and transplant sites), or hypertrophic/keloidal with some cases demonstrating several centimeters of protrusion from the surrounding skin (Figs. 14.3 and 14.4).

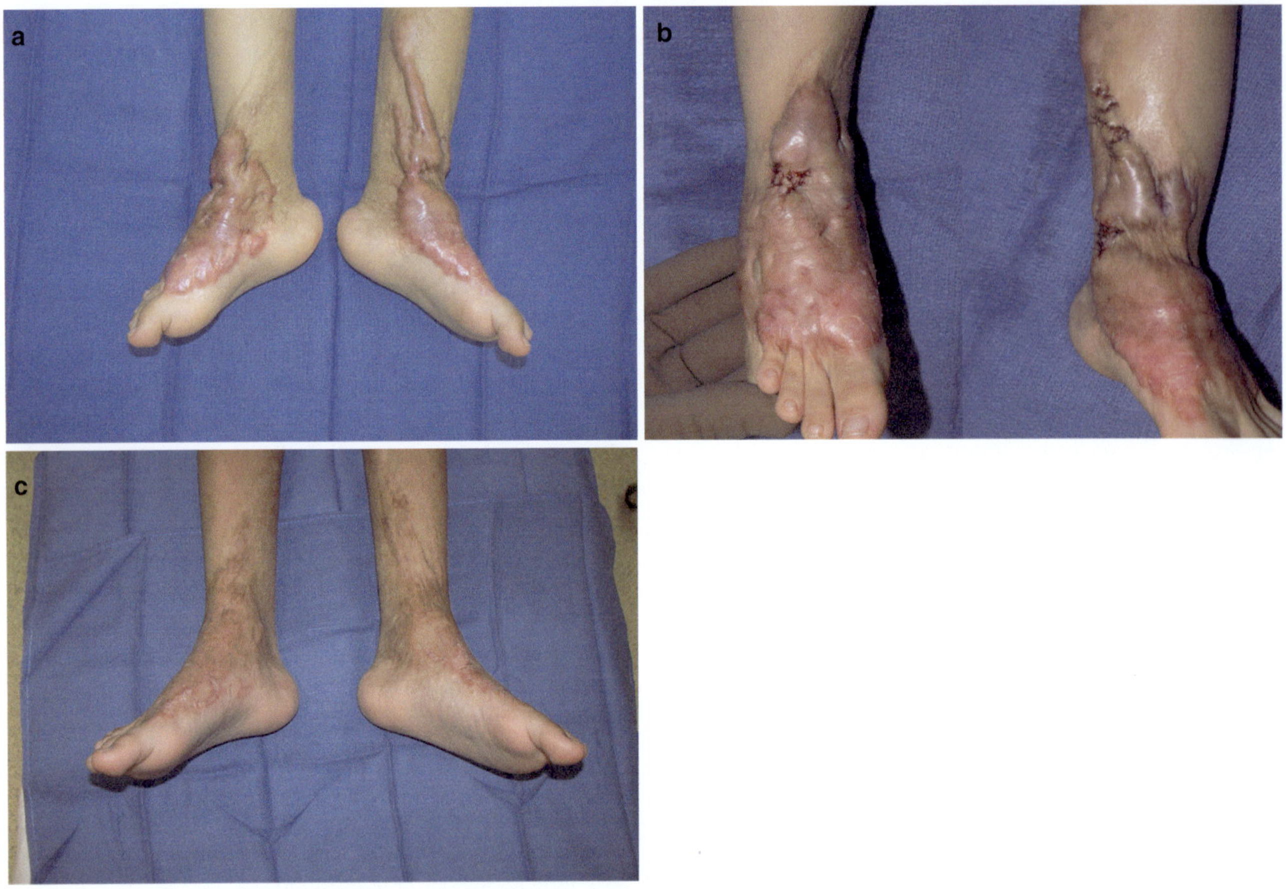

Fig. 14.3 (**a**) Massive hypertrophic burn scars on the lower legs, ankles, and feet 1 year following a scald burn injury. The erythema and pruritus were treated initially with PDL. (**b**) Tension across the ankle joints was relieved by performing small z-plasties. (**c**) Five years later, after 12 laser treatments with the CO_2 AFL and topical corticosteroids, the hypertrophic scarring has completely resolved. No scar tissue was excised

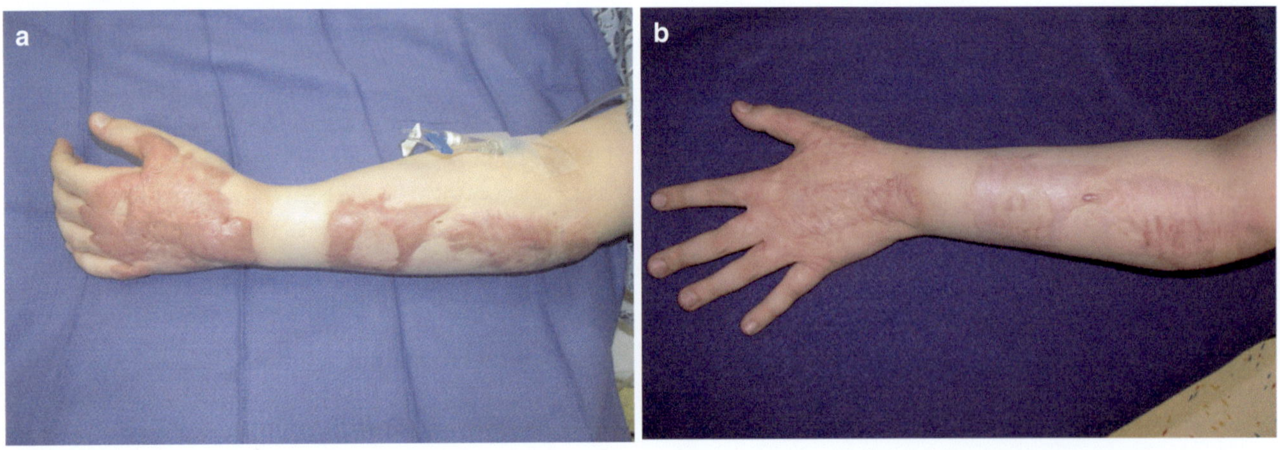

Fig. 14.4 (**a**) Hyperemic and hypertrophic burn scars of the arm and hand 11 months after a 16% flame burn injury in a 10-year-old male patient. The scars project 1.0–1.5 cm above the adjacent uninjured skin. (**b**) Five years later, after 2 PDL and 11 CO_2 AFL treatments, the erythema is eliminated and the hypertrophy is essentially resolved. The two PDL treatments were performed simultaneously with first two AFL treatments. Topical triamcinolone was applied after all AFLs to decrease post-treatment symptoms and enhance treatment outcome. Scar excision was never indicated

Scar thickness, particularly in the case of hypertrophic or keloidal scars, determines the depth at which the laser energy needs to penetrate in order to have the desired clinical effect. Although physician experience is often relied upon to determine this depth, objective measurement devices do exist for this purpose, including high-frequency ultrasound devices. The current literature suggests that the laser energy should penetrate at least 80% into the full thickness of the scar [33, 34].

The last consideration in the initial assessment is the appropriate treatment setting for each patient. Lasers commonly employed in the treatment of scars are relatively mobile devices that can be carefully wheeled between the clinic and operating room (OR). The size of the treatment area, the patient's age and maturity level, and the specific modality of laser therapy all factor into the decision to treat in the clinic versus the OR. Strategies used by the authors for in-clinic treatments include pharmacologic anxiolysis (only after signature of the consent form in the case of an adult patient), topical anesthetic agents [e.g., eutectic mixture of local anesthetics (EMLA), benzocaine-lidocaine-tetracaine (BLT)], infiltration with local anesthetics (including tumescent lidocaine), and nerve blocks. Ultimately, a discussion between the physician and consenting party will direct the ideal strategy for each patient.

14.7.2.2 Evidence-Based Literature

Fully ablative resurfacing with carbon dioxide or erbium:YAG laser was commonly performed for cosmetic reasons in the 1990s. However, full ablation of the skin carried with it a significant side effect profile to include prolonged post-procedural erythema, hyperpigmentation, herpes simplex virus (HSV) reactivation, and delayed hypopigmentation [35]. Fractional photothermolysis, the concept behind AFL and NAFL, was developed in 2004 to mitigate the side effect profile of full ablation while still maintaining the desired results that ablation provided [36]. The principle of fractional photothermolysis centers around the creation of the microscopic thermal zones (MTZs) of either ablation or thermal injury (coagulation) in a geometric pattern at a density specified by the laser surgeon [36]. The diameter of each MTZ is a function of the laser wavelength, pulse width, and beam optics, whereas the depth is a function of the fluence [37].

The MTZs of ablation are repopulated by epidermal stem cells in the nontreated adjacent skin and adnexal structures resulting in controlled collagen remodeling [38]. Fractional photothermolysis has been shown to generate diffuse localized collagen remodeling, despite a relatively small percentage of the cutaneous surface being treated during each session [39]. Whether utilizing AFL or NAFL, the selected chromophore is intracellular water.

Scars are biologically active even at the point of clinical maturity. AFL creates physical channels in the treatment area by means of tissue ablation [36]. AFL influences the biologic activity of scar tissue at the cellular level by altering fibroblast activity and upregulating matrix metalloproteinases [40]. The collagen profile of scar tissue treated with AFL begins to approximate normal skin with continued treatment [41]. Subsequent improvements in pliability, contracture, symptoms, and overall appearance occur in hypertrophic scars [42, 43]. These improvements have been illustrated by objective measures of extensibility and elasticity [34, 44]. In addition, improvements in the volume and appearance of atrophic scars have been reported [45, 46]. Despite numerous case reports and series, correlation of subjective improvement with objective measures has yet to be well established, causing some to question the utility of AFL in certain scar populations [47]. In recently reported data from a prospective trial presented at a national conference, objective improvements in scar thickness and elastic properties were well correlated with subjective improvements [12]. Further study of these correlations will serve to solidify what has been clinically apparent to clinicians and patients for over a decade.

NAFL creates MTZs via coagulation of tissue through the transfer of thermal energy at a sub-ablative energy level [48]. This thermal damage caused by NAFL stimulates neocollagenesis and scar remodeling akin to the changes induced by AFL [49, 50]. However, the molecular changes have been shown to be less robust in NAFL-treated scars compared to AFL, which likely explains the necessity for an increased number of overall treatments with NAFL [51]. Although the majority of the literature surrounding NAFL focuses on the treatment of atrophic scars, at least one study of normotrophic and hypertrophic burn scars demonstrated improvement after three treatment sessions [52]. Overall, NAFL has been established as an effective and relatively safe treatment for atrophic scars, but additional data is needed to fully evaluate its role in the treatment of hypertrophic scars.

14.7.2.3 Treatment Approaches

Hypertrophy

Ablative Fractional Laser (AFL)

The two commonly used AFL platforms utilize carbon dioxide (CO_2, 10600 nm) or erbium-doped yttrium aluminum garnet (Er:YAG, 2940 nm) as their laser-generating media. AFL can be used for a variety of indications including atrophic, normotrophic, and hypertrophic scarring. Although the authors primarily use a CO_2-based platform as described below, the literature does not support a distinction in effects between CO_2 and Er:YAG for hypertrophic scarring.

The authors use the 10,600 nm UltraPulse CO_2 laser platform (Lumenis, Yokne'am, Israel). AFL platforms have a fixed pulse width for each MTZ created in order to promote uniformity within the treatment area. For example, the UltraPulse has a fixed pulse width of 0.8 ms per MTZ, which approximates, but does not exceed, the thermal relaxation time of the skin, which is approximately 1 ms [53, 54]. This precision ensures targeted delivery of energy without excess damage to surrounding skin. Each MTZ generated by the UltraPulse has a diameter of approximately 120 microns [54]. The density and frequency of MTZ delivery are determined by the physician. The physician must also select the energy (in milliJoules) which determines the depth of treatment. The UltraPulse is capable of achieving a skin penetration depth of up to 4 mm [54]. Many modern AFL platforms indicate the depth anticipated with each energy setting selected on the user interface. Physicians should familiarize themselves with these settings prior to treatment.

The UltraPulse is capable of both superficial (ActiveFx handpiece) and deep (DeepFx/SCAAR Fx handpiece) fractional ablation, which is deployed in a stamping fashion using the handpiece with pulses activated via footpedal [54]. Deep AFL is used initially in the treatment of scars to address the specific issues of scar projection and thickness. Superficial AFL addresses surface textural irregularities and helps blend the treatment area into the surrounding normal skin. Without appropriate deep AFL to induce collagen remodeling of dermal scar tissue, superficial AFL alone is unlikely to result in adequate clinical improvement. When both modalities are used over multiple treatments, the resolution of hypertrophy and improvement in appearance of scars demonstrates a transformational benefit to patients. (Figs. 14.3 and 14.4).

After cleansing the treatment area with alcohol or acetone to remove all cosmetics and/or topical anesthetics, the authors initiate treatment with the UltraPulse DeepFx with energy set to target at least 80% thickness of the scar. A density of 5–10% and frequency of 250 Hz are typically selected. Increasing density and frequency may lead to increased tissue injury and bulk heating with subsequent dyspigmentation. To achieve a 10% density, two passes at 5% density may be utilized to minimize these risks. The authors then proceed to pass over the same treatment area with the ActiveFx setting for superficial AFL. Although the UltraPulse is capable of full ablation on the ActiveFx setting, the authors recommend an initially conservative approach with a starting treatment level of 2, which corresponds to a 55% density. Depending on the body site and thickness of the scar, energy levels of 80–125 mJ (corresponding to depths of 55–115 microns) are typically used.

It is important to avoid overlapping pulses during both superficial and deep AFL. In addition, including a 2 mm margin of surrounding normal skin during treatment allows for greater blending of the scar tissue and unaffected tissue. A thin layer of petrolatum or topical corticosteroid ointment is applied immediately after the procedure. The authors provide patients with a handout at their consultation appointment addressing home care. An antiseptic solution consisting of 1 teaspoon of white vinegar and 1 cup of water should be applied 3–4 times daily for 4–5 days. A towel soaked in the solution or a spray bottle kept in the refrigerator may be utilized for application. Petrolatum should be reapplied after each cleansing. Patients must be counseled on the importance of direct sun avoidance for 1–2 weeks after the procedure. Furthermore, patients should also be encouraged to consistently use sunscreen once re-epithelialization has occurred (typically 4–5 days post-treatment). Treatment of facial or abdominal/pelvic scarring should be accompanied by HSV prophylaxis. The authors prescribe valacyclovir 1 g for 10 days to be started the day prior to the procedure. Because full collagen remodeling takes several weeks to months, treatments are repeated at 12-week intervals.

Atrophy

Non-ablative Fractional Laser (NAFL)

Commonly used NAFL platforms utilize erbium-doped glass to generate a laser beam with a wavelength in the 1540–1565 nm range. The authors use the 1550 nm erbium-doped glass Fraxel system (Solta Medical, Pleasanton, CA) for NAFL. This system utilizes a rolling handpiece to deliver laser energy with either built-in or external forced-air cooling. This particular system allows for up to a 1.4 mm depth of penetration into the skin at the 70 mJ setting [55]. Density is determined by treatment level selected. For Fitzpatrick Skin Type (FST) III-V patients, treatment levels of 3–4, corresponding to a density of 9–11%, are typically initiated. Higher treatment levels can be used for lighter skin tones (FSTI-II) due to a decreased risk of post-treatment dyspigmentation. Treatment levels of 6–7, corresponding to a density of 17–20%, can be safely used in these patients. A foot pedal is engaged to allow firing of the laser; however, the laser will only fire if the rollers of the handpiece tip are in contact with the skin and rotating.

The treatment area is cleansed with alcohol or acetone to remove all cosmetics and/or topical anesthetics prior to treatment. An energy of 65–70 mJ is typically selected, as this depth of penetration will provide maximal benefit without increased risk for harm given the mechanism of injury induced by the laser. The density selected is delivered in a fractionated way based on the number of passes selected by the clinician. A standard number of passes to deliver the energy is 8 for patient comfort. One unidirectional movement across a treatment area counts as a single pass. The typical back-and-forth motion across each treatment area counts, then, as two passes. In the case of a full-face treatment, each cosmetic subunit should be treated with two passes prior to repeating any one subunit to avoid bulk heating. If only a small area is being treated, a 1–2-min respite between passes is sufficient to allow for cooling. For each group of two passes across a treatment area, the direction of travel of the handpiece (e.g., up-and-down, side-to-side) should be alternated. The Fraxel system has auditory feedback built in to alert the physician if the laser is firing (relatively lower pitched beeping) and if the handpiece is moving too quickly for optimal energy delivery (relatively higher pitched beeping).

Because of the lack of ablation and preservation of the skin barrier, infection prophylaxis and antiseptic measures are not required for NAFL. Again, a thin layer of petrolatum is applied after the procedure. Patients must still be warned to avoid direct sunlight for a minimum of 3–4 days immediately following treatment. Total downtime for the patient is typically only a few days. Although the collagen remodeling of NAFL occurs over the same time period as AFL, treatments may occur more frequently due to the relatively low side effect profile. Physicians may repeat treatments every 4–6 weeks for 4–6 months in order to maximize benefit from this treatment modality. Expected improvement with treatment varies between 30% and 70% in NAFL-treated atrophic scars 2–3 months after concluding treatment (Fig. 14.5).

14.7.3 Hyperpigmentation

The literature on the treatment of scar hyperpigmentation is sparse. Some have reported that fractional photothermolysis (AFL and NAFL) alone improves hyperpigmentation [56]. Recently, there have been reports of improvement after treatment with the 1927 nm thulium-doped glass laser (2–5 treatments, 10 mJ, 30% density, 4–8 passes) [57]. Additional lasers that target melanin, such as Q-switched or picosecond alexandrite and Nd:YAG laser platforms, may also be trialed in refractory scar hyperpigmentation.

14.7.4 Hair-Bearing Areas

If scarring occurs in hair-bearing areas, depending on the mechanism of injury, viable hair follicles may become entrapped in the involved area. Continued hair growth then may lead to chronic irritation and pain [58]. Laser hair removal has the capability to alleviate this complication. The 755 nm alexandrite laser is typically used in lower (I-II) FSTs. The 1064 nm Nd:YAG laser is typically used in higher (III-VI) FSTs. The longer wavelength of the Nd:YAG laser allows for deeper penetration of the laser energy which avoids targeting the higher melanin content at the basal epidermal layer of patients with higher FSTs.

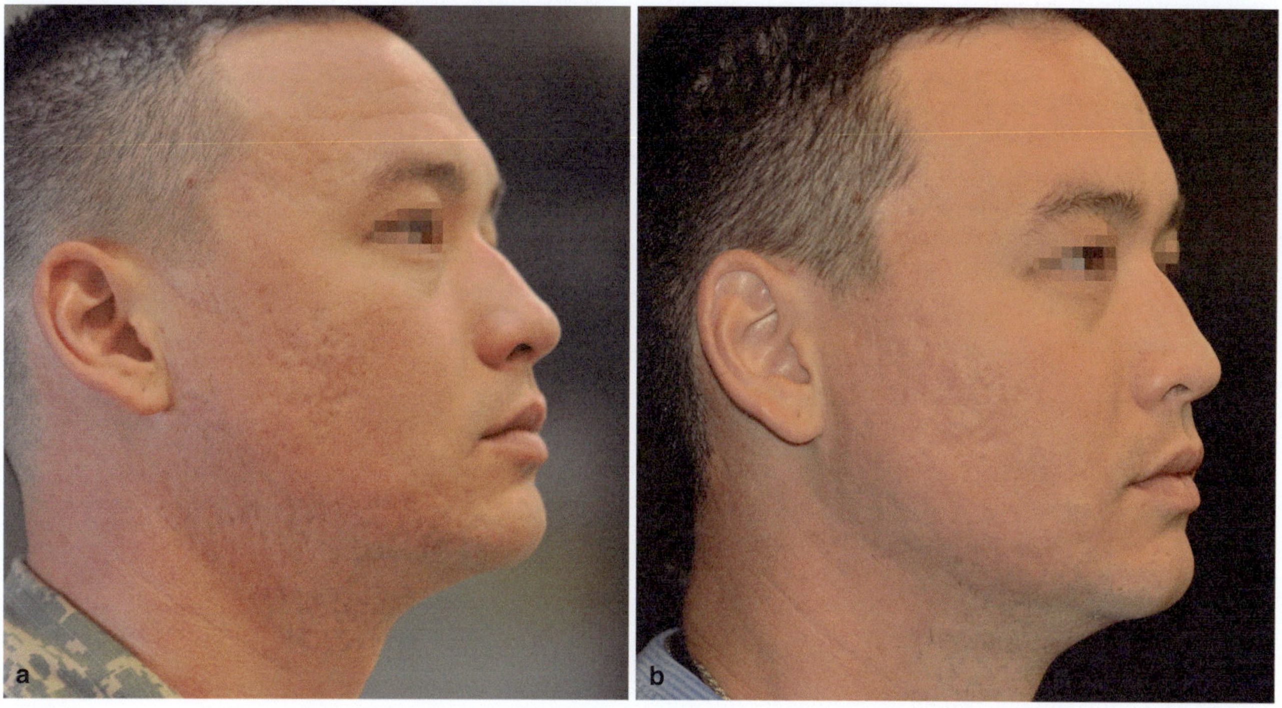

Fig. 14.5 (**a**) Atrophic boxcar and rolling acne scars on the temple, cheek, and neck of a FST III patient before non-ablative fractional laser (NAFL). (**b**) Significant atrophic acne scar improvement 3 months after three treatments of non-ablative fractional laser therapy

14.8 Laser-Assisted Drug Delivery

Because laser therapy, specifically AFL, can create discrete channels into scars via MTZs, it allows for direct access and delivery of intralesional medicine through simple topical application and massage. This technique of laser-assisted drug delivery (LADD) has been shown to have beneficial effects in both adult and pediatric populations with hypertrophic and keloidal scars treated with corticosteroids [59, 60]. In addition, pain scores have been reported as lower with LADD versus traditional intralesional injection for keloids [61]. LADD of 5-fluorouracil has also been reported as beneficial in the treatment of scars of varying etiologies [62, 63]. Poly-L-lactic acid filler material has been reported as useful via LADD for atrophic acne scars [64]. LADD may also play a role in the future of treating scar hypopigmentation, a concept still in its research infancy [65].

14.9 Laser Safety

Several resources exist to assist the physician, assisting staff, and patients in maintaining safety measures during laser therapy. The Occupational Safety and Health Administration (OSHA) as well as the American National Standard Institute (ANSI) Z136.1 guidelines serve to minimize hazards with respect to medical laser usage [66, 67]. Injuries to the eye, aerosolized carcinogens and infectious agents, and laser-induced fires, as well as accidental injuries from misdirected laser energy can all be mitigated with appropriate precautions and checklists. Please refer to the above noted resources to develop your clinic's laser safety protocols. When treating in the operating room, special precautions need to be taken around the endotracheal tube. Careful attention to the treatment, reduction of the oxygen saturation to room air concentrations, and wrapping of the endotracheal tube with wet gauze minimize the risk of combustion. The laser surgeon should be sure to have a bucket filled with sterile water and wet 4 × 4 gauze readily available.

14.10 Conclusion

Scars, regardless of the inciting mechanism, are often an underappreciated and undertreated problem. Reasons for this shortcoming include a lack of access to skilled care in many areas of the world and the denial of insurance coverage in most countries. Scarring is often considered a "cosmetic problem" despite the overwhelming evidence of the negative effects it has on the health and lives of injured patients. Shakespeare brilliantly summed up the reasons for this attitude in Romeo and Juliet: "He jests at scars that never felt a wound." Many payers and government providers of health services who have not been directly affected by the emotional and physical impact of scars are reluctant to pay for an aggressive, effective, multidisciplinary approach to scar therapy. Laser therapy, with its diverse mechanisms of action and targeted delivery of energy, provides a unique methodology in the treatment of scars of varying etiologies and clinical appearance. Abundant evidence now exists that it is state of the art and standard of care for the best scar management. Combining the direct action of laser energy on chromophores, the induced remodeling of scar tissue, and the creation of channels for medication delivery, laser therapy has transformed the treatment of scars. Advances in wound healing science and laser technology have enabled the scar tissue to be viewed as natural resource for the patient rather than as an obstruction that must be removed to facilitate improvement. Opportunities exist for the rehabilitation of scars and scar tissue, which could not have been imagined 25 years ago. Improving the patient's own damaged autologous tissue in its indigenous location is superior to excision and autologous replacement with associated iatrogenic deformities. Laser technology has become an essential tool to give scarred patients the best possible outcomes. Every practitioner involved with the treatment of scars should be knowledgeable and expert in the indications and usage of lasers.

References

1. Leblebici B, Adam M, Bağiş S, Tarim AM, Noyan T, Akman MN, et al. Quality of life after burn injury: the impact of joint contracture. J Burn Care Res. 2006;27(6):864–8.
2. Stekelenburg CM, Marck RE, Tuinebreijer WE, de Vet HC, Ogawa R, van Zuijlen PP. A systematic review on burn scar contracture treatment: searching for evidence. J Burn Care Res. 2015;36(3):e153–61. https://doi.org/10.1097/BCR.0000000000000106.
3. Bijlard E, Uiterwaal L, Kouwenberg CA, Mureau MA, Hovius SE, Huygen FJ. A systematic review on the prevalence, etiology, and pathophysiology of intrinsic pain in dermal scar tissue. Pain Physician. 2017;20(2):1–13.
4. Parnell LKS. Itching for knowledge about wound and scar pruritus. Wounds. 2018;30(1):17–36.
5. Van Loey NE, Van Son MJ. Psychopathology and psychological problems in patients with burn scars: epidemiology and management. Am J Clin Dermatol. 2003;4(4):245–72.
6. Stoddard FJ Jr, Ryan CM, Schneider JC. Physical and psychiatric recovery from burns. Surg Clin North Am. 2014;94(4):863–78. https://doi.org/10.1016/j.suc.2014.05.007.
7. Bock O, Schmid-Ott G, Malewski P, Mrowietz U. Quality of life of patients with keloid and hypertrophic scarring. Arch Dermatol Res. 2006;297(10):433–8. https://doi.org/10.1097/01.BCR.0000245652.26648.36.
8. Brown BC, McKenna SP, Siddhi K, McGrouther DA, Bayat A. The hidden cost of skin scars: quality of life after skin scarring. J Plast Reconstr Aesthet Surg. 2008;61(9):1049–58. https://doi.org/10.1016/j.bjps.2008.03.020.
9. Bijlard E, Kouwenberg CA, Timman R, Hovius SE, Busschbach JJ, Mureau MA. Burden of keloid disease: a cross-sectional health-related quality of life assessment. Acta Derm Venereol. 2017;97(2):225–9. https://doi.org/10.2340/00015555-2498.

10. Donelan MB, Parrett BM, Sheridan RL. Pulsed dye laser therapy and Z-plasty for facial burn scars: the alternative to excision. Ann Plast Surg. 2008;60:480–6.
11. Levi B, Ibrahim A, Mathews K, Wojcik B, Gomez J, Fagan S, et al. The use of CO2 fractional photothermolysis for the treatment of burn scars. J Burn Care Res. 2016;37(2):106–14. https://doi.org/10.1097/BCR.0000000000000285.
12. Miletta N, Siwy K, Hivnor C, Clark J, Shofner J, David Z, Rox Anderson R, Lee K, Donelan M. Fractional ablative laser therapy is an effective treatment for hypertrophic burn scars: A prospective study of objective and subjective outcomes. Ann Surg. 2019; https://doi.org/10.1097/SLA.0000000000003576. [Epub ahead of print].
13. Issler-Fisher AC, Fischer OM, Smialkowski AO, Li F, van Schalkwyk CP, Haertsch P, et al. Ablative fractional CO2 laser for burn scar reconstruction: an extensive subjective and objective short-term outcome analysis of a prospective treatment cohort. Burns. 2017;43(3):573–82. https://doi.org/10.1016/j.burns.2016.09.014.
14. Einstein A. On the quantum theory of radiation. Physikal Zeitschr. 1917;18:121.
15. Nelson JS. An introduction to lasers and laser-tissue interactions in dermatology. In: Kauvar ANB, Hruza GJ, editors. Principles and practices in cutaneous laser surgery. Boca Raton: Taylor & Francis Group; 2005. p. 59–78.
16. Anderson RR, Parrish JA. Selective photothermolysis: precise microsurgery by selective absorption of pulsed radiation. Science. 1983;220:524–7.
17. Alster TS. Improvement of erythematous and hypertrophic scars by the 585-nm flashlamp-pumped pulsed dye laser. Ann Plast Surg. 1994;32(2):186–90.25.
18. Allison KP, Kiernan MN, Waters RA, Clement RM. Pulsed dye laser treatment of burn scars. Alleviation or irritation? Burns. 2003;29:207–13.
19. Nast A, Eming S, Fluhr J, Fritz K, Gauglitz G, Hohenleutner S, et al. German S2k guidelines for the therapy of pathological scars (hypertrophic scars and keloids). J Dtsch Dermatol Ges. 2012;10(10):747–62. https://doi.org/10.1111/j.1610-0387.2012.08012.x.
20. de las Alas JM, Siripunvarapon AH, Dofitas BL. Pulsed dye laser for the treatment of keloid and hypertrophic scars: a systematic review. Expert Rev Med Devices. 2012;9(6):641–50. https://doi.org/10.1586/erd.12.56.
21. Kuo YR, Wu WS, Jeng SF, Huang HC, Yang KD, Sacks JM, et al. Activation of ERK and p38 kinase mediated keloid fibroblast apoptosis after flashlamp pulsed-dye laser treatment. Lasers Surg Med. 2005;36(1):31–7. https://doi.org/10.1002/lsm.20129.
22. Syneron Candela. VBeam Perfecta system specification. https://syneroncandela.com/int/product/877/system_specifications. Accessed 7 Oct 2018.
23. Keaney TC, Tanzi E, Alster T. Comparison of 532 nm potassium titanyl phosphate laser and 595 nm pulsed dye laser in the treatment of erythematous surgical scars: a randomized, controlled, open-label study. Dermatol Surg. 2016;42(1):70–6. https://doi.org/10.1097/DSS.0000000000000582.
24. Lee Y, Kim W. Combination laser treatment for immediate post-surgical scars: a retrospective analysis of 33 immature scars. Lasers Med Sci. 2017;32(5):1111–9. https://doi.org/10.1007/s10103-017-2215-9. Epub 2017 May 2.
25. Raulin C, Weiss RA, Schönermark MP. Treatment of essential telangiectasias with an intense pulsed light source (PhotoDerm VL). Dermatol Surg. 1997;23(10):941–5. discussion 945–6.
26. Hultman CS, Edkins RE, Lee CN, Calvert CT, Cairns BA. Shine on: review of laser- and light-based therapies for the treatment of burn scars. Dermatol Res Pract. 2012;2012:243,651. https://doi.org/10.1155/2012/243651.
27. Kim DY, Park HS, Yoon HS, Cho S. Efficacy of IPL device combined with intralesional corticosteroid injection for the treatment of keloids and hypertrophic scars with regards to the recovery of skin barrier function: a pilot study. J Dermatolog Treat. 2015;26(5):481–4. https://doi.org/10.3109/09546634.2015.1024598. Epub 2015 Sep 4.
28. Quarato D, Pascali M, Carinci F. Traumatic and surgical scars: successful treatment with a 1,565nm erbium-glass NAFL combined with IPL. J Biol Regul Homeost Agents. 2018;32(2 Suppl. 1):159–65.
29. Peng L, Tang S, Li Q. Intense pulsed light and laser treatment regimen improves scar evolution after cleft lip repair surgery. J Cosmet Dermatol. 2018; https://doi.org/10.1111/jocd.12684. [Epub ahead of print].
30. Wanner M, Sakamoto FH, Avram MM, Chan HH, Alam M, Tannous Z, et al. Immediate skin responses to laser and light treatments. Therapeutic endpoints: how to obtain efficacy. J Am Acad Dermatol. 2016;74(5):821–33. https://doi.org/10.1016/j.jaad.2015.06.026.
31. Iyer S, Fitzpatrick RE. Long-pulsed dye laser treatment for facial telangiectasias and erythema: evolution of a single purpuric pass versus multiple subpurpuric passes. Dermatol Surg. 2005;31(8 Pt 1):898–903. https://doi.org/10.1111/j.1524-4725.2005.31802.
32. Srinivas CR, Kumaresan M. Lasers for vascular lesions: standard guidelines of care. Indian J Dermatol Venereol Leprol. 2011;77(3):349–68. https://doi.org/10.4103/0378-6323.79728.
33. Cheng W, Saing H, Zhou H, Han Y, Peh W, Tam PK. Ultrasound assessment of scald scars in Asian children receiving pressure garment therapy. J Pediatr Surg. 2001;36(3):466–9.
34. Lee KC, Dretzke J, Grover L, Logan A, Moiemen N. A systematic review of objective burn scar measurements. Burns Trauma. 2016;4:14. https://doi.org/10.1186/s41038-016-0036-x. eCollection 2016.
35. Nanni CA, Alster TS. Complications of carbon dioxide laser resurfacing. An evaluation of 500 patients. Dermatol Surg. 1998;24(3):315–20.
36. Manstein D, Herron GS, Sink RK, Tanner H, Anderson RR. Fractional photothermolysis: a new concept for cutaneous remodeling using microscopic patterns of thermal injury. Lasers Surg Med. 2004;34(5):426–38. https://doi.org/10.1002/lsm.20048.
37. Miletta NR, Beachkofsky TM, Donelan MB, Kaiser SE, Hivnor CM. Lasers for burns and trauma. In: Kantor J, editor. Dermatologic surgery. New York: McGraw Hill Education; 2018. p. 1065–90.
38. Laubach HJ, Tannous Z, Anderson RR, Manstein D. Skin responses to fractional photothermolysis. Lasers Surg Med. 2006;38(2):142–9. https://doi.org/10.1002/lsm.20254.
39. Azzam OA, Bassiouny DA, El-Hawary MS, El Maadawi ZM, Sobhi RM, El-Mesidy MS. Treatment of hypertrophic scars and keloids by fractional carbon dioxide laser: a clinical, histological, and immunohistochemical study. Lasers Med Sci. 2015;31(1):9–18. https://doi.org/10.1007/s10103-015-1824-4.
40. Qu L, Liu A, Zhou L, He C, Grossman PH, Moy RL, et al. Clinical and molecular effects on mature burn scars after treatment with a fractional CO(2) laser. Lasers Surg Med. 2012;44(7):517–24. https://doi.org/10.1002/lsm.22055.
41. Ozog DM, Liu A, Chaffins ML, Ormsby AH, Fincher EF, Chipps LK, et al. Evaluation of clinical results, histological architecture, and collagen expression following treatment of mature burn scars with a fractional carbon dioxide laser. JAMA Dermatol. 2013;149(1):50–7. https://doi.org/10.1001/2013.jamadermatol.668.
42. Hultman CS, Friedstat JS, Edkins RE, Cairns BA, Meyer AA. Laser resurfacing and remodeling of hypertrophic burn scars: results of a large prospective, before-after cohort study with long term follow-up. Ann Surg. 2014;260(3):519–29. https://doi.org/10.1097/SLA.0000000000000893.
43. Waibel J, Beer K. Ablative fractional laser resurfacing for the treatment of a third-degree burn. J Drugs Dermatol. 2009;8(3):294–7.
44. Kimura U, Kinoshita A, Osawa A, Negi O, Haruna K, Mizuno Y, et al. Biophysical evaluation of fractional laser skin resurfacing

with an Er:YSGG laser device in Japanese skin. J Drugs Dermatol. 2012;11(5):637–42.
45. Weiss ET, Chapas A, Brightman L, Hunzeker C, Hale EK, Karen JK, et al. Successful treatment of atrophic postoperative and traumatic scarring with carbon dioxide ablative fractional resurfacing: quantitative volumetric scar improvement. Arch Dermatol. 2010;146(2):133–40. https://doi.org/10.1001/archdermatol.2009.358.
46. Bhargava S, Cunha PR, Lee J, Kroumpouzos G. Acne scarring management: systematic review and evaluation of the evidence. Am J Clin Dermatol. 2018;19(4):459–77. https://doi.org/10.1007/s40257-018-0358-5.
47. Zuccaro J, Ziolkowski N, Fish J. A systematic review of the effectiveness of laser therapy for hypertrophic burn scars. Clin Plast Surg. 2017;44(4):767–79. https://doi.org/10.1016/j.cps.2017.05.008. Epub 2017 Jul 10.
48. Bass LS. Rejuvenation of the aging face using Fraxel laser treatment. Aesthet Surg J. 2005;25(3):307–9. https://doi.org/10.1016/j.asj.2005.03.003.
49. Vasily DB, Cerino ME, Ziselman EM, Zeina ST. Non-ablative fractional resurfacing of surgical and post-traumatic scars. J Drugs Dermatol. 2009;8(11):998–1005.
50. de Sica RC, Rodrigues CJ, Maria DA, Cuce LC. Study of 1550-nm Erbium glass laser fractional non-ablative treatment of photoaging: comparative clinical effects, histopathology, electron microscopy, and immunohistochemistry. J Cosmet Laser Ther. 2016;18(4):193–203. https://doi.org/10.3109/14764172.2015.1114645. Epub 2016 Mar 8.
51. Min S, Park SY, Moon J, Kwon HH, Yoon JY, Suh DH. Comparison between Er:YAG laser and bipolar radiofrequency combined with infrared diode laser for the treatment of acne scars: differential expression of fibrogenetic biomolecules may be associated with differences in efficacy between ablative and non-ablative laser treatment. Lasers Surg Med. 2017;49(4):341–7. https://doi.org/10.1002/lsm.22607. Epub 2016 Nov 2.
52. Taudorf EH, Danielsen PL, Paulsen IF, Togsverd-Bo K, Dierickx C, Paasch U, et al. Non-ablative fractional laser provides long-term improvement of mature burn scars—a randomized controlled trial with histological assessment. Lasers Surg Med. 2015;47(2):141–7. https://doi.org/10.1002/lsm.22289. Epub 2014 Aug 22.
53. Omi T, Numano K. The role of the CO2 laser and fractional CO2 laser in dermatology. Laser Ther. 2014;23(1):49–60. https://doi.org/10.5978/islsm.14-RE-01.
54. Lumenis. UltraPulse. https://lumenis.com/wp-content/uploads/2018/07/UltraPulse-Brochure-for-web_PB-1124760_RevD_A4_250117_web.pdf. Accessed 8 Oct 2018.
55. Solta Medical. Fraxel. https://www.fraxel.com/hcp#the-fraxel-system. Accessed 8 Oct 2018.
56. Tierney EP, Hanke CW. Review of the literature: treatment of dyspigmentation with fractionated resurfacing. Dermatol Surg. 2010;36(10):1499–508. https://doi.org/10.1111/j.1524-4725.2010.01672.x.
57. Tao J, Champlain A, Weddington C, Moy L, Tung R. Treatment of burn scars in Fitzpatrick phototype III patients with a combination of pulsed dye laser and non-ablative fractional resurfacing 1550 nm erbium:glass/1927 nm thulium laser devices. Scars Burn Heal. 2018;4:2059513118758510. https://doi.org/10.1177/2059513118758510. eCollection 2018 Jan–Dec.
58. Royston S, Tiernan E, Wright P. Post-burn non-emergent hair in the male moustache area. Burns. 2012;38(4):615–6. https://doi.org/10.1016/j.burns.2011.12.024. Epub 2012 Feb 22.
59. Waibel JS, Wulkan AJ, Shumaker PR. Treatment of hypertrophic scars using laser and laser assisted corticosteroid delivery. Lasers Surg Med. 2013;45(3):135–40. https://doi.org/10.1002/lsm.22120. Epub 2013 Mar 4.
60. Greywal T, Krakowski AC. Pediatric dermatology procedures and pearls: multimodal revision of earlobe keloids. Pediatr Dermatol. 2018;35(2):268–70. https://doi.org/10.1111/pde.13374. Epub 2017 Dec 20.
61. Park J, Chun J, Lee JH. Laser-assisted topical corticosteroid delivery for the treatment of keloids. Lasers Med Sci. 2017;32(3):601–8. https://doi.org/10.1007/s10103-017-2154-5. Epub 2017 Jan 26.
62. Prince GT, Cameron MC, Fathi R, Alkousakis T. Intralesional and laser-assisted 5-fluorouracil in dermatologic disease: a systematic review. J Drugs Dermatol. 2018;17(3):274–80.
63. Lee BW, Levitt AE, Erickson BP, Ko AC, Nikpoor N, Ezuddin N, et al. Ablative fractional laser resurfacing with laser-assisted delivery of 5-fluorouracil for the treatment of cicatricial ectropion and periocular scarring. Ophthal Plast Reconstr Surg. 2018;34(3):274–9. https://doi.org/10.1097/IOP.0000000000000948.
64. Rkein A, Ozog D, Waibel JS. Treatment of atrophic scars with fractionated CO2 laser facilitating delivery of topically applied poly-L-lactic acid. Dermatol Surg. 2014;40(6):624–31. https://doi.org/10.1111/dsu.0000000000000010.
65. Carney BC, McKesey JP, Rosenthal DS, Shupp JW. Treatment strategies for hypopigmentation in the context of burn hypertrophic scars. Plast Reconstr Surg Glob Open. 2018;6(1):e1642. https://doi.org/10.1097/GOX.0000000000001642. eCollection 2018 Jan.
66. Occupational Safety & Health Administration. Surgical Suite Use of Medical Lasers. https://www.osha.gov/SLTC/etools/hospital/surgical/lasers.html. Accessed 8 Oct 2018.
67. American National Standards Institute. ANSI Z136.1: American National Standard for Safe Use of Lasers; 2014. http://webstore.ansi.org/RecordDetail.aspx?sku=ANSI+Z136.1-2014&source=blog. Accessed 8 Oct 2018.

MIX
Papier aus verantwortungsvollen Quellen
Paper from responsible sources
FSC® C105338

If you have any concerns about our products,
you can contact us on
ProductSafety@springernature.com

In case Publisher is established outside the EU,
the EU authorized representative is:
Springer Nature Customer Service Center GmbH
Europaplatz 3, 69115 Heidelberg, Germany

Printed by Libri Plureos GmbH
in Hamburg, Germany